Men'sHealth

MAXIMUM
MUSCLE PLAN

MensHealth
MAXIMUM
MUSCLE PLAN

THE HIGH-EFFICIENCY WORKOUT PROGRAM TO INCREASE YOUR STRENGTH AND MUSCLE SIZE IN JUST 12 WEEKS

THOMAS INCLEDON, CSCS, RD
MATTHEW HOFFMAN

RODALE

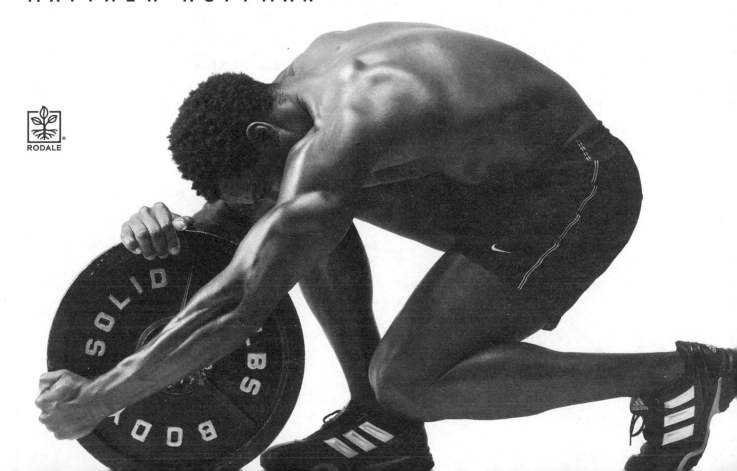

© 2005 by Thomas Incledon and Matthew Hoffman
Photographs © 2005 by Rodale Inc.

Printed in the United States of America
Rodale Inc. makes every effort to use acid-free ∞, recycled paper ♻.

Book design by Chris Rhoads

Interior photography by Mitch Mandel/Rodale Images

Library of Congress Cataloging-in-Publication Data

Incledon, Thomas.
   Men's health maximum muscle plan : the high-efficiency workout program to increase your strength and muscle size in just 12 weeks / Thomas Incledon and Matthew Hoffman.
      p.   cm.
   Includes index.
   ISBN-13 978–1–59486–306–6 hardcover
   ISBN-10 1–59486–306–7 hardcover
   ISBN-13 978–1–59486–314–1 paperback
   ISBN-10 1–59486–314–8 paperback
   1. Bodybuilding.   2. Physical fitness for men.   I. Hoffman, Matthew, date.   II. Men's health (Magazine)   III. Title.
   GV546.5.I53   2005
   613.7'13—dc22   2005021114

         2   4   6   8   10   9   7   5   3   hardcover

         2   4   6   8   10   9   7   5   3   1   paperback

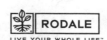

To my family and friends:

Thanks for your continued support and encouragement.

Set your goals high and let nothing stand in the way of accomplishing them.

CONTENTS

PART 4: THE CARDIO EDGE

PART 5: HARD-BODY EATING

INTRODUCTION

Most of my friends lift weights. At some point they made the commitment to stay in shape and do solid workouts at least a few days a week. That alone puts them in an elite group. Every man wants the kind of build that gets noticed. It takes real motivation to go from *wanting* to *getting.* The guys I know put in the hours and the sweat.

And yet . . . even these guys aren't where they should be. A lot of them look almost the same today as they did when they first started lifting. They're probably a little stronger. They have a little more endurance. Their builds are okay. But they've never made any *real* progress. They're (commendably) committed to exercise quantity. They're less committed to quality.

Total mistake. Without quality workouts—taking advantage of the latest scientific principles in training, nutrition, rest periods, and so on—any gains they make are invariably second rate.

Weight training is a science. Intuition can get you started, but it won't take you very far. In the past few years, sports physiologists have essentially rewritten the rules of lifting. They know exactly what it takes to maximize muscle breakdown and growth, the twin pillars of achieving maximum size. But what looks impressive in a university laboratory doesn't always play out in the gym. A lot of interesting theories get knocked out of the ring when real-live men in real-world gyms find that those theories are not very practical—or, for that matter, not very effective.

I'm lucky enough to have a foot in each world. With five college degrees, I'm one of the top sports and health scientists in the world. As CEO of Human Performance Specialists, I work with people from all over the world to optimize their health and improve their performance. I work with men (and women) who want to push themselves to the top levels of health and fitness. That's the academic side of my life.

Then there's the fun stuff. I'm nationally ranked in powerlifting, weight lifting, and strongman competitions. When I first started out, I never would have guessed I'd eventually hit 187 pounds in the one-arm snatch, 352 pounds in the power clean and jerk, and 615 pounds in the deadlift. I've also set a few national records in strongman competitions, including 19 reps in the 200-pound axle press.

This book, **Men's Health® Maximum Muscle Plan,** incorporates elements from both of these worlds: the latest scientific breakthroughs, plus real-life programs that put these principles to work. A lot of this information is so new that gym trainers haven't caught on yet. The guys at the gym? Forget it. Their techniques are so out of date that they should be preserved in a museum of ancient history.

Here's the bottom line: Forget just about everything you know (or were taught) about strength training. Whether you are just starting out or have been lifting for years, there's a good chance that most of your techniques are flat-out wrong. **Men's Health** *Maximum Muscle Plan* explains exactly how the science of muscle building has changed. More important, it shows how to use this information to achieve fast gains in size and strength—gains that would have been considered impossible just a few years ago. Here are just a few of the highlights.

- Ways to add 50 pounds to your bench weight in less than 3 months

- A 13-week plan for doing pushups for *180 seconds straight*—one of the best ways to develop a massive chest and win any bar bet

- Workout programs for every fitness level, from beginning to advanced

- Muscle-building nutrition plans, including the lowdown on meal timing and supplements

- Rest-and-recovery plans to optimize strength gains

- Workouts tailored for different body types

This book is *complete*. If you've never picked up a barbell in your life, you'll find complete instructions on doing it right—and avoiding a lifetime of bad habits that can shove future progress into the slow lane. If you're an experienced lifter, you'll find hundreds of advanced techniques that can blast you to the next level.

This isn't a small book. It couldn't be. You'll find a total of more than 190 exercises, many of which I bet you've never seen before. Advice on combining isolation movements with compound exercises. The latest and greatest news about supplements that accelerate muscle breakdown and regrowth. Tips on adjusting workouts—even changes in handgrip can make a huge difference—to get over the hump of plateaus. And a heck of a lot more.

Men's Health *Maximum Muscle Plan* is the ultimate workout guide for men who want to get bigger and stronger, faster. It skewers the myths and highlights the science. This stuff *is* a science. Take advantage of it. The result will be faster gains. The build you want. More energy and stamina. And progress that won't quit—ever.

—Thomas Incledon, CSCS, RD

PART 1

THE SCIENCE OF
SIZE

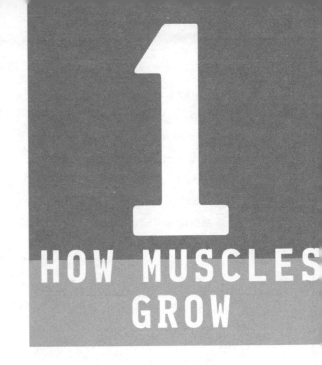

For years, the focus of strength-training science was almost entirely on building bulk. But the latest research shows that you can't reach optimal size unless you bring other factors into play. Organizing your workouts around movement patterns, a concept we'll talk about throughout this book, is one key factor. Another is developing the network of nerve fibers that thread through muscles and eventually snake back to the brain. Every time you lift, the body releases chemicals that thicken individual muscle fibers so they contract with more force. Lifting increases the supply of capillaries, the tiny networks of

blood vessels that carry in nutrients and cart away wastes. At the same time, the endless repetition of lifting conditions nerve fibers and improves their efficiency at firing muscles into action. That's why a tall, lean man who lifts smart and develops a finely honed nervous system might be stronger than the stocky man with tree-trunk legs and a barrel chest.

What you want, of course, is to bring all these factors into play. Even if you lift for practical reasons—to protect your back, say, or build endurance for weekend sports—there's a lot to be said for developing a physique that not only works well, but gets *noticed*. That's what this book is all about.

BREAK 'EM DOWN, BUILD 'EM UP

Every man has a mix of slow-twitch and fast-twitch muscle fibers. Fast-twitch fibers are the ones that

contract powerfully and give pure strength. They fatigue quickly, which is why you might be able to curl a 50-pound dumbbell just a few times. The slow-twitch fibers are made for endurance. They can't propel the kinds of force generated by fast-twitch fibers, but they can go just about forever.

Each of your skeletal muscles is made up of water, protein, fat, and carbohydrates, along with glycogen (the stored form of blood sugar) and a host of amino acids and chemical compounds. All of the usual lifestyle factors—good nutrition, good sleep, adequate rest between workouts, and so on—are critically important in any lifting plan. Men who optimize these factors while maintaining a tough workout regimen can achieve steroidlike results without ever touching those noxious drugs.

There's another factor, not related to lifestyle, that can take you from merely fit to *built*. It's called muscle damage. We're not talking about pain or post-workout soreness, though those are pretty good indicators of what's happening beneath the surface. At the level of individual muscle fibers, damage and destruction are your best friends.

Strip away all the scientific jargon. Weight lifting boils down to what trainers call the *progressive overload* of skeletal muscles—in other words, pushing those muscles harder than they're accustomed to working.

Every time you lift, you produce tiny tears in the muscle fibers. Depending on your level of fitness and how hard you work, the tears can be as small as just a few molecules across, or large enough to affect entire muscle cells (along with the supporting connective tissue). The body then responds to tears in muscle fibers by making bigger proteins as well as more proteins, which translates into bigger muscles.

You obviously don't want to lift yourself into traction. But you need some damage, and that means pushing yourself. A man who never taxes his muscles to their uppermost limits can lift every day for years without gaining appreciably in size. Conversely, the man who *overloads* his muscles the right way will get bigger much faster.

The process of tearing down and rebuilding muscle is incredibly complex. Basically, here's what happens.

- When you lift, damaged muscle tissues release signaling factors, substances that attract neutrophils, macrophages, and other immune cells to the damaged site.

- The immune cells trigger inflammation. This process is designed to remove damaged tissue from around the torn fibers. If you've overdone it, the inflammation might be painful. If you're lifting smart, however, you'll just feel a pleasant tightness.

- The immune cells release substances that stimulate the production of cells called satellite cells. The satellite cells, stimulated by hormones and other anabolic chemicals, then merge with the muscle cells as part of the repair process.

At the end of the process, the muscle tear is repaired. But the muscle itself isn't quite the same one you had before because it's gained additional and larger cells. It's like nailing a 2-by-4 to a shaky gate. The structure is stronger—and bulkier—than it was before.

The traditional thinking was that muscles in-

MORE REPS OR MORE WEIGHT?

It's probably the oldest locker room debate, and still the most common: Do you get optimal results using the heaviest possible weight, even if you can only finish 1 repetition? Or is it better to stack up the reps using lower weights? The definitive answer: It depends.

If your goal is to boost endurance, higher reps at lower weights make sense. But most men want to gain muscle and definition. To do that, you need to push serious iron.

A recent report compared the effects of different training loads on strength and muscular hypertrophy (increased size). Men who lifted 80 percent to 95 percent of their *1 repetition maximum*—the heaviest weight they could lift *once* at full-out exertion—had greater increases in size than those who stuck with lower weights.

THE "TERMINATOR" GENE

Men are undergoing record numbers of appearance-enhancing procedures these days, but at some point, we might look back on hair replacement and chest implants as relics from the Dark Ages. On the horizon: the ability to manipulate a man's genetic material to create massive size without a hint of sweat.

Scientists have discovered some of the genes that control muscle growth. Some genes limit size; others enhance it—sometimes to a startling degree. When scientists blocked the myostatin gene, mice and cows developed *double* the usual amount of muscle. Other genetic pathways, such as the Akt/p70S6 kinase protein synthesis pathway, may cause an increase in muscle growth and an accelerated rate of fat burning.

Leaner and bigger without lifting a finger, let alone lifting weights? It's a tantalizing possibility, though light-years from reality at this point. The studies have been done on animals, not humans. And genetic tinkering is always risky. It's impossible to predict what might happen when genes are artificially switched on or off. The genes that control muscle growth might turn out to control other things, as well.

So, don't give up your gym membership yet. Even if it were possible today to get that genetic edge, the men who work out hard would still be a step ahead.

---

variably reached the point at which increases in size basically stop. New research suggests that doesn't happen. It's possible that once muscle fibers reach a certain size, they split like twigs on a tree, creating more muscle fibers. Each of these new fibers will grow until it reaches maximum size, then it will split again. This could mean that every man can keep getting bigger, no matter how long he's been lifting.

BIGGER, FASTER

The ripped physiques and hard-core musculatures that most men would kill to have don't come quickly. But you can get there a lot faster than you probably think. Scientists have known for almost 50 years that muscular strength increases rapidly when men start a lifting program. Gains in maximal force of up to 15 percent have been measured after a *single* training session.

Obviously, no one becomes Schwarzeneggeresque in a few days—or a few months. That kind of build takes work, a lot of it. But the initial "quick jumps" in strength when you start lifting, or bump up your workouts another notch, have relatively little to do with muscle size. They're mainly due to neural factors—alterations in the nervous system that increase force and power in an astonishingly short time. Think of these gains as confidence builders. You'll move up in weights very quickly. The heavier weights take you further into the realm of muscle overload, and that's the secret to size.

Nothing increases muscle mass faster than lifting, not even steroids. In a 10-week study that directly compared weight lifting with steroids for muscle gain, guys on a lifting program increased their bench weight by 22 pounds, compared to the 19-pound gain among men taking steroids. The lifters increased their squat poundage 55 pounds, compared to a scant 28 pounds in the steroid group.

Nor will combining aerobic exercise and strength training increase your muscle gains. Aerobic workouts can get the heart and lungs working like a bass drum. Aerobic exercise also boosts endurance, burns more fat calories, reduces the risk of dozens of diseases, and generally makes you healthier. What it won't do is make you bigger. In fact, it has just the opposite effect.

Researchers looked at gains in strength and muscle size in three groups of men: those who lifted, those who did endurance workouts, and those who combined both. Men in the strength-training group showed greater muscle gains than those in either of the other groups. Endurance training actually limited increases in strength and muscle size.

This is because skeletal muscle can't adapt to both strength and endurance training simultaneously. Put another way, the muscle changes that you experience when you run, for example, are the opposite of the changes needed for maximum size. The muscles simply can't adapt to both activities simultaneously. Running before a weight-lifting session produces muscle fatigue that makes it impossible to generate the necessary muscle tension to reach peak power.

This doesn't mean you should blow off running, swimming, or other endurance sports. They're good for you. But if your primary goal is to get bigger, focus on the weights first. To keep the heart rate up and the calories burning, keep moving when you lift, with nonstop motion from one exercise to another.

LIFELONG POWER

Most men will never compete on the bodybuilding circuit or line up to be the year's top male model. Guys lift because it makes them look and feel better. They're stronger generally, which makes the ho-hum, practical details of living, like hoisting a 50-pound bag of dog food out of the car, a little easier.

If you keep lifting—not just this week or next year, but over the decades—you'll see payoffs such as a much lower risk of obesity, diabetes, high blood pressure, and heart disease. You'll also have a physique that other men will envy. The sad truth is that most men lose a lot of muscle as they age. Weight lifting is by far the best way to reverse muscle declines. Older men who lift just a few times a week don't lose muscle at all. They *gain* mass as well as strength.

Most of us aren't satisfied with the status quo. We want *more*—bigger arms, a stronger chest, that elusive washboard gut. You can have all this and more. But there's no lazy way out. Remember the term *progressive overload*. Push your muscles hard, and push them often. We'll show you how.

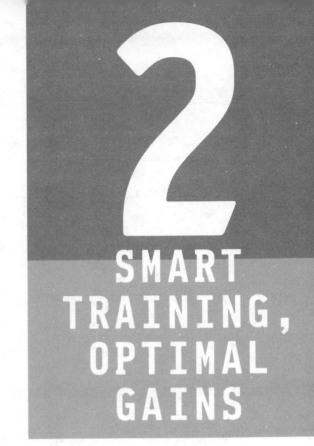

2
SMART TRAINING, OPTIMAL GAINS

I f you're reading this book, you're probably an experienced lifter already. You don't need an extensive primer on avoiding injury, basic lifting techniques, or other Gym 101 strategies. We'll touch on some of these issues because everyone can use reminders. But the focus of this chapter—indeed, of the entire book—is how to tweak your current workouts so that you reach levels of size, strength, and fitness that you didn't reach before.

FOCUS YOUR WORKOUTS

Anyone who's serious about lifting eventually hits a time crunch: Choose between the hours needed to stay in shape or keep up with the zillions of responsibilities that never seem to stop. Unless you're prepared to throw it all away and open a surf shop in Mexico, there's probably not a lot you can do to simplify your life. What you can do is make your workouts more efficient so you get the same or better results in less time.

A lot of guys spend *unnecessary* hours at the gym. We're not talking about the occasional half-hour of locker room jawing. The real issue is how well your workouts line up with your ultimate goals. You can bet that the guy who spends 30 minutes on the treadmill, 45 minutes on the weight floor, and another hour on a yoga mat is in okay shape. But he won't be in top shape because his workouts are really too scattered to achieve any one fitness goal.

It's a fact of physiology: Muscles can only do so much. Train them for endurance *and* strength *and* growth, and they'll settle into a comfortable middle ground—okay at everything, excellent at nothing. They do a lot better when they specialize.

Scientists generally identify muscle cells, or myocytes, as either type 1 (slow-twitch cells) or type 2 (fast-twitch cells). A trained endurance athlete has a higher proportion of slow-twitch fibers that can keep producing power for a long time. A trained power athlete has a lot more fast-twitch fibers that can't perform as long as slow-twitch fibers but are capable of great strength and explosive force.

In reality this is an oversimplification. All muscle fibers have varying degrees of both properties. Muscle is a plastic tissue, meaning it adapts and changes in response to different types of stress. These adaptive qualities are known as *shifting*. For example, you can choose a workout that promotes changes within fast-twitch fibers that increase their endurance or work capacity. They're still fast-twitch

HOW GOOD ARE STABILITY BALLS?

The rationale for so-called balance training using stability balls or wobble boards is that it helps people develop, well, better balance. There's some truth to this approach: Rehab programs use stability balls and wobble boards to help clients recover from injuries. But if you aren't injured or don't have balance problems, should you bother with this approach when doing crunches, dumbbell curls, or whatever?

Probably not. Studies show that lifting weights while lying on a stability ball reduces force output. You have to lift lighter weights, which retards the stimulus for muscle growth. There's also evidence that men burn fewer calories when they use this approach.

That's not to say you can't take advantage of wobble boards or stability balls. They might be useful when:

• You want to give your body a break from lifting. Trainers often recommend a 1- or 2-week *unloading period* a couple of times a year.

• You want to warm up before launching into your regular lifting routine.

Otherwise, don't bother.

fibers, but they can be shifted somewhat to slow-twitch types of work.

This has practical applications in the gym. It's always better to focus your workouts—to push your muscles in the direction you want them to go. A man who's mainly interested in looking better on the beach will want to choose workouts that put the most stress on the powerful (and size-enhancing) fast-twitch fibers. A man looking to run a marathon will want to emphasize workouts that stress the slow-twitch fibers. A workout that combines both types of exercise will obviously promote gains in both directions. But you'll only get *peak* gains when you choose one type of workout over the other.

GET THE HORMONAL EDGE

The fact that testosterone and other hormones influence muscle size is nothing new. What is new is the knowledge that you can optimize your hormonal environment to achieve greater (and faster) gains in size.

If you've been lifting for years and can't see any real progress in size, definition, or strength, you can bet that you haven't been doing everything you can to shift your hormonal balance in your favor. Mainly, of course, we're talking about testosterone, a steroid hormone produced by the testes. Other hormones that directly affect muscle growth include growth hormone (GH), produced by the pituitary gland, and insulin-like growth factor-1 (IGF-1), mainly produced by the liver and to some degree by other cells.

These are the big three when it comes to muscle size and strength. Testosterone, GH, and IGF-1 are categorized as anabolic hormones because they stimulate protein synthesis in muscles, causing them to get bigger. Cortisol, on the other hand, is a catabolic hormone that breaks down muscle. When you're trying to get bigger, you want the highest possible levels of anabolic hormones and lower levels of catabolic hormones such as cortisol. You can hit the right balance with smart training.

Concentrate on weights. Lifting increases muscle-building levels of anabolic hormones much more than endurance workouts do. Serious endurance athletes have *lower* levels of testosterone than resistance-trained athletes. If your main goal is getting bigger, spend more of your gym time in the weight room. Keep the endurance workouts as a sideline.

Lift late. Levels of both testosterone and cortisol are highest in the mornings and lowest in the evenings. Trainers used to advise men to lift early in the day to take advantage of the higher testosterone. The problem with this approach is that the higher levels of cortisol that occur at the same time offset some of the benefits. You're better off lifting later in the day. Lifting weights at 6:00 p.m. has been shown to optimize the hormonal environment by elevating testosterone proportionally more than cortisol. Evening workouts minimize catabolic activity, which means more muscle growth in less time.

Get enough fat. There are good health reasons to eat less fat, but if you're trying to get bigger, you need adequate levels to increase testosterone and promote muscle growth. Sports nutritionists advise men to get roughly 25 percent of their total daily calories from fat. They agree with cardiologists that saturated fat, found mainly in red meats as well as in some processed foods, is as likely to add bulk to the arteries as to the muscles. Avoid it—or at least limit red meat servings to three or four a week. But don't skimp on monounsaturated fat, found in olive, canola, and safflower oils, as well as in nuts and seeds. Along with the healthful oils in fish, it has the same testosterone-boosting effects as saturated fats, but is a lot better for your cardiovascular plumbing.

Don't go crazy with protein. A lot of serious lifters are convinced that they need massive amounts of protein to promote muscle growth. Not true. You do need extra protein to stimulate muscle growth and repair (and to help burn body fat and suppress appetite), but it doesn't take a whole lot. For most men, the amount of protein in a normal diet—5 to 20 percent of daily calories—is enough.

POSITIVE SIZE FROM NEGATIVE WORK

Lifting has two phases: the positive, or concentric phase, in which you lift the weight; and the negative, or eccentric phase, when the weight lowers. Eccentric training is often used in rehab programs to help athletes recover from injuries and return to competition. It also turns out to be a superb shortcut that helps healthy men get bigger faster.

Even though fast lifting is advisable for all sorts of reasons, you might want to experiment with lowering weights more slowly than usual. Studies show that this technique can greatly increase strength in trained as well as untrained men. It's especially effective when you combine it with a program to improve the rate of force development—for example, by alternating speed workouts with strength workouts (where eccentric loading is emphasized).

Eccentric training puts tremendous stress on the muscles, however, and can generate post-workout soreness. It's usually recommended only for men who have a lot of lifting experience and are already in good shape.

There aren't any hard and fast rules for how slowly you should lower weights to get the most benefit. You'll have to see what feels best. Move as quickly as you can (while maintaining full control) during the concentric phase, then take 4 to 8 seconds to complete the eccentric phase. If you have excessive soreness the next day, back off a bit and lower the weights more quickly.

If you're doing hard-core workouts, protein should compose roughly 20 to 25 percent of your total daily calories. Getting more may be counterproductive because it's linked to drops in testosterone. Here's an easy formula: Each day, take 1 gram of protein powder for every pound of body weight.

REFRESH YOUR TECHNIQUE

Unless you're lucky enough to have a workout partner who doubles as a trainer and keeps an eye on your form, you probably do exercises today the same way that you did when you first learned them. The habits we establish early are the ones that stick with us. And nine out of 10 times, they're not as effective as they should be—or may even be flat-out wrong. Whether you're a new lifter or have been doing it for years, it's worth reexamining your technique occasionally. You can always make small refinements that will give better results in a lot less time.

Check what the pros are doing. There are dozens of superb exercise books written (and photographed) by the top names in lifting. Keep them around the house and check out the workouts every now and then. Or get on the Internet (check out the exercise video clips at www.thomasincledon.com). You might find that you've been doing exercises inefficiently. At the very least, you'll pick up some tips for getting more juice from every lift you do. Good technique develops the neuropathways that determine intramuscular coordination as well as size. Without it, you won't progress the way you should—and you're more likely to get hurt.

Adjust technique to your goals. Suppose your main goal is to add as much bulk as you can. If you're doing barbell rows, you'll maximize muscular hypertrophy when you isolate the muscles and minimize the use of your lower body. But what if you're more interested in power and strength than sheer size? You'll want to move the weight explosively, and that means using your lower body as much as possible. (That's why barbell rows are sometimes called "power rows" when they're used in this phase of training.)

There are dozens of potential ways to get effective results from any given exercise or workout. Lifting techniques can vary greatly, depending on your ultimate goals. That's why it's a good idea to work with a trainer now and then.

Stay in your range of motion. Forcing yourself to do any exercise that pushes your joints beyond their *current* range of motion guarantees a world of hurt. Even if you aren't yet at the point where you can hit the full range of extension (or contraction), you always want to maintain the proper mechanical position. Joint flexibility and mobility improve quickly. Don't rush it. If you notice any pain when you go beyond a certain point, stop and back off a little.

You should definitely back off if you've had a recent injury. If you've hurt your knee, for example, and it hurts to do full leg presses, try partial leg presses for a while. Decrease the amount of weight, as well. As your knee heals, experiment with extending your *pain-free* range of motion. Lifting should never hurt. If it does, either you're doing something wrong or you need to back off. If it still hurts, you need to see a competent doctor or physical therapist.

TRAINING TOOLS

You probably spend most of your gym time in the weight area. That's where you want to be when you're working on size and strength. But if you look around in some of the less used corners of the gym, you'll see pieces of equipment that deserve a second look, if not a whole lot of your time.

Other gear to consider:

- Body-weight platforms: pullup bars, dip bars, and so on. They're great for intermediate or beginning lifters. However, once you're strong

FREE WEIGHTS VERSUS MACHINES

Do machine weights give the same oomph as free weights? For the most part, no. Free weights are superb for overloading muscles, the main step in breaking down muscle tissue and bringing it back larger and stronger. As a bonus, free weights improve coordination because the only thing holding them level and upright is your body.

Don't ignore the machines, though. They aren't just for beginners. Unlike free weights, which generally bring a lot of muscles into play, machines can be engineered to isolate just a few muscles. You can concentrate the tension right where you want. They're a good choice if you aren't quite strong enough for body-weight exercises, such as pullups. A lot of men use machines as an intermediate step; when one barbell or dumbbell weight has gotten too easy, but you aren't quite ready to move up to the next size, you can often find an in-between zone on machines.

enough to lift your own body weight, you can't progress any more. The workouts then become muscular endurance exercises and offer relatively little for strength or size gains.

- Elastic tubing and bands. You can use them to design workouts that create unique movement patterns that stretch and strengthen various muscle groups. You can certainly get a good workout using elastic tubing or bands, but they don't provide a way to measure different levels of resistance. That means there's no way to measure progress—a motivation killer, for most men. Throughout the book, we'll show you how to incorporate tubing or bands into free weight exercises for a greater challenge.

- Weight belts. If you're a competitive lifter, you need a weight belt. With upper-limit loads, a properly fitted belt helps keep your spine where it should be—like attached to your back. If you aren't at this level of lifting, don't bother. The belt doesn't do much of anything except make your back sweat. Besides, you should be strengthening your back muscles when you train. That's all the support you need.

- Weight-lifting shoes. They have a harder sole than regular gym shoes. The sole doesn't com-

press as much when you lift, which can improve traction and stability. The heels are also designed to make it easier (and safer) to do squats. Like weight belts, though, they really aren't necessary for most men.

- Chalk. Nothing is more frustrating, and potentially dangerous, than feeling a heavy weight start to slip out of your grip. A dusting of chalk makes it a lot easier to grip the weights. Definitely consider using chalk when you're doing deadlifts or other pulling movements.

- A spotter. Okay, a spotter isn't exactly gear, but a good one is worth his weight in gold. A spotter is the guy who stands by while you push yourself a little harder than usual, and is ready to give just a nudge of assistance while you finish that last rep—or to call 911 when you drop a 250-pound load on your chest.

  A good spotter pays attention. He instinctively knows when to help and when to stand back. He doesn't get distracted. He keeps an eye on you all the time.

  When do you need a spotter? Usually when you're doing forced reps—pushing yourself all the way to your limit. He'll help you complete movements when you can't quite go all the way yourself. He'll also help you rack the weight if you can't complete that final movement.

Some spotters are overzealous and start touching the weight while you're lifting. This isn't what you want. Unless you're doing negatives—lowering massive amounts of weight—the spotter should only touch the bar when you can't possibly lift it on your own. Talk about what you want before you start your set. Make sure your spotter knows what you want him to do and when to do it.

HOW MANY WEEKLY WORKOUTS?

There's no right answer to this question. It really depends on your recovery time. A guy who recovers quickly can work out more than one who doesn't. Family and work responsibilities also come into play. It doesn't make sense to insist that men have to work out at least 5 days a week, for example, when doing so would land them in divorce court or in the unemployment line.

- On *average,* plan on lifting a minimum of 2 days a week. This is enough to make solid gains, as long as your workout includes at least 8 sets per muscle group, and you're lifting at least 85 percent of your repetition maximum (RM) to the point of muscle failure. The most repetitions you can complete is your RM.

- It's safe for experienced lifters to work out three to five times a day, every day. Of course, it's not very practical unless you have a trust fund and a very understanding spouse.

- Most men who are serious, but not fanatical, about lifting go to the gym once a day, 4 to 6 days a week. A few times a year, they can push themselves a little harder by working out twice a day for a week or two, then sliding back to the once-a-day schedule.

- The fanatics do work out all 7 days of the week—sometimes even twice a week.

HOW MANY REPETITIONS?

A repetition is one complete movement of an exercise. Does it really matter if you complete 1 rep or 100? You bet it does. Our bodies adapt very specifically to what we do.

- If you use light weights and complete 12 repetitions, you'll primarily develop muscular endurance.

- If you use heavier weights and do fewer reps—say, 6 to 12—you'll primarily develop muscle size and power.

Men who really want to get bigger push their weight loads to the max, even if they complete 6 or fewer repetitions.

WHAT'S THE BEST LIFTING SPEED?

Nothing beats speed for unadulterated, muscle-gain efficiency. You want to move the weights as fast as you can *while maintaining total control* of the bar or dumbbells. Fast lifting causes the greatest improvements in size and strength, as well as explosive power. (Some exercises, such as power cleans and snatches, can only be done explosively because they require the entire body to coordinate to achieve joint extension.)

Suppose you're lying on the bench below an unloaded bar (45 pounds). You lift and lower the bar as fast as possible. If you add a small amount of weight (say, 10 pounds) to the bar, you can still move it just as quickly as you did when it was empty. At a certain point, however, you add enough weight that you can no longer move the bar as fast. When the weight gets heavier, your body calls on more muscle fibers. You can only recruit so many

A WORLD OF HURT

COLLAR THE BAR

Every barbell comes with collars or clamps, devices that prevent plates from slipping should the bar tip to one side. Yet these sensible safety devices invariably get left on the floor—and every now and then a 45-pound plate goes airborne, and some poor guy hobbles around in a cast for the rest of the month.

Always use collars, even if you've been lifting for years without a mishap. There will come a day when the bar tips, either because you're not paying attention or because muscles on one side of your body unexpectedly give out. Not using collars is among the top causes of gym injuries. You're threatening not only yourself but the guy working out next to you.

fibers at a time, and their contraction speed has limits.

Hitting your top lifting speed is among the most important benchmarks when you're trying to build muscle fast. The faster you move a weight, the more muscle fibers you stimulate, and the greater the potential for muscle growth. At the same time, this approach improves your speed and reaction times overall. You'll literally move faster—partly because the muscles get bigger and also because you're intensifying nerve signals that zap the muscles into action. Sports physiologists call this concept the "rate of force development," and it's one of the cornerstones of modern weight-lifting science. Men who lift quickly and improve their rate of force development lift heavier weights, throw balls farther, punch faster, and hit golf balls farther. In other words, when you move fast, you get better at moving faster.

So how fast is fast enough?

Lifting and lowering a load in 1 to 2 seconds for each movement has a lot of advantages. Mainly, it develops the ability to move faster overall, while improving size, strength, and general neuromuscular conditioning.

Unless you work with a trainer or have a lot of experience, though, that kind of speed might not be comfortable—or safe. So plan on raising weights to a 1–2 count, and lowering them to a count of 3 or 4.

This rate of lifting is fast enough to train your body into the speed zone and slow enough to eliminate residual momentum and isolate the muscles you want to work. The speed of lifting is less important than your level of control. You always want to precisely control the weight, without jerking or swaying. Don't let gravity take over—say, by letting a barbell drop toward your chest. You want to feel the tension all the way.

HOW GOOD ARE GLOVES?

There are a few reasons to consider wearing those fingerless lifting gloves. They can improve your grip on slippery, sweat-streaked bars, and they keep your hands from getting callused. But they're hardly a necessary accoutrement. In fact, they have a few significant drawbacks.

For one thing, gloves are a pain to pull on and off, especially after a sweaty workout. Also, gyms are very dirty places. Have you ever seen anyone scrub a barbell or dumbbell? All that dirt ends up on your gloves, which provide a perfect environment for bacterial growth.

If you do wear gloves, wash them every week or two. Or give them up entirely. You can get a perfectly good grip with your bare hands, especially if you use a paper towel to swab the sweat off bars and dumbbells.

WHEN SHOULD I SLOW DOWN?

Muscle fibers do only two things: contract and relax. The contraction phase—the movement with the most exertion—is the big one. That's when the tension within muscle fibers stimulates growth.

Men who are serious about getting big usually lift quickly. Yet during different phases of training, they slow w-a-a-a-y down. Completing repetitions slowly—for example, taking a weight that you normally lift for 8 to 10 reps and moving it more slowly for 5 or 6 reps—increases the time that muscle fibers are under tension. This in turn stimulates rapid muscle growth.

Adding variety to your workouts is always a good thing. You might lift at your normal pace for a week or two, then set aside a few days for slow lifting. And of course, if you're recovering from an injury, you'll naturally move slower, if only to control the weight and minimize momentum and stress on connective tissues.

HOW MANY SETS?

The war between single sets versus multiple sets will never end, even though the facts make it pretty simple to sort out.

- A healthy man should do single sets for up to 16 weeks after he first starts a lifting program. Doing more than this greatly increases the risk of post-workout soreness—and a total crash in motivation. If you have orthopedic problems, such as a bad back, you might stay with single sets indefinitely.

- After 16 weeks, bump up your sets. Plan on 3 to 6 sets per exercise. Men who lift at this level will show significant gains in size as well as strength.

The workouts in this book include single-set programs for beginners or men facing a real time crunch, as well as multiset programs for advanced lifters.

HOW MUCH WEIGHT?

Trainers call this intensity, and there are all sorts of formulas for figuring out what intensity is right for you. Numbers aside, you can trust your intuition. Use a weight that's heavy enough to challenge you, but not so heavy that it makes you compromise proper form and control. If you're twisting, heaving, jerking, or otherwise distorting your body to complete a movement, you're lifting too much weight.

Now for the numbers. The intensity of an exercise is determined by the 1RM. That stands for "1 repetition maximum," the absolute top weight that you can lift one time.

- The *minimal* intensity that will give measurable increases in size and strength is 60 to 65 percent of the 1RM. If the most you can lift one time is 100 pounds, the minimal 1RM for strength gain is 60 to 65 pounds.

- For maximal gains in strength and muscle size, use weights at 80 percent to 90 percent of your 1RM. If you can lift 100 pounds, this means you'll usually be using 80 to 90 pounds in your workouts.

- Weights below these thresholds are fine for building endurance. You might want to incorporate lighter weights now and then—to give your muscles a break and also to improve their ability to generate strength for longer periods.

HOW MUCH VOLUME?

Volume is a measure of the amount of work performed. Sports scientists calculate volume by measuring the number of reps performed, the amount and distance lifted, and the number of exercises. All of this gets multiplied to identify the work volume.

The level of precision needed for laboratory studies isn't necessary in the gym, of course. You can calculate your volume of work by counting sets, counting repetitions, or counting the total amount of weight lifted.

- Using a rep-based volume system, multiply the number of reps per set by the number of sets to get a total rep count. If you're doing 5 reps and a total of 8 sets, your total rep count is 40. That's the volume.

- Using a weight-based volume system, you'd multiply the number of reps by the weight used in each set, then multiply that by the number of sets. Five reps of 100 pounds is 500 pounds. If you do 8 sets, multiply again to get your volume—in this case, 4,000 pounds.

Keeping track of volume is a good gauge of progress. Higher training volumes (without overtraining) stimulate more muscle strength and growth, so you want to see that number climb over time.

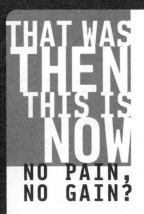

THAT WAS THEN THIS IS NOW
NO PAIN, NO GAIN?

For a long time, trainers and coaches exhorted men to, well, hurt themselves. If you weren't hurting after a workout, the thinking went, you weren't trying hard enough. You were a slacker. A weenie. Which may explain why a lot of men never touched a piece of exercise gear after escaping from high school gym.

Pushing your body to the limit invariably causes occasional aches and pains. But pain isn't a badge of honor. It means you're not training smart—and, if it's bad enough, it can totally derail your workouts.

Bottom line: You *never* want to experience pain when you're lifting. If you do, back off on the weights or do a different exercise or movement.

Soreness is a little different. It's normal to feel a little sore after a really hard workout. But soreness shouldn't reach the level of real pain. If you hurt so much you can't exercise, it means you overdid it and have experienced significant muscle damage. That's called overtraining, and it *slows* muscle growth and development.

BREATHE BETTER, LIFT MORE

Natural breathing—randomly sucking air in and blowing it out—isn't good enough for weight training. Men who inhale and exhale at the right times can dramatically increase their weight loads.

The breathing pattern that seems to provide the best internal pressure for lifting maximal weights is to inhale, hold your breath, lift the weight past the point of toughest resistance, then exhale. The problem with this technique is that it can send blood pressure through the ceiling—bad news for men with hypertension or risk factors for stroke or cardiovascular disease.

A safer technique, and one that also increases lifting capacity, is to exhale hard during the exertion phase, then inhale while lowering the weights. It's not quite as effective for increasing weight loads as holding your breath, but it's a lot safer.

WHAT IS PROGRESSION?

Progression is the planned increase in weight, reps, or volume—or any combination of the three—for a workout. Your workouts should progress just enough to stimulate maximal muscle growth, but not so much that you're at risk of overtraining or injury.

The programs throughout this book are designed with progression built in. For example, we'll recommend that certain phases of training be done with a given weight, a given number of reps, and a given number of sets. The number of sets will be increased each week for 4 weeks, then you'll cut back to the starting number of sets. This approach not only stimulates muscle growth but also allows for recovery after higher volumes of training. The combination of these two factors—high workout loads followed by recovery—is ideal for achieving maximum size.

Of course, every workout should allow for plenty of flexibility. You don't want to do the same things every time. Vary the exercises, the order in which you do them, the number of repetitions and sets, and so on.

HOW MUCH REST BETWEEN SETS?

This is another one of those "on the one hand, on the other hand" issues. The amount of rest between sets depends on your goals.

- Beginning lifters should rest 3 to 5 minutes between sets to minimize muscle stress and soreness.

- Advanced lifters going after strength and power should rest 3 to 5 minutes between sets, assuming the sets include 3 to 6 repetitions.

- Advanced lifters going after muscle size should do 6 to 12 repetitions and rest 1 to 2 minutes between sets.

- Advanced lifters who want maximum endurance should rest 30 to 45 seconds between sets, assuming the sets include 15 to 20 reps.

It's fine to estimate your rest periods, but time estimates are notoriously inaccurate. That doesn't matter if you're lifting just to get in better shape overall. It will make a difference if you're going for peak conditioning. You might want to wear a watch with a second hand or carry a stopwatch.

Another way to gauge rest periods is to use a heart rate monitor. When your heart rate drops to 105 to 110 beats per minute, start the next set. This is actually the best approach—and one used by a lot of serious lifters—because your rest periods will be based on what's happening in your body, rather than an absolute time measurement that doesn't allow for individual variability.

HOW MUCH REST BETWEEN EXERCISES?

Follow the same recovery rules that you did for sets. Men who are new to lifting should rest 3 minutes between exercises. Advanced lifters who want maximum strength and power should rest 3 to 5 minutes between exercises, assuming the exercises include 3 to 6 repetitions. For high-intensity conditioning, rest 1 to 2 minutes between exercises with 6 to 12 repetitions. To build endurance, rest 30 to 45 seconds between exercises, with 15 to 20 repetitions.

HOW MUCH REST BETWEEN WORKOUTS?

This is another area that's rife with disagreement. A lot of it is intuitive. If you feel good the day after a hard workout, without soreness, you can assume you're recovered and ready to go again. If you're sore or stiff, you need to take the day off.

Most beginning lifters can plan on getting three workouts a week, with a day off in between. You'll probably experience some soreness for the first few weeks; that's normal. It will stop once you start getting into shape.

Men who are dead serious about lifting can train every day, or even twice a day. In fact, they should—it's optimal for increasing muscle size and strength. However, don't work the same muscles in the same ways if you're working out this often. Do different exercises, and vary the repetitions and set schemes when doing daily or twice-a-day workouts.

MORE MUSCLES, LESS PAIN

There are literally hundreds of exercises you can do with weights, including movements that work single muscles that most of us have never heard of. This kind of tweaking makes sense if you're competing on the bodybuilder circuit, but it isn't necessary for most strength programs—and it can do a lot of muscle damage if you don't know exactly what you're doing.

There are two main types of exercises. *Compound exercises,* such as the bench press and squat, involve multiple joints. *Isolation exercises,* such as chest flies and shoulder raises, target only one joint.

Compound exercises are a better choice for beginners. They work a lot of muscles and are less likely to cause injury. Advanced lifters mainly do compound exercises, as well. However, they'll supplement their basic plan with isolation exercises to develop weaker muscle groups. If your goal is massive size, this is a good approach. Stick with compound exercises and add the occasional isolation movement to build up areas that need more work.

HOW MUCH VARIETY?

Have you been doing the same workout for years? Maybe when doing upper-body workouts you always start on the bench, then wander over to the dumbbell rack for a few sets of incline flies. Or start with squats for lower-body workouts, then move on to lunges or leg extensions.

Routines are great. They make it easy to remember the exercises you want to do. Doing the same movements also improves neural efficiency and yields the best strength gains. But sticking with the same routine—doing the same exercises in the same order, with the same number of reps and sets—is a problem. Muscles need change in order to grow.

Shake up your workouts every 3 to 4 weeks. Add new exercises, or scramble the order in which you do them. Do extra sets of one exercise, or fewer of another. Change forces muscles and nerves to adapt to new movements—the key to optimal gains in size and strength.

WHAT IS PERIODIZATION?

This is another way to shake up your workout. Rather than changing your exercise routine without a plan, with periodization you plan variety in training volume and intensity. Classic strength-training programs typically are divided into periodization cycles, in which you gradually increase training intensity (the amount of weight lifted) while decreasing training volume (the number of exercises multiplied by the number of sets and reps).

Periodization can get incredibly complex. For day-to-day purposes, you can keep it pretty basic. On Monday, for example, you might practice a high-volume, low-intensity workout by doing 12 to 15 repetitions of some exercises. As the week progresses, you'll do fewer reps, but work with heavier weights.

These frequent changes, called undulating periodization, are ideal for muscle-building stimulation.

SHOULD I TRAIN TO FAILURE?

For beginners, the answer is probably not. Doing new movements until the point of failure—where the muscles in play absolutely give out—may make you too sore to move for the next 2 to 3 days. It's hard to get bigger and stronger when you can't move.

For advanced guys, the answer is a little more debatable. You don't always have to train to failure, but you do have to progressively increase what you are doing. The easiest way to accomplish this really is to train to failure. This means pushing and pushing until you're physically incapable of completing one more movement. If you keep lifting more weight at the same reps, or doing more reps at the same weight, you will be getting bigger and stronger—no one disagrees about this.

Naturally, sports scientists break it down even more. Lifting a weight as many times as possible until you can no longer lift it is called training to momentary *positive* muscular failure. Lifting until you can no longer *lower* the weight with control is called training to momentary *negative* muscular failure.

Training to muscle failure is advanced stuff. Beginners shouldn't push themselves quite that hard. To prevent soreness and injury, they should wrap up an exercise 1 to 2 repetitions *before* positive muscle failure occurs.

Advanced lifters can go all the way. They should train to positive muscle failure during most workouts, and only occasionally train to momentary negative muscular failure.

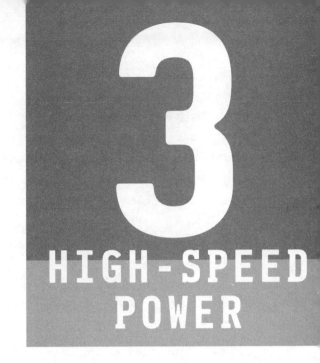

3
HIGH-SPEED POWER

A few decades ago, long workouts were thought to be the only way to produce the muscle breakdown required to promote bulk and better definition. Since then, research has shown that *efficient* workouts can provide the same or better results in a fraction of the time. For most men, a 30- to 45-minute workout two to three times a week will give them the physiques they want. Progress comes faster if you extend that to 4 to 6 days a week—but each workout can still be trimmed to as little as 30 minutes.

Of course, this will only happen if you streamline your workouts and make every gym minute count. Here are some ways to do that.

HIGH-SPEED SUPERSETS

Supersetting is a technique in which you do one set each of two (or more) different exercises back-to-back, without any rest in between the sets.

- New lifters usually do supersets for opposite muscle groups—chest and back, for example. One muscle group rests while the other works. This allows you to pack twice as much exercise into the same workout time.

- More advanced lifters can do supersets for the same muscles. In 30 minutes, you can work your muscles to total exhaustion and get an incredible amount of muscle-building stimulus.

- If your goal is to improve endurance or high-intensity conditioning, you'll probably do supersets for the same muscle groups—for example, a bench press followed by chest flies.

- If your goal is maximal size and strength, you'll want to do supersets for opposing, or antagonistic, muscle groups—for example, a barbell row followed by a bench press.

Remember, one muscle group is recovering while you're training the other muscle group. You save time and allow for more recovery. More recovery means you'll be lifting heavier weights and adding muscle fast.

COMBINATION EXERCISES

The concept is similar to supersets in that you do multiple exercises without any rest in between. That's a time-saver by itself. In addition, combination exercises—as opposed to isolation exercises—work multiple muscle groups with the same movements. That shaves even more time off your workouts.

For example, you might do a dumbbell curl for the biceps, followed by a dumbbell press for the shoulders and triceps. As with supersets, you'll probably combine exercises that train different muscle groups. Ideally, you'll pick workout combinations that don't require changing weights or equipment—and that means even more time saved.

There are probably hundreds of combination exercises. Some of the most popular include the following.

FOR DEVELOPING POWER TRANSFER FROM THE LOWER TO THE UPPER BODY. Combine front squats (page 224) with barbell shoulder presses (page 138). Or combine barbell squats (page 220) with barbell shoulder press from behind the neck (no photos).

FOR POWER CONDITIONING. Perform a one-arm dumbbell snatch with the right hand (page 202), shuffle sideways 10 feet, and snatch with the left hand. Or combine one-arm snatches with kick-out-into-pushups (page 127). After performing a dumbbell snatch, place both hands on the floor in front of your feet and kick out (backward) with your feet so that you end up in a pushup position. Perform the desired reps and kick back into place and proceed to do a dumbbell snatch with the other arm.

FOR BUILDING MUSCLE SIZE AND STRENGTH. Combine pushups (page 127) with two-arm dumbbell rows (page 171). For better results, keep the dumbbells in your hands for both exercises. Or combine upright rows (page 146) with dumbbell presses (page 139).

BODY-WEIGHT EXERCISES

Work some body-weight exercises into your program. You don't need any equipment beyond what nature has already given you, and you can do them in your office, hotel room, or a convention center hallway.

Moving your body weight is surprisingly tough at first. If you haven't worked out for a long time, take it easy: Doing more than a few pushups or squats will make you sore in places you probably forgot existed. The workouts get easier quickly. When that happens, you can make them harder by working one arm or leg at a time. In fact, there are all sorts of refinements for adapting body-weight workouts to your current fitness level.

DUMBBELL SQUAT (PAGE 223). Make it easier by going only halfway down, or by holding on to something stable. Make it harder by squatting on the balls of your feet, or by standing on one leg.

SINGLE LEG SQUAT (PAGE 232). Make it easier by going only halfway down or holding on to something stable. Make it harder by squatting all the way down s-l-o-w-l-y, holding the tension for a few seconds at the bottom, then jumping up.

BULGARIAN SPLIT SQUAT (PAGE 222). Make it easier by holding on to something stable. Make it harder by squatting on the balls of your feet.

PUSHUP (PAGE 127). Make it easier by letting your knees touch the floor, or by spreading your feet farther apart. Make it harder by using one arm, or moving against an elastic band.

TWO-ARM DUMBBELL ROW (PAGE 171). Use books or other objects for resistance. Make it easier by raising your torso above parallel with the floor. Make it harder by holding the objects at the top position.

VERTICAL LEG CRUNCH (PAGE 64). Make it easier by bending your knees or crossing your arms on your chest. Make it harder by keeping your legs straight and holding a book or object between your feet.

ELBOW BRIDGE (PAGE 44). Make it easier by spreading your feet wider or bending your knees. Make it harder by keeping your feet closer together or extending your arms.

A HIGH-SPEED PROGRAM

We designed this workout with two things in mind: You can do it anywhere, without any equipment at all; and you can do it in 30 minutes or less. Start out by doing two to three complete circuits. That means repeating the series of exercises two or three times. If you want, do it at least 3 days a week.

To keep your motivation high, set benchmarks—then try to break them. For example, the first week you might try to hold the Plank for 30 seconds. The second week, progress to 35 seconds. Add 5 seconds each week. Or try to complete 5 to 10 reps of other exercises the first week, then progress to as many as you can manage the second week. Don't progress too fast or you'll wind up with a lot of residual soreness.

The chart below summarizes the workout. You can find more information on this and other quick training programs at www.thomasincledon.com.

EXERCISE	TIME OR REPS
PLANK	30 SEC
SIDE PLANK	30 SEC EACH SIDE
HIP-THIGH EXTENSIONS	AS MANY REPS AS POSSIBLE
PARTIAL SPLIT SQUATS	AS MANY REPS AS POSSIBLE
T-PUSHUP	AS MANY REPS AS POSSIBLE
STEPUP	AS MANY REPS AS POSSIBLE
REPEAT CIRCUIT	

PLANK

This exercise is designed to strengthen the abdominals and other muscles that stabilize your spine. It will also improve stability around your wrists and make your triceps beg for mercy.

Start in a pushup position. Your ankles, knees, hips, and head should be in a straight line. Hold the pose for 30 seconds to start; increase the hold time if it gets too easy.

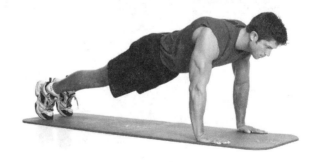

SIDE PLANK

This is a powerful strengthening movement for spinal stabilizers. And because you have to balance on one arm, it's superb for improving arm and wrist strength.

A Balance on your left arm and foot, with your trunk and legs at a 45-degree angle to the floor. Your right foot should be on top of your left. Don't position the supporting arm directly under the shoulder. Position it slightly forward of the shoulder. Your right arm extends out in a straight line from the left hand and elbow (keep the same angle).

B Straighten the supporting arm by contracting the triceps muscle. Press your index finger firmly on the floor. Align your body so that it's in a diagonal line, from the heels to the top of your head. Hold the pose for 30 seconds to start; increase the hold time if it gets too easy. Repeat.

A

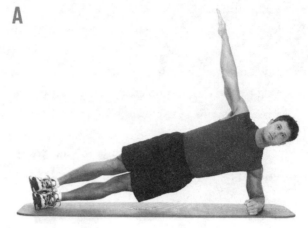

B

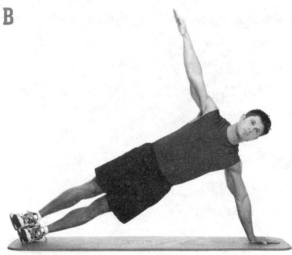

HIP-THIGH EXTENSIONS

This exercise is designed to strengthen your hip muscles and build that hard butt women love to see in jeans.

A Lie faceup on the floor. Bend your left leg to a 90-degree angle, keeping your right leg straight. Your arms should be extended at a 45-degree angle from the body, palms up. Raise your body about 1 inch by pushing off with your left foot.

B Continue to lift until your entire body is in a straight line and your thighs are parallel to each other. Only your arms, upper back, and left foot should be in contact with the floor. Pause at the top of the movement, lower to within 1 inch of the floor, then repeat. Do as many reps as possible. Then repeat on the other side.

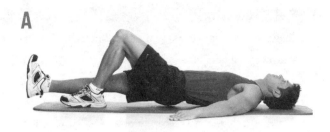

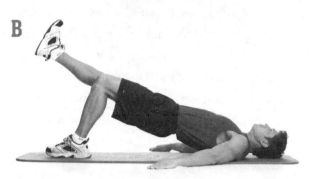

PARTIAL SPLIT SQUAT

This exercise will blast your thighs to new growth and strengthen your knees.

A Step forward with your left leg, taking a bigger-than-normal step. Keep your upper body upright and your arms at your sides. Bend your left leg to 90 degrees, keeping your left knee in line with your ankle. Lower your back leg (right leg) until your knee touches the floor. Place your right hand on the inside of the front (left) knee, and put your left hand on the butt muscle of the left leg. Raise your back knee 1 inch off the floor. This is the starting position.

B Raise yourself up by extending both legs; you'll feel tension in your knee and butt. The movement is completed when you no longer feel these muscles contracting. Pause, then return to the starting position, with your knee 1 inch off the floor. Complete a set, then repeat on the other side.

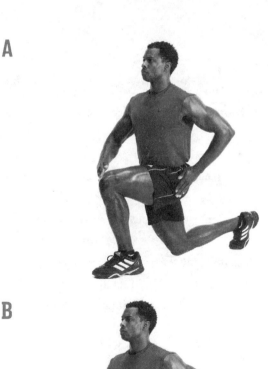

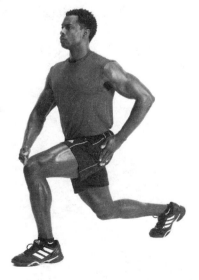

T-PUSHUP

This exercise works the chest and arms. It helps build rotational strength in your core.

A Assume a normal pushup position. From the lowered position, push yourself up.

B When you reach the top, elbows-locked position, transfer your body weight to your right arm and rotate your body to the right. Reach up and behind you with your left hand. Keep both feet on the floor initially. If you can, lift your left foot off the floor at the end of the movement. You'll make an X shape with your arms and legs. Return to the starting position, and repeat on the other side. Then perform as many reps as possible.

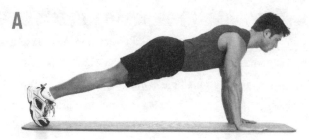

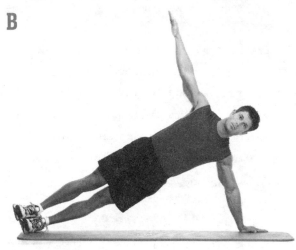

STEPUP

This is another leg exercise that will strengthen your hips and knees.

A Stand while facing a bench or the seat of a chair; the bench or chair should be slightly above knee height. Place your left foot on the bench or chair.

B Push up through the heel of the raised foot until you can stand on the bench or chair. Slowly lower yourself down, keeping the left foot on the bench or chair; keep your right foot suspended in the air. Return to the starting position, switch legs, and repeat. Then repeat as many times as possible.

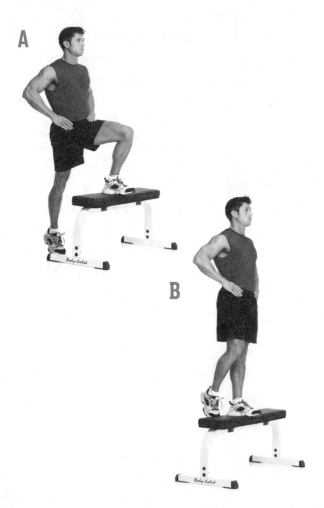

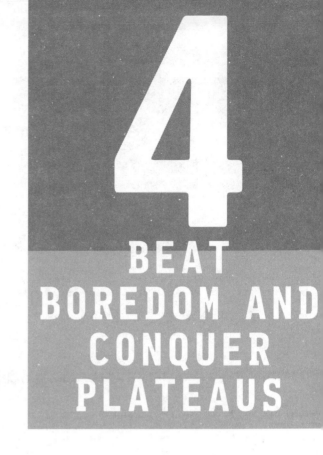

4

BEAT BOREDOM AND CONQUER PLATEAUS

Lifting is work. Hard work. No matter how much you enjoy it, it's still a repetitive, body-hammering activity that's easy to skip when other things get in the way.

Another, more insidious trap is plateauing. No matter how long you've been lifting, there will come a time when the exciting, initial progress grinds to a halt. You've been lifting the same weight loads for what seems like forever. You can't see significant changes in the mirror. You feel good and look good—but honestly, no different than you

felt or looked last week. You get complacent or, let's be honest, lazy. Why work so hard, you tell yourself, when nothing's happening?

This is the critical juncture at which a lot of men get discouraged, give up, and drop out. About half of all men who start lifting quit somewhere between 6 months and a year into their program. This is less likely to happen with men who already have a lot of lifting history under their belts, but they, too, have to deal with the motivation traps.

PLANNING YOUR MOVES

Researchers have found that athletes who measure themselves against themselves, who focus on increasing their own competence and strength, do a lot better overall than the ones who are always competing against others. No matter how long you've been lifting, there will always be guys who are bigger

and better defined. Your motivation will take a hit if you measure your own progress (or shortcomings) against them. The men who focus only on their own improvement, who look at what they're doing today compared to last month, have built-in motivators that keep them going.

Set clear, realistic training goals. Most of us like a good challenge. Even if you don't think of yourself as a competitive type, nothing beats the feeling of setting a new personal record. That's pretty easy in the initial months. A man who starts out benching 100 pounds can easily progress to 150 in about 12 weeks. That's powerful motivation to keep going!

Advanced weight lifters won't make those kinds of rapid gains, of course. Some guys hit a wall and get discouraged. Smart lifters get around it by setting more distant but still tangible goals: moving up a plate size by a certain date, for example, or completing 10 reps instead of 8.

The goals you set should be realistic. Maybe you want to increase your bench weight by 25 pounds. Break it down into increments: 5 pounds by the end of the month, another 5 pounds the month after that, and so on. You might move faster than that. But if you don't, you'll still know you reached your targets—and have additional goals to shoot for.

Just as important, make sure that goals you set are things you can actually control. You might or might not be able to increase your bench weight 25 pounds in X amount of time. That's out of your control. You can control how many sets you do, how challenging you make the exercises, and how many hours you commit to your workouts. Don't just think about your program. Write it down where you'll see it. Put a sticky note on your computer: "5 more pounds this month." The more you see it, the more you think it—and do it.

Keep a training log. Write down the exercises, weights, sets, reps, length of rest, and all the other variables that influence your progress. Competitive lifters almost always keep a log of some kind; it's the only way to keep track of where you are, especially as your workouts get more complex.

Another advantage of a written log is that it allows you to jot down goals for each training cycle and to keep track of changes. A lot of men have started using computer spreadsheets to track training. Others carry a notebook to the gym. It doesn't matter what you use. The idea is to put your program somewhere you can *see* it.

Build in variety. A varied workout means you can shift your mental and physical gears. There will be days when you don't feel like lifting or running or whatever. That's when a lot of guys simply blow off their workouts. Do that a few times and you start to lose momentum. You always need pleasurable alternatives. Stretch when you don't feel like lifting. Lift when you don't feel like riding your bike. *Keep the habit going.*

Get the most from your membership. Even the lowest-rent gyms these days offer a lot of classes. Commit to trying something new at least once a month. Maybe yoga. Pilates. Kickboxing. Classes are fun. You get top-flight instruction, and you don't feel like you're out there on your own. If you don't like the class, don't take it again. But at least you've got more options to choose from.

Take a look at other gyms in your area. Some men still prefer the dark, messy look of old-style gyms. Sports-oriented men tend to prefer athletic training center designs with provisions for sports medicine, sports psychology, massage therapy, strength training, and training analysis. Men in business might gravitate to a club where they can train as well as socialize and look at potential deals. Just getting into a new environment, whatever your preference, might be the kick-start you need.

YOUR WORKOUTS, YOUR LIFE

Guys who are serious about lifting and getting in shape know that workouts don't start and stop at the gym door. It's about balance: incorporating every conceivable type of movement into every corner of your life. Muscles and nerves adapt to change as well as to things like intensity and frequency. You only pack so much into an hour in the weight room. Men who attain optimal levels of fitness are *always* working out.

Move and keep moving. You should be moving every day of your life, even if that only means taking stairs instead of elevators or cycling to work instead of driving. Muscles, joints, and nerves require a lot of movement for peak efficiency. At the very least, staying physically active in day-to-day ways improves joint lubrication and the muscle and joint flexibility that you need to work out *hard*. Just as important, it keeps you focused on your long-term goal of getting—and staying—in top shape.

Don't depend on gear. Every man should know how to exercise without equipment. It takes care of those days you can't get to the gym. It also means you can do something new, on the spot, when you're tired of the same old routine. Bored with bench presses? Drop down and do some pushups. Close your office door and do a few sets of squats, lunges, or crunches.

Set a schedule and keep to it. We're all creatures of habit. Men who always work out at the same times every day are the ones who are still doing it years later. Part of this is mental, but it's also physiology. Once you establish a schedule, your body's hormones adjust and kick in at the appropriate time. That means you can train more efficiently and with less fatigue.

QUALITY BEATS QUANTITY

Never use time (or the lack of it) as an excuse not to train. Use it to be more creative.

- Research shows evening is the best time to exercise. That makes a difference in research labs, but it's not that important for most guys. If you have time in the mornings, use it.

- Workouts are most efficient when they last 20 to 60 minutes—but hey, some is better than none. Five-minute blasts spread throughout the day can do pretty much the same job as 30 minutes of concentrated lifting.

- Push hard on days you have more time. Other days, do what you can—walk to the store, hike around the park, work in the yard. *Everything* you do burns calories and gets you where you want to be.

Work with a training partner. It's almost always better to work out with someone than to do it alone. Why? A partner depends on you to show up—a good push when you really don't feel like going to the gym. A partner keeps you company, creates friendly competition, and pushes you to push yourself.

While you're in a social frame of mind, think about lining up a trainer for a few sessions. *Every* serious lifter does it. It's impossible to watch yourself in any detail while you're lifting. A trainer can see exactly what you're doing and make the kinds of minor (or not so minor) adjustments that translate into substantial muscle gains.

SHAKE IT UP

We explained in earlier chapters that change is the cornerstone of lifting. You have to keep your muscles challenged. If you keep putting them through the same paces over and over again, eventually the muscle fibers adapt. They get bored and complacent. They go through the motions, but no longer have the incentives to get bigger. And you find yourself on a plateau.

Some men are perfectly happy to stay on a plateau indefinitely. Their goal is to maintain the level of conditioning they already have. If this sounds like you, fine. The plateau is an okay place to be.

But most men want to see progress. That's why they lift. For them, the plateau is an uncomfortable place to be. They want to get off it as quickly as possible. And there are some pretty simple fixes.

Change your routine. Beginners can get away with doing the same program for up to 6 months before they start to plateau. The more experience you have lifting, the more frequently you have to change your training. A good rule of thumb is to overhaul your workout every 3 to 4 weeks.

It doesn't matter what changes you make. You can reverse the order in which you do your exercises. If you usually start with bench presses, you may want to switch to an incline press. Even though both exercises work the chest, shoulders, and triceps, the slightly different movements involved activate additional muscle fibers for greater stimulus.

Or suppose you hit a wall doing 3 sets of each exercise. Try switching to 1 set while using more weight and maintaining better form. You can increase the intensity of exercises, change the reps, or change the frequency of workouts or rest periods.

OVERTRAINING WON'T PURGE PLATEAUS

One of the prevailing myths about plateaus is that a few superhard workouts will somehow whip recalcitrant muscles into shape and, in essence, show them the errors of their ways. The first problem with this concept is that men who overlift don't get stronger. They get hurt. The second problem is that it doesn't work. Muscles need change. A *smart* increase in intensity or frequency is one way to achieve that. Pounding muscles into submission isn't the answer.

In fact, men who overtrain generally can't get *off* plateaus. They get cranky and irritable. They can't sleep. Their blood pressure rises. They get so sore they can't move. They essentially break down from the inside out. This is not to be confused with workout progress.

HOW TO VARY YOUR WORKOUTS

Changing your training routine is the best and quickest way to get off a plateau. The potential variations are endless. Don't be one of those guys who does only barbell bench presses and barbell curls—always in the same order. Look around the gym. Be creative, for cripe's sake!

If you want to add size to your chest, for example, you might start out with dumbbell bench presses and medicine ball pushups for 4 weeks. The next 4 weeks, switch to incline barbell presses and one-arm pushups. Follow that with 4 weeks of bench presses and one-arm stability ball pushups. Do this kind of thing all the time, and you can say good-bye to plateaus.

Other good changeups include the following:

- Change your technique. Lift fast and lower slowly. Then switch to slow lifting and slow lowering. Then to fast lifting and fast lowering.

- Change your mechanics. For example, use your legs (when appropriate) for added power. Then quit using your legs for more isolation.

- Change body-part groupings. Work your chest and back on the same days. Later, combine chest, shoulder, and triceps workouts.

- Change the exercise order. Start with a bench press followed by flies. Then reverse the order.

- Change the order of muscle groups. Do chest workouts followed by back workouts. Then start with back workouts and follow with chest exercises.

- Change rep and set numbers.

- Change the amount of rest between sets—anywhere from 30 seconds to 3 minutes.

- Change equipment. Stick to free weights for a while. Then switch to machines.

The bottom line is that *any* change will get you off the plateau.

Use the sawtooth solution. Also called periodization programs, sawtooth training mixes hard stretches of training with periods of active rest. Suppose you like to do 3 sets of bench presses with 200 pounds. For a week, drop it down to 2 sets with 150 pounds—this is the beginning of the active rest phase. A week later, gradually build it back up, going to 3 sets with 170 pounds for the first workout, 180 pounds for the second, 190 for the third. After that, you are ready to return to where you started—and then move on to the next higher level.

The rest periods allow muscles to fully recover from the initial exertion, often with dramatic results. A lot of men who try this get a surge of progress that takes them beyond the plateau.

Pyramid the weights. This tough technique is another way of tricking your muscles into exerting more effort than they're used to. By lifting heavier and heavier weights in progressive sets, you push the muscles beyond the point they've adapted to. You could, for example, start with biceps curls, using weights that are a little lighter than usual. Do fewer reps than you're accustomed to (5 instead of 10, for example), then do another set with the next size up, again doing 5 reps. Keep going until you reach a weight that's too heavy to curl 5 times. Then work your way *back down* through the weights.

Don't let injuries hold you back. You need to cut way back on your workouts when you're hurt or sick. But that doesn't mean giving them up altogether. Unless you're truly, seriously sick, work *around* your injury. Got a shoulder pull? Train your legs. Knee out of whack? Work your upper body. Remind yourself how hard it was to get into the lifting habit in the first place. Keep going to the gym. Even if you don't do anything more strenuous than floor stretches, at least you'll keep the habit going.

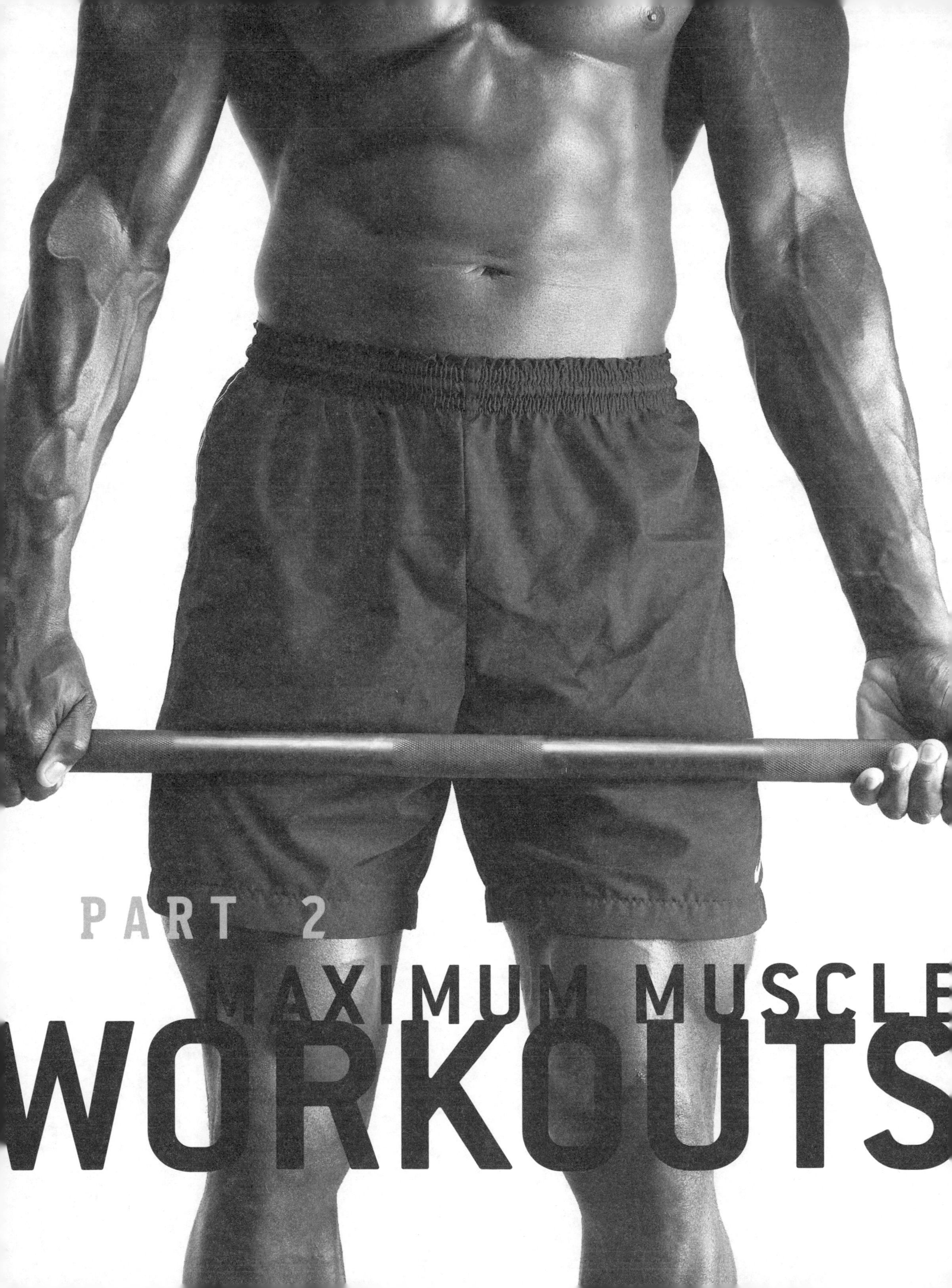

PART 2

MAXIMUM MUSCLE
WORKOUTS

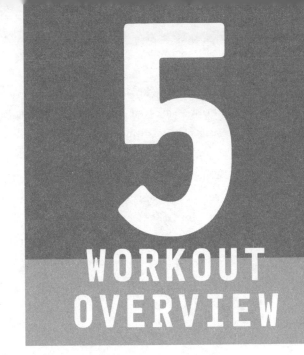

5

WORKOUT OVERVIEW

It's time to get down to the business of working out. This section of the book offers specific programs for each of your favorite muscle groups: abs, arms, chest, shoulders and neck, back, hips and glutes, and legs. There's also a total-body program, plus a flexibility program. If you're serious about building a particular muscle group, the program concentrating on that group will get you where you want to be. The more exercises you incorporate in your workouts, the more quickly you'll force the breakdown and growth of the targeted muscles. Of course, the full-body training and conditioning

program in chapter 13 provides the fastest, most efficient way to achieve optimal strength and size. Remember, you want balanced, full-body workouts for overall fitness. However, individual muscle-group workouts are superb for concentrating your workouts on weak areas.

WORKOUT CHECKLIST

1. Work out 3 days a week.
2. Warm up with the dynamic warmup program starting on page 285.
3. Choose your resistance carefully. In Level 1 workouts, since you are just starting out, make your weights easy. You can always add more weight later. If you can't complete the body-weight exercises initially, it's fine to shorten the range of motion to make them easier. Then increase the range of motion as you get in better shape.

4. Before working out, perform a full-body warmup, followed by a dynamic warmup, followed by an exercise-specific warmup.
5. Hold weights with your thumb wrapped around the grip.
6. Take advantage of safety racks—and use a spotter when possible.
7. When doing dumbbell exercises, keep rubber mats on the floor by your sides. The mats will absorb some of the impact if you drop the weights.
8. If possible, lift in front of a mirror so that you can watch your form.
9. Make sure your body is balanced and stable before starting the movement. Keep your feet anchored or firmly planted on the ground for better stability.
10. Always perform each movement with *total control*. Don't heave or jerk. The positive (lifting)

phase should be done with a little speed, but not all out—say, to a count of 2. The negative (lowering) phase should be done more slowly—say, to a count of 4.

11. Breathe in during the negative (lowering) phase. Breathe out during the positive (lifting) phase.

12. Sip a lot of water to stay hydrated. And keep a towel handy to wipe sweat off equipment.

13. After your workout, cool down with the static flexibility program starting on page 289.

14. Allow at least 1 day of rest between workouts.

15. The workout programs for each muscle group, as well as the total-body program, are each divided into three levels. Level 1 focuses on building muscle mass, level 2 is devoted to increasing strength, and level 3 features hybrid training, a combination of size and strength. For any given program, stick with each level for 12 weeks before moving on to the next. Once you've performed level 3 for 12 weeks, add additional exercises and programs to your workouts.

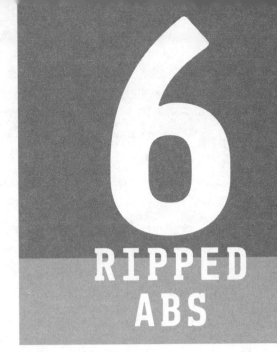

6

RIPPED ABS

There's a reason that *Men's Health*® and other fitness magazines feature cover models with ripped abs: That's the look men want most. Strong arms and a broad chest might represent the masculine ideal, but nothing says "I'm serious about my body" more than a washboard gut.

So why do so many men devote so little time to abdominal workouts? Partly because of the work involved. Those muscles aren't used to heavy lifting. When you first put them through their paces, they're going to complain—a lot. The average guy with an average degree of self-preservation will naturally gravitate to biceps curls or other exercises that actually feel good.

Then there's the "so what?" factor. Ab workouts by themselves won't make a dramatic difference in how your gut actually looks. Unlike bench presses, say, which produce visible changes in as little as a few weeks, crunches and other abdominal exercises produce more subtle results. The muscles get bigger and stronger the more you work them. They don't necessarily get any more ripped.

The *only* way those muscles will ever reveal themselves is to trim body fat. Period. You can do crunches and situps from dawn until dusk, but until you strip away those surface layers of fat, the muscles themselves stay out of sight. The best fitness models know this. On top of hours in the gym (and, in most cases, the blessings of genetic good luck), they watch calories and eat the kinds of foods that are an integral part of any total-body conditioning program.

That said, the workouts you choose will go a long way toward building the abs and bringing them into sharp relief.

ABS EXPLAINED

The abdominal muscles are primarily involved in moving the spine (spinal flexion). This is the movement that allows you to bring your chin to your knees or, more practically, to turn and see what's going on around you. They also protect the spine when you lift. Strong abdominals make you look lean and fit. More important, they can help you play harder and stay injury-free longer.

The abs consist of a series of six muscles:

- The rectus abdominis, responsible for flexing the trunk

- The internal and external obliques (which have right and left sides), responsible for rotation, lateral (to the side) flexion, and flexion of the spine
- The transverse abdominis, responsible for holding your internal organs in place

Virtually every abdominal exercise works the rectus abdominis. It's the main muscle, and the biggest one. You can fine-tune your workouts to bring more of the other muscles into play.

THE TOTAL AB WORKOUT

Abdominal training is rife with myths and misconceptions. For example, men with bad backs are often advised to strengthen their abs with high-repetition workouts. This is nonsense. Studies have found *no* difference in abdominal use, from exercise or anything else, between men with chronic lower-back pain and men without. The concept of high-repetition workouts is similarly misguided. High reps are good for muscular endurance, not strength. The standard advice almost guarantees a bad back *and* weak abs. (For the record: Men with back pain should focus on exercises that strengthen the lower back. Working the abs is less critical.)

Then there's the latest trend to put guys on stability balls for crunch workouts. There's nothing wrong with this approach, but it doesn't work as well as you might think. It's certainly not in the same league as traditional ab workouts.

This doesn't mean you should ignore stability balls, wobble boards, elastic tubing, or other gadgets. Like machine weights, free weights, and simple body-weight exercises, they're useful tools—good for some things, not so good for others. Training the muscles of the trunk without weights (such as on a stability ball) requires different muscle activity than using weights or machines for resistance.

An ideal program has a little bit of everything.

To get the most out of any ab workout, here are some points to keep in mind.

Do ab exercises at the end of your workout. You'll never achieve the cut look unless you integrate abdominal exercises into a whole-body strengthening plan. Ab workouts are hard work. Training them first may cause you to fatigue prematurely and reduce the effectiveness of the rest of your workout.

On the other hand, if you're new to abdominal training, there's something to be said for doing the exercises at the beginning of your workout, when you're refreshed and ready. And if you're one of those guys who truly hates ab exercise and always finds an excuse to do something else, *anything* else, that's another good reason to train them first.

Remember progression. If you're working on machines or with free weights, start with weights that are easy to handle. Increase weights gradually—initially, usually by about 5 pounds a week.

Take your feet off the floor. It's the best way to blast your abs hard when doing crunches and situp movements. The exception is when you're working the hip flexor muscles, in which case you should not only keep your feet planted on the floor but anchor them to keep them from moving.

Curl in the correct sequence. Start curls by lifting the shoulders, then the upper back, then the lower back.

Don't sit up to an upright position. Raise your torso no more than 30 degrees. Hold momentarily, then lower back down.

Don't forget flexibility. Finish the workout by stretching the abdominals.

If you're pressed for time, eliminate the ab workouts. No kidding. Heavy squats, deadlifts, and cleans do more for strengthening the abdominals than dedicated ab exercises.

AB ROTATION

This exercise uses resistance to put serious strain on the oblique (side) muscles, while also increasing core stability and strength.

A Attach stretch tubing or a cable to a post or other stationary object at chest height. Stand with your shoulders lined up with the fixed object; your face will be at a right angle to it. Grip the tubing or cable handles with both hands. Step arm's length away, with your legs shoulder width apart, and knees slightly bent, arms extended in front of you.

B Rotate your torso, using your abdominal muscles to work against the resistance. Work from left to right until you finish the set; then do the same number of reps from right to left.

MAKE IT EASIER

- Don't rotate all the way through your potential range of motion. Move only as far as you comfortably can, while maintaining total control.
- Keep your hands close to your body during the rotations.

DO IT HARDER

- Rotate faster through your complete range of motion.

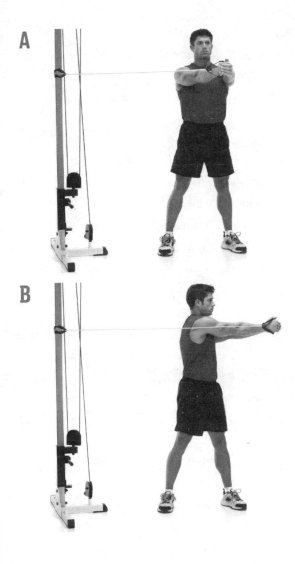

BALL FORWARD CRUNCH (OR PIKE ROLL OUT AND IN)

Working out on an exercise ball puts tension on muscles in your midsection, hips, and thighs, while keeping your torso stable.

A Lie on your stomach. Position the ball under your shins or ankles. Support your upper body on your hands in a pushup position.

B Roll the ball in toward the chest, contracting the abs and keeping your back straight. Roll the ball back out, then repeat.

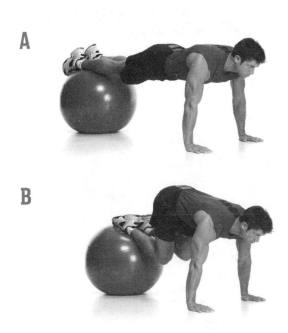

MAKE IT EASIER

- Use a bigger ball. It puts more tension on your hands and less on your abs.
- Hold on to a bench or rack for increased support.

DO IT HARDER

- Use a smaller ball. It puts less tension on your hands and more on your abs.
- Hook an ankle strap on your ankles, and use a cable or tubing attached to a stationary object behind you for more resistance.

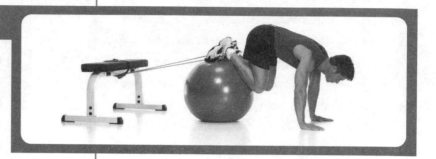

BICYCLE MANEUVER

This exercise works the oblique (side) muscles, with an added rotational movement that improves balance, stability, and core strength.

A Lie on your back with your hands clasped lightly behind your head. Bend your knees to about a 90-degree angle; your shins will be parallel to the ceiling.

B Lift your shoulders off the floor, bring your left knee to your right elbow, and straighten your right leg.

C Using a bicycle-pedaling motion, straighten your left knee while bringing the right knee in toward the left elbow. Extend your legs out only as far as is comfortable without arching your back. Alternate sides, keeping the movement slow and controlled.

MAKE IT EASIER

- Don't lift your knees up all the way.
- Keep your hands under your butt instead of behind your head.

A

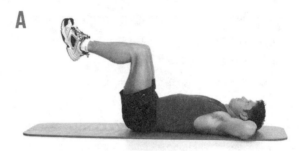

B

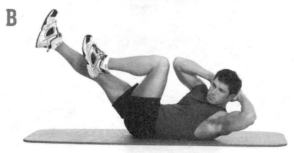

C

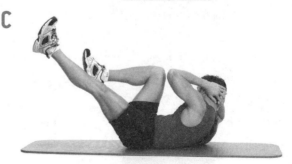

DO IT HARDER

- Attach tubing to a stationary object behind you, holding each end in your hands for more resistance when you lift your shoulders off the floor.
- Use ankle weights to increase muscle load.

CABLE CRUNCH

This is a good general exercise that works all of the abdominal muscles—the upper, lower, and oblique (side) abs. Using a cable pulley machine allows you to increase the resistance as your training permits.

A Kneel on the floor, facing away from a high pulley with a rope handle on the cable. Bend your legs at a 45-degree angle. Grab the rope handle with both hands and hold it at about forehead level.

B Contract your abdominal muscles and slowly curl your torso in, pulling the handle forward. (Use only your abs, not your upper body.) Curl as far in as you can without moving the handle from your forehead. Hold for a second, then slowly return to the starting position.

MAKE IT EASIER

- Keep the handle close to your body.
- Get closer to the cable machine when assuming the initial position.

DO IT HARDER

- Keep the handle farther from your body.
- Get farther away from the cable machine when assuming the initial position.

A

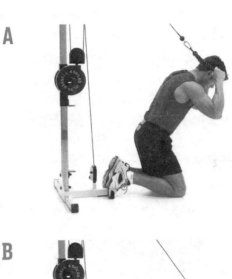

B

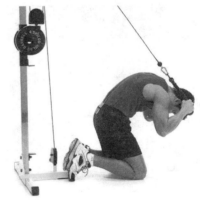

CABLE CURLUP

This exercise works both the upper and lower abs.

A Lie flat on your back in the crunch position in front of a low pulley cable with a Y-shaped rope handle. Your head should point toward the pulley. Keep one knee bent and one leg straight to maintain a neutral hip position. Grab one end of the handle with each hand. Your hands should be just behind your ears.

B Curl your upper torso in toward your lower body, pressing your lower back to the floor and raising your shoulder blades as high off the floor as you can. Don't pull your head up with your hands. Move your torso all the way up to a count of 2. Concentrate on contracting your abdominal muscles. Hold for a second, then count to 2 again as you return to the starting position.

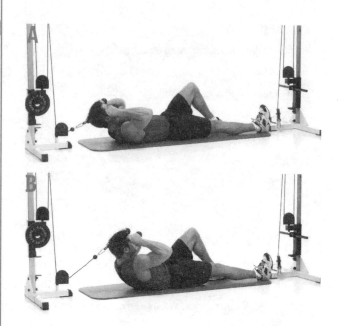

MAKE IT EASIER

- Anchor your feet to provide more support.
- Get closer to the cable when assuming the initial position.

DO IT HARDER

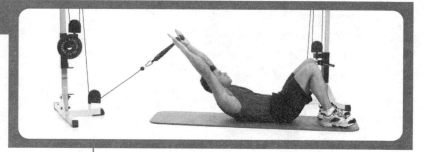

- Set up farther away from the cable, with your knees bent, which prevents the weight plates from touching.
- Extend your arms and shoulders away from your body. As you curl up, keep your arms, shoulders, and spine moving as one unit. This will make your abs work much harder.

CABLE SIDE BEND

In addition to the oblique (side) muscles, this exercise also works your upper and lower abs.

A Stand sideways next to a D-handle low pulley cable. Your right side should be closest to the machine. Grab the handle with your right hand, using an overhand grip, palm facing in. Keep your left hand on your left hip. Your feet should be shoulder width apart.

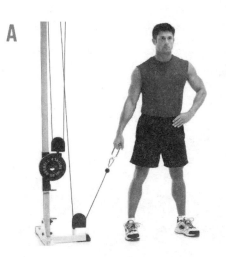

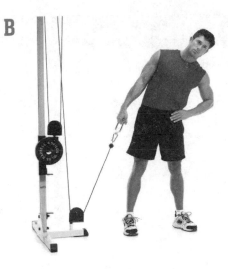

B Slowly bend sideways to the left. Keep your body facing forward; don't turn into the bend. Go as far as you can, then slowly return to an upright position. Don't rest between repetitions; keep your abs and oblique (side) muscles contracted. Finish a set, then repeat on the other side.

MAKE IT EASIER

- Set the pulley higher.
- Stand closer to the cable to shorten the range of motion.
- Keep your arm at a 45- to 60-degree angle from your side.

DO IT HARDER

- Stand farther away from the cable to increase the range of motion.
- Keep your arm close to your side.

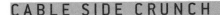

CABLE SIDE CRUNCH

Definitely make time for this exercise. It will give your oblique (side) abs a great workout and help eliminate love handles. It works the internal and external obliques, which run along the sides of the upper and lower abdomen.

A Stand sideways under a D-handle, overhead pulley cable. Your right side should be closest to the machine. With your right hand, grab the handle with an underhand grip. Keep your left hand on your hip. Pull the handle down until your right hand is roughly between your shoulder and your nose.

B Without moving your arm, slowly crunch toward the weight stack. You should feel your obliques contracting forcefully. If you use the proper form and crunch to the side rather than to the front, you'll move only a few inches. Hold for 2 seconds, slowly return to the starting position. Finish the set, then repeat on the other side.

MAKE IT EASIER

- Keep the handle close to your body.
- Set up closer to the cable machine.

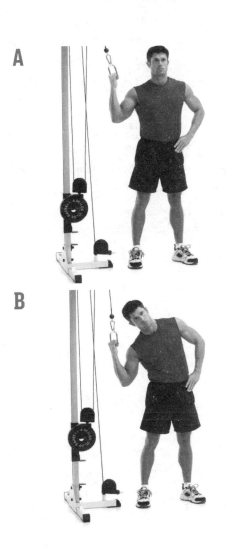

DO IT HARDER

- Keep the handle or weight farther away from your body.
- Set up farther away from the cable machine.

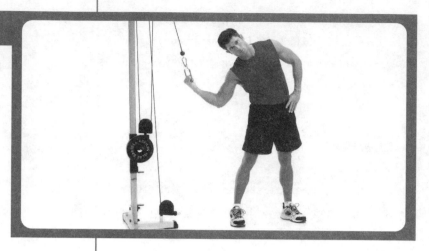

CURLUP

Slightly more difficult than a crunch, but safer than a situp, the curlup involves curling your torso into your body (crunches push your upper body straight up).

A Lie flat on your back with your hands cupped behind your ears and your elbows out. Bend one knee about a 45-degree angle, about 6 inches from your butt, and keep your other leg straight.

B Curl your upper torso in toward your knees, pressing your lower back to the floor and raising your shoulder blades as high off the floor as you can get them. Keep your knees in line with your feet—and don't use your hands to pull your head up. Move your torso all the way up to a count of 2. Concentrate on contracting your abdominal muscles. Hold for a second, then count to 2 again as you return to the starting position.

MAKE IT EASIER

- Cross your hands in front of your chest.

DO IT HARDER

- Keep your hands farther away from your body.

A

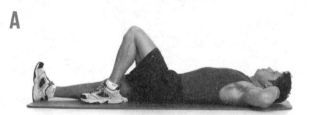

B

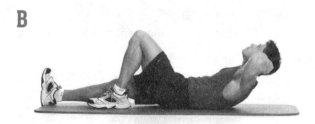

DUMBBELL SIDE BEND

This oblique builder will strengthen the muscles responsible for side-to-side torso movements.

A Stand upright with a dumbbell in your right hand. Your feet should be about shoulder width apart. Keep your left hand on your hip.

B Slowly bend to the right side, allowing the dumbbell on the right side to ride up your hip. You should feel your oblique (side) muscles working. Keep your body facing forward; don't turn your torso into the bend. Bend to the side as far as possible, then slowly bend to the right side as far as possible. Finish the set, then repeat on the other side.

MAKE IT EASIER

• Spread your feet wider than shoulder width apart.

DO IT HARDER

• Stand with your feet closer together; your feet and legs should be touching.
• Keep the hand with the dumbbell farther away from your side.

A
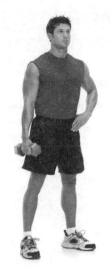

B
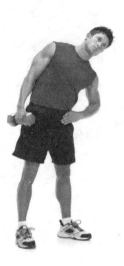

ELBOW BRIDGE

This exercise looks easy, but it's not. It puts a lot of tension on the deep abdominal muscles and the lower back.

A Lie facedown, supporting your upper body on your forearms with your elbows on a mat or towel and your legs extended behind you.

B Lift your body off the floor and rest on your forefeet and elbows. Maintain a planklike position; don't let your butt drop or rise. Only your forefeet and elbows should be on the floor—not your chest or lower arms. Hold for 15 to 30 seconds, rest, then repeat.

MAKE IT EASIER

- Spread your feet wider.
- Hold for only 10 seconds.

DO IT HARDER

- Keep your feet close together.
- Extend your arms, so that only your forefeet and hands are in contact with the floor.

B

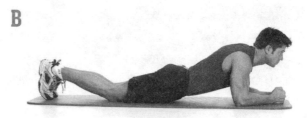

A

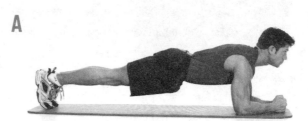

KEEP YOUR HIPS UP

The elbow bridge looks simple, but it can put tremendous strain on your lower back—especially if you have weak "core" muscles. To save your back, don't let your hips drop when doing this workout. If you have trouble keeping your hips horizontal, forget elbow bridges at first. Build up your core first with crunches, curlups, and other, less stressful exercises.

FORWARD BALL ROLL

This difficult exercise works the abdominals and improves the core strength needed to maintain good balance.

A Kneel behind an exercise ball. Place your hands on top of the ball.

B Contract the abdominals and extend forward from the hips as you roll the ball away from you with your hands. Roll forward as far as possible, keeping the tailbone tucked under, abs tight, and back straight. Pause, then roll back to the starting position.

MAKE IT EASIER

- Use a bigger ball.
- Do the exercise near a wall. The ball will rest against the wall at the end of the range of motion.

A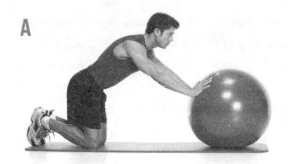

B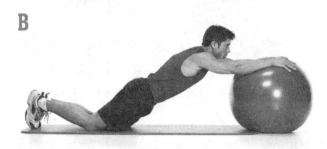

DO IT HARDER

- Use a smaller ball.
- Do the exercise while in a pushup position.

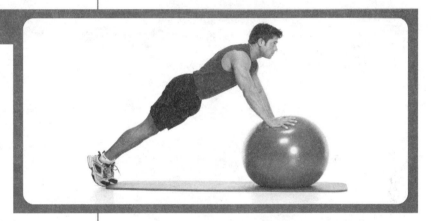

HANGING KNEE RAISE

This multipurpose exercise strengthens the upper, lower, and oblique (side) abdominal muscles, as well as muscles in the front hip (hip flexors). It also gives your back and shoulders a great stretch. You'll need a strong grip—possibly with the help of lifting gloves or a wrist strap—to prolong your hang time.

A Hang from a bar with your legs extended.

A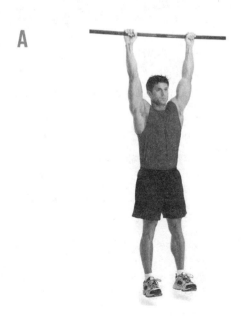

B Using your lower abdominal muscles, bend your knees and raise them as high as you can in a smooth, controlled movement. Your hips will naturally move forward slightly, but don't let the momentum swing your body. Hold for a second, then slowly return to the starting position.

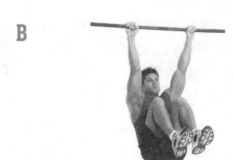

MAKE IT EASIER

- Just bring your knees up to 90 degrees.
- Hang from ab straps.

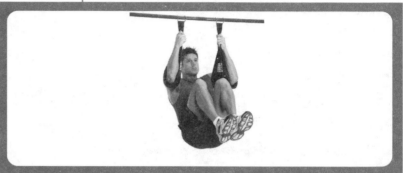

DO IT HARDER

- Raise your legs while keeping them straight.
- Hold a dumbbell between your feet.

SAVE YOUR BACK

Lifting should *never* cause lower-back pain. If it does, you can bet you're doing something wrong. This happens a lot when men do hanging knee raises. You'll see a lot of guys jerking the knees up, or letting the hip flexors collapse when they lower their knees. These mistakes result in excessive arching, or hyperextension—extending the spine beyond its normal range of motion.

Want to know real pain? Arching your back too much during this exercise increases compression in the lower back. Result: sprained ligaments or, worse, a herniated disk, either of which can put you out of commission for 12 weeks, or longer.

Stay in your *pain-free* range of motion when doing hanging knee raises—and perform the exercise under total control.

HANGING KNEE RAISE CROSSOVER

As the abs become stronger, you may want an additional challenge. This gut-buster will work not only your lower and upper abs, but also your oblique (side) muscles.

A Hang fully extended from a chinning bar, with your hands a little more than shoulder width apart. Your palms should face out, and your feet should lightly touch the floor.

B Keeping your legs together, slowly lift your knees toward one shoulder. Go as high as you can. Thrust your pelvis slightly forward, but don't rock or sway for momentum. Hold for a second at the top, then slowly lower your knees. Repeat on the other side. Don't rest between repetitions. Keep your abdominal muscles tight.

MAKE IT EASIER

- Just bring your knees up to 90 degrees.
- Hang from ab straps.

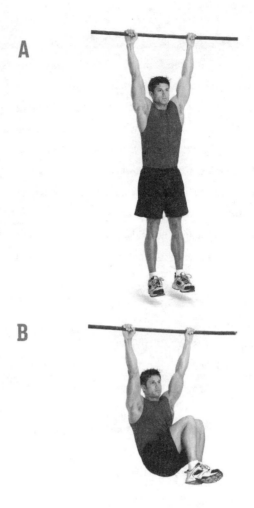

A

B

DO IT HARDER

- Lift your legs instead of just your knees. Keeping your feet together, without bending your knees, lift toward one shoulder, going as high as you can. You'll need to tilt your pelvis slightly forward to complete the movement.

- Hold a dumbbell between your feet. Start by lifting your knees. When this begins to feel easy, try holding the dumbbell between your feet and lifting your legs without bending your knees.

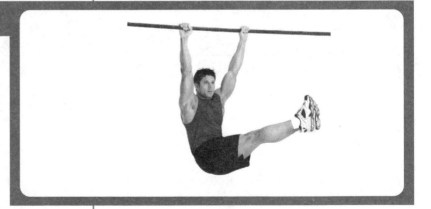

HANGING LEG RAISE

The straight-leg version of this popular exercise increases the workload to the hip flexors as well as the abs.

A   Hang fully extended from a chinning bar, with your hands a little more than shoulder width apart. Your palms should face out, and your feet should lightly touch the floor.

B   Keeping your feet together, slowly lift your legs as high as you can without bending your knees. You'll need to tilt your pelvis slightly forward, but don't rock or sway for momentum. Hold for a second at the top, then slowly lower your legs and repeat. Don't rest between repetitions. Keep your abdominal muscles tight.

MAKE IT EASIER

- Just bring your legs up to 90 degrees.
- Hang from ab straps.

DO IT HARDER

- Hang from a bar that's high enough so that your feet don't touch the floor.
- Hold a dumbbell between your feet.

HIP RAISE

This exercise works the lower abs as well as the gluteal (butt) muscles. Adding ankle weights will allow you to work the quadriceps muscles in the thighs.

A   Lie flat on your back with your legs in the air. Your knees should be unlocked, and your toes pointed. Place your hands at your sides, palms down.

B   Contract your lower abdominal muscles, shift your weight toward your shoulders, and slowly lift your hips off the floor. Keep your legs in a vertical position throughout the exercise. Hold for a second, then slowly return to the starting position.

MAKE IT EASIER

- Anchor your upper body by holding on to a bench or other stable object behind your head for support.
- Only move up 1 to 2 inches. Lift your hips higher as you get stronger.

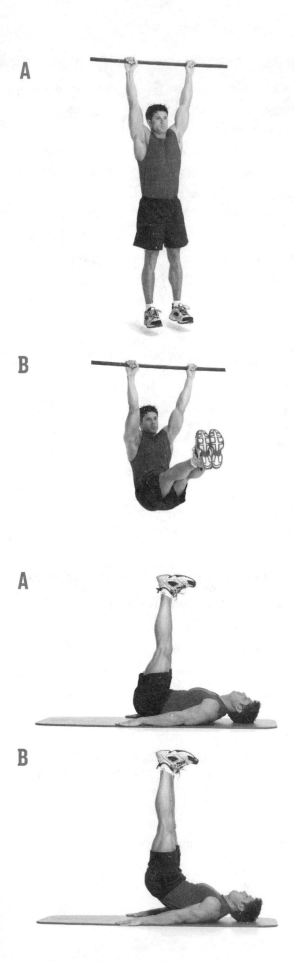

DO IT HARDER

- Do the exercise on a bench and attach tubing to your ankles with the other end attached to the bench for more resistance.
- Hold a small dumbbell between your feet.

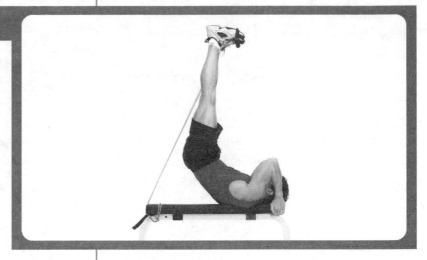

HIP ROLL

Hip rolls mainly work the oblique (side) muscles. They're a good choice for beginners.

A Lie on your back with your hands by your sides, palms down, and bend your hips and knees to 90-degree angles.

B Lower the knees to one side, turning at the waist. Lower your knees until the thighs touch the floor. Then repeat in the opposite direction.

MAKE IT EASIER

- Don't rotate all the way. Move only as far as you comfortably can, while maintaining total control.
- Hold on to a fixed object like a bench or rack with hands above and behind your head (instead of at your sides).

DO IT HARDER

- Straighten your legs, reaching for the floor with your toes instead of your knees.
- Hold a small dumbbell between your feet and do the exercise with straight legs.

A

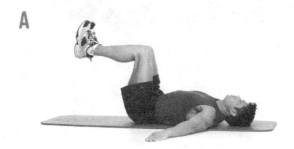

B

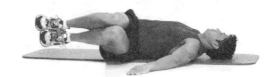

JACKKNIFE KNEE TO CHEST

This exercise improves core stabilization by working the legs and abs.

A Lie on your back, with your arms straight behind your head.

B Bend at the waist while raising your legs and arms so that they meet in a jackknife position. Hold for a moment, then slowly lower your arms and legs back to the starting position. Keep your elbows and knees locked throughout the movement.

MAKE IT EASIER

- Don't come up all the way.
- Keep your arms close to your head.

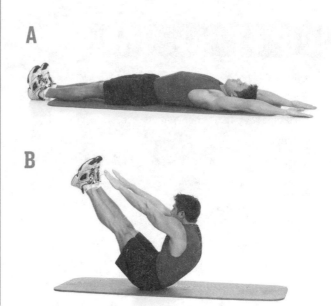

DO IT HARDER

- Anchor one end of tubing to a stationary object behind you and hold the other end in your hands for more resistance. Attach one end of a second tube to your feet, with the other end fixed to another stationary object.
- Hold small dumbbells between your hands and feet.

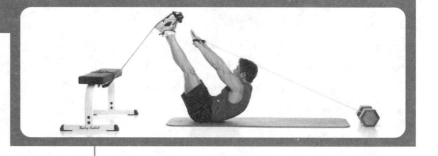

LONG ARM CRUNCH

This move generates 19 percent more activity for the rectus abdominis muscle than the traditional crunch—and is correspondingly more difficult.

A Lie on your back with your knees bent, feet flat on the floor. Extend your arms overhead.

B Slowly raise your arms, head, shoulders, and upper back about 30 degrees off the floor. Hold, then slowly lower. Keep your arms straight, next to your ears, and in line with your head. Don't generate momentum by throwing your arms forward.

MAKE IT EASIER

- Don't come up all the way. Move only as far as you comfortably can, while maintaining total control.

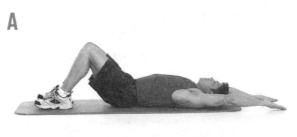

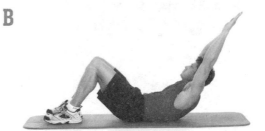

DO IT HARDER

- Anchor one end of tubing to a stationary object behind you and hold the other end in your hands for more resistance.
- Hold your feet up off the ground.

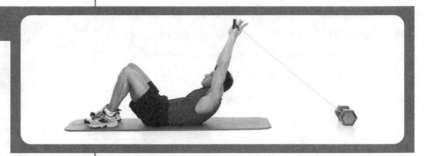

LYING LEG RAISE

This is a good, all-purpose abdominal exercise. For additional resistance, fasten a weight around each ankle.

A Lie on your back on a bench, with your hips near the end. Grip the corners of the bench next to your hips. Extend your legs straight out, toes pointed toward the ceiling.

B Keeping your legs together with your knees unlocked, slowly raise your legs to a vertical position, pressing your lower back into the bench. Hold for a second, then slowly lower your legs until your body is horizontal.

MAKE IT EASIER

- Don't come down all the way. Move only as far as you comfortably can.
- Grip the bench farther back behind the hips.

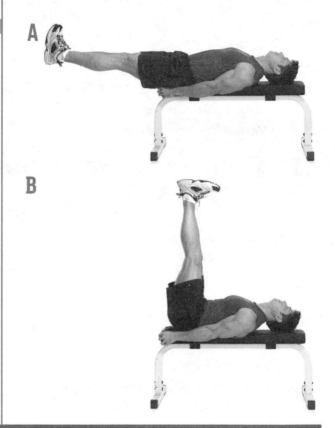

DO IT HARDER

- Anchor tubing to a stationary object in front of you and hold or attach the other end to your feet.
- Hold your legs out in front of you at the bottom of each rep; this maintains muscle tension for a longer period of time.

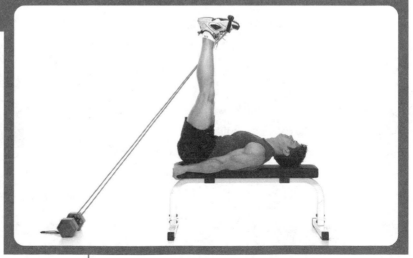

MACHINE CRUNCH

This is a great finishing exercise to wrap up your ab routine. The abdominal crunch machine can be found in most gyms. Be sure to correctly adjust the seat height. Your head should stay flush against the headrest throughout the exercise.

A After adjusting the seat, grab the handles.

B Crunch your body down so that your elbows and knees come toward each other. Exhale on the way down, pause for a moment, then return to the starting position, inhaling on the way up.

MAKE IT EASIER

- Shorten the range of motion by setting the pin in the weight stack at a higher setting.
- Keep your hands closer to your body.

DO IT HARDER

- Pause at the end of the crunch to put additional tension on your abs.
- Keep your hands farther away from your body.

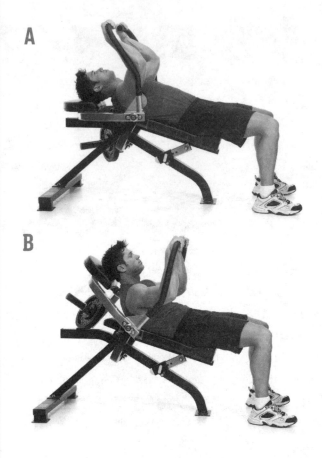

NEGATIVE SITUP

The point of "negatives" is to stay in the zone where the muscles lengthen, but still remain tense. Unlike traditional situps, this exercise makes muscles longer as well as bulkier.

A Sit on the floor with your knees bent and your feet flat on the floor, shoulder width apart. Place your feet under a support—the base of a weight machine, for example, or even your couch—to stabilize your lower body. Begin with your upper body at slightly less than a 90-degree angle to the floor.

B Slowly lower your upper body toward the floor with your abdominal muscles contracted, curling your torso forward and rounding your lower back. When your body reaches a 45-degree angle to the floor, slowly return to the starting position.

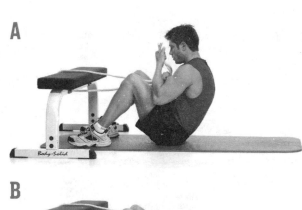

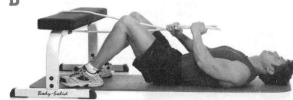

MAKE IT EASIER

- Don't come down all the way.
- Attach a jump rope to a stationary object in front of you and pull yourself up to the start position, or use just one hand to pull your body forward.

DO IT HARDER

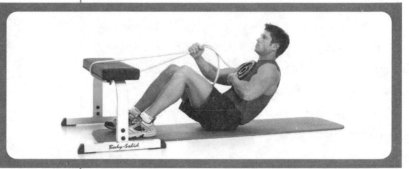

- Lower yourself to a count of 12.
- Stop at three different positions on the way down.
- Hold a weight plate to your chest.

ONE-ARM ROTATION

This is similar to ab rotations, except you use only one arm at a time. This exercise works the oblique (side) muscles, used for rotational movements in most sports.

A Attach stretch tubing to a stationary object or a cable to weights at chest height. Stand with your legs shoulder width apart and knees slightly bent. Your right shoulder should be in line with the fixed object. Grip the tubing or the pulley handle in your right hand and extend your arm out in front of you.

B Rotate your torso to the left. Use your abdominal muscles to work against the resistance. Finish a set, then repeat on the other side.

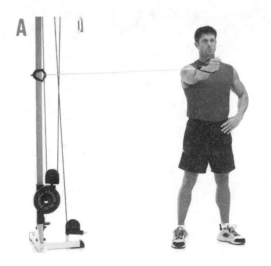

MAKE IT EASIER

- Stand closer to the stationary object to decrease resistance.
- Stand with your feet farther apart.

DO IT HARDER

- Stand farther away from the stationary object to increase resistance.
- Narrow your stance; stand with your legs hip width apart.

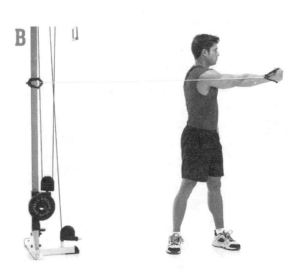

ONE-LEGGED ANTERIOR REACH

If you want to train the abs in a very explosive fashion—perfect for generating muscle size as well as strength—this exercise is for you.

A Face away from a weight stack. Grab the high pulley handle and extend your arms overhead, while balancing on one leg.

B With your arms extended overhead, use your abdominal muscles to flex your trunk. Keep your arms in the same plane as your torso. Don't allow your shoulders and arms to do all the work. After flexing forward, return to the starting position. Use your abs to slow your movement; don't allow momentum to make it easy.

MAKE IT EASIER

- Stand on both legs initially; gradually put more weight on one leg.
- Bend your elbows to bring your hands closer to your head.

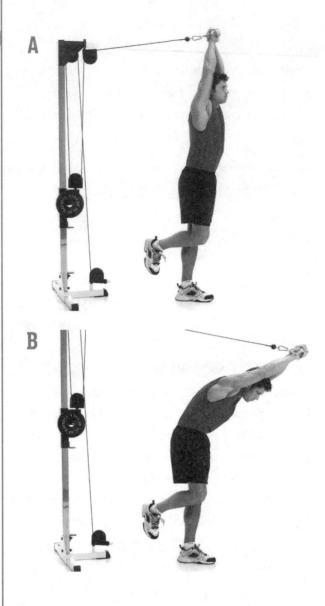

DO IT HARDER

- Stand sideways to the cable and rotate toward the opposite cable.
- Stand on an air cushion or other balance device.

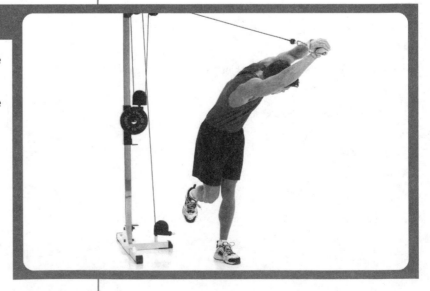

REVERSE CRUNCH

This exercise works the lower abs.

A Lie on your back on a weight bench. Grip the top of the bench to anchor your body. Bend your knees 90 degrees and bring them toward your head until your lower back starts to flatten.

B Raise your hips toward your chest. Keep going until you feel your abs fully contract. Hold a second, then return to the starting position.

MAKE IT EASIER

- Let your feet rest between reps.
- Keep your hands on your sides.

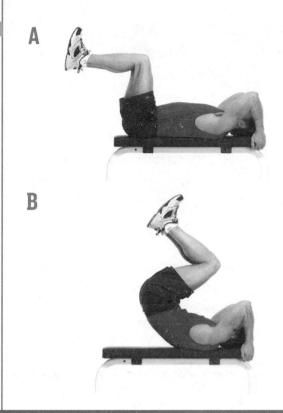

A

B

DO IT HARDER

- Attach tubing to the bench and your ankles for more resistance.
- Hold small dumbbells between your hands and feet, or place a medicine ball between your knees or feet.

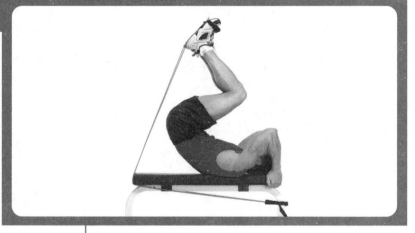

ROWING CRUNCH

This exercise works all the abdominal muscles. To achieve the most benefit, maintain tension on your abs until the end of the set. Keep your back straight when returning to the starting position.

A Sit on the end of a bench with your knees bent and your feet flat on the floor. Hold the sides of the bench for support. Lean back at about a 45-degree angle. Keeping your knees slightly bent, extend your legs and raise them a few inches off the floor.

B While bringing your upper body to an upright position, slowly pull your knees in to your chest. Hold for a second. Then, keeping your back straight, slowly return your upper body to the starting position.

MAKE IT EASIER

- Place a mat or towel under your butt to reduce pressure on the glutes.
- Use a sturdy bench that has a wide base of support and doesn't rock back and forth.

DO IT HARDER

- Lift your legs straight up toward your head instead of pulling your knees in.
- Anchor tubing to the bench and attach it to your feet to provide additional resistance.

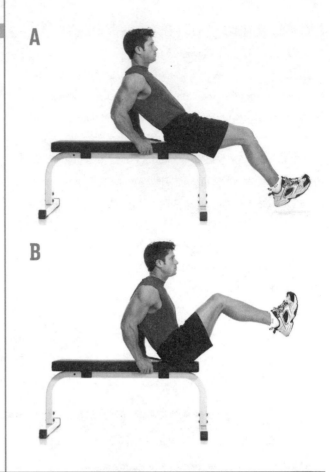

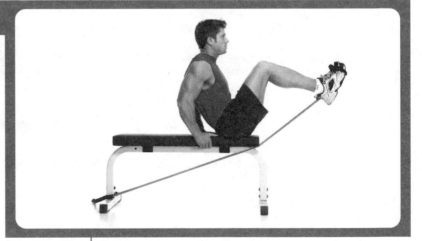

RUSSIAN TWIST

This beginner-to-intermediate exercise works the oblique (side) muscles as well as the upper and lower abs.

A Sit with your torso at a 45- to 60-degree angle to the floor, as though you're halfway through a situp. Your arms should be raised and extended in front of you, hands clasped, and your heels should rest on the floor. Keep your knees bent and your feet "free" rather than anchored to anything.

B While maintaining the torso angle, rotate as far as possible to one side. Move your arms with your torso so that they reach out to the side. Without pausing, rotate to the other side, then repeat, using continuous motions.

MAKE IT EASIER

- Don't rotate all the way.
- Anchor your feet for more support.

DO IT HARDER

- Hold your legs up off the floor.
- Hold a small medicine ball between your hands.

A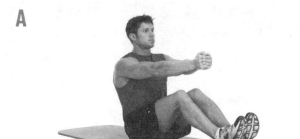

B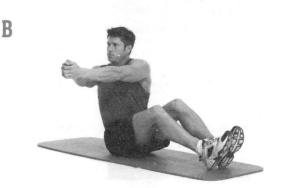

NO KIDDING?

WHO NEEDS AB DEVICES?

You've seen those infomercials with hot-body men and women rolling and crunching their way to perfect abs using all sorts of just-four-easy-payments-of-$29.99 contraptions. Do the devices really work? Do they do anything that regular crunches don't?

Researchers have studied this. They found, for example, that there is no difference in the muscle activity generated by a traditional crunch, the Ab Roller Plus, and a Torso Track 2. (The AB-DOer, low-resistance Torso Track model, and Perfect Abs provided significantly *less* activity than a traditional crunch.) Some of the devices, however, provided *more* of a workout than a crunch when used in certain positions or with varying degrees of resistance. Portable abdominal devices can be extremely effective when they not only mimic the mechanics of a traditional crunch, but also provide external resistance. When they're used without resistance, on the other hand, they don't do anything that a regular crunch won't—and often do less.

If you like gadgets and want to make your workouts a little harder, the devices aren't a bad choice. Even at their best, however, they provide only a marginal benefit over crunches—which you can do anywhere, anytime, without spending a dime.

RUSSIAN TWIST ON STABILITY BALL

This movement strengthens the oblique (side) muscles and helps protect the body from injury during twisting motions or sports that require rotation, such as golf or tennis.

A Rest your upper back, shoulders, and head on a stability ball, with your hips parallel to the floor. Grab a medicine ball with both hands, keeping your arms straight overhead.

B Rotate your trunk from the center to one side, back to center, then to the other side. Move quickly enough that you roll onto your shoulder on each side. Don't let your hips drop. Try to keep your chest, hips, and knees in a straight line.

MAKE IT EASIER

- Get more of your body on the ball for extra support.
- Keep your hands close to your head by bending your elbows.

DO IT HARDER

- Keep more of your body off the ball for less support.
- Hold a dumbbell instead of the medicine ball between your hands for extra resistance.

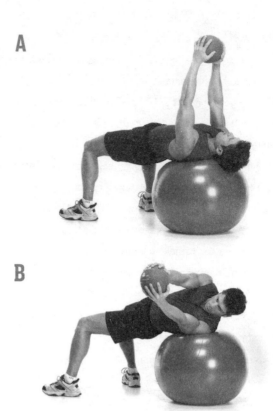

SIDE-LYING HIP LIFT

This seemingly simple exercise strengthens the deep abdominal muscles and the lower back. Careful, it's harder than it looks.

A Lie on your side, with one hand on your upper hip. Balance on your forearm, with your legs and feet stacked on top of each other.

B Keeping your trunk steady, slowly contract your abs and lift your hip off the floor. Your body should form a straight line from the head to the ankles; don't let your weight sink into your shoulder. Breathe regularly and try to hold the position for 30 to 45 seconds. Return to the starting position, and finish the set. Then repeat on the other side.

MAKE IT EASIER

- Bend your knees.
- Place a ball under your hip to use as a guide before you begin.

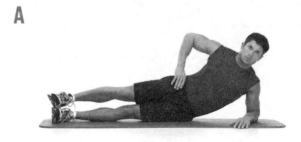

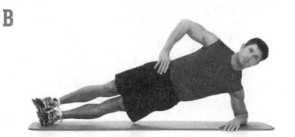

DO IT HARDER

- Balance on your hand by straightening your arm.
- Hold a weight plate on your hip.

STABILITY BALL CRUNCH

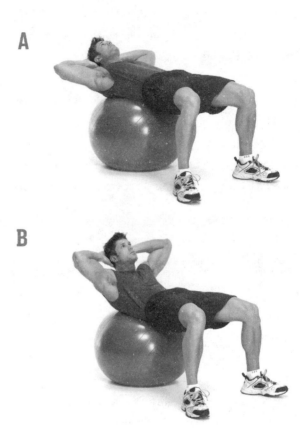

If regular crunches no longer feel challenging, try this variation. The ball will add as much as 15 degrees to your range of motion and improve your balance. You can add weight by holding a dumbbell under your chin. Keep your head and neck aligned by keeping a fist's distance between your chin and chest.

A Lie with your back across the ball, with your feet flat on the floor. Your thighs and torso should be parallel with the floor. Put your hands behind your head.

B Use your upper abs to bring your rib cage toward your pelvis. Raise your shoulders off the ball. Don't raise your torso more than 45 degrees. Hold for a second, then slowly return to the starting position.

MAKE IT EASIER

- Slightly flatten an exercise ball by letting some of the air out.
- Cross your arms on your chest.

DO IT HARDER

- Use a fully inflated ball. The rounder ball will allow you to increase your range of motion.
- Hold your arms straight and in line with your spine; the farther the hands are from the body, the harder the movement.
- Hold a weight plate on your chest.

STRAIGHT-ARM BAR ROLLOUT

This exercise works the abs, shoulders, and lower back. Starting from a kneeling position puts less stress on the lower back than the standing, forward-bend position.

A Kneel behind a barbell loaded with 25-pound plates. Put your hands on the bar, slightly wider than shoulder width apart. Tilt your pelvis so that your lower back is flat, not arched.

B Roll the barbell forward, keeping your back flat. Move forward until your body is almost parallel to the floor. Your upper body should be in a straight line. Don't allow any part of your upper body to touch the floor. Pause briefly, then contract your abs and roll the barbell back to the starting position.

MAKE IT EASIER

- Place a mat or towel under your knees to reduce friction.
- Set up closer to a wall so that the plates hit the wall. This allows you to increase your range of motion as you get stronger.

DO IT HARDER

- Start with your legs straight from a pushup position. You'll need to tilt your pelvis slightly forward to complete the movement.
- Use more or heavier plates to provide additional resistance.

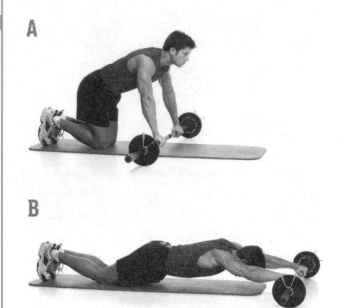

TRUNK ROTATION

This exercise works the upper and lower abs. Do it in one slow, continuous motion. You can increase the difficulty by cupping your hands behind your ears, elbows out to the sides.

A Sit on the floor with your hands crossed over your chest, your knees bent. Place your feet under a support, such as a barbell, the base of a weight machine, or a heavy piece of furniture, to stabilize your lower body. Hold your torso at a 45-degree angle to the floor.

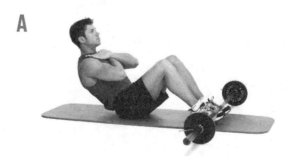

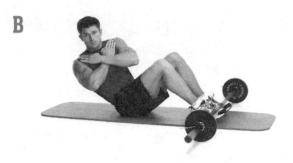

B Start by moving your torso to the left. Stay to the left as you lower your back to the floor. Completing a clockwise rotation, raise your torso to the right side. Then repeat the exercise, this time moving down your right side and around to your left.

MAKE IT EASIER

- Don't go all the way down.
- Bend your knees more.

DO IT HARDER

- Hold a weight plate on your chest.
- Keep your legs straighter, but still slightly bent.

TRUNK ROTATION WITH CABLE

Also known as a lying crossover cable crunch, this exercise will strengthen all of your abdominal muscles.

A Lie in a crunch position in front of a low pulley cable with a Y-shaped rope handle. Your head should be pointed toward the pulley. Bend your hips and knees to 90-degree angles. Grab one end of the handle with each hand so the rope is behind your head, with your hands a bit more than shoulder width apart.

B Slowly lift your shoulders and shoulder blades off the floor. Instead of pausing at the top, slightly twist toward one of your knees. Hold for a second, then slowly lower to the starting position. Without resting, lift and twist toward your other knee.

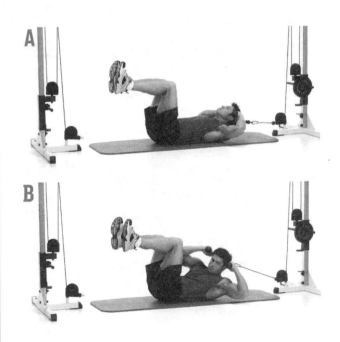

MAKE IT EASIER

- Set up closer to the cable to shorten the range of motion.
- Keep your hands close to your head.

DO IT HARDER

- Set up farther away from the cable to increase the range of motion.
- Keep your arms extended away from your head.

TRUNK TWIST

In addition to working the upper and lower abs, trunk twists also target the love-handle area (the obliques).

A Grab a stick or a light bar. It should be about the length of a broomstick. While seated, rest the bar behind your head, across your shoulders. Place your hands as close to the ends as you can, keeping your elbows slightly bent.

B Use your oblique muscles to smoothly twist your torso as far to the right as you can, while keeping your hips stationary. Your head should move with your torso. Repeat the movement to the left. Continue to rotate right and left, without pausing, until completing a set.

MAKE IT EASIER

- Do the exercise while standing.
- Have a partner help with the rotation.

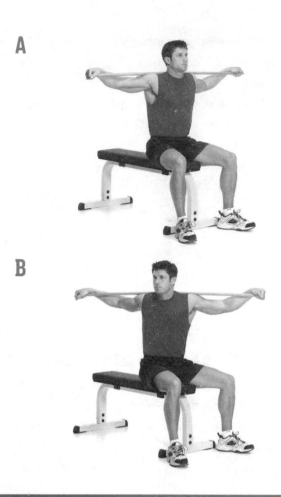

DO IT HARDER

- Attach tubing to one end of the stick and a stationary object for more resistance. Switch sides to work both sides of the body.
- Do this while lying in a Roman chair or across a bench in a horizontal position.

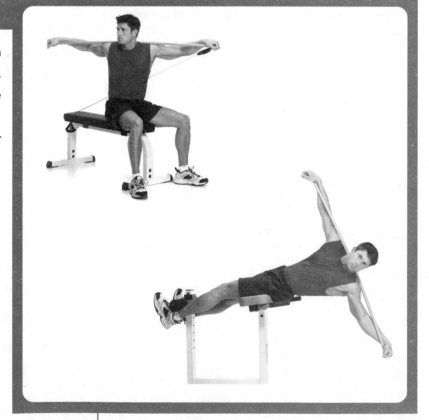

TRUNK TWIST WITH DUMBBELLS

This exercise works the internal and external oblique (side) abdominals and is often recommended for men who participate in activities that involve trunk rotation, such as tennis and golf. Because it keeps the arms at constant tension, your biceps and forearms also benefit.

A Sit at the end of a bench with your feet flat on the floor. Keep your chest out and your head aligned with your torso. Hold a dumbbell in both hands, extending your arms out in front of you.

B Slowly and smoothly twist your torso to the right as far as you can comfortably go. When you reach the end of your range of motion, hold for a second, then slowly return to the starting position. Repeat to the left. Continue alternating right and left until your muscles are fatigued.

MAKE IT EASIER

- Do the exercise while standing.
- Have a partner help with the rotation.

DO IT HARDER

- Attach tubing to one hand and a stationary object for more resistance. Switch sides to work both sides of the body equally.
- Do this while lying across a bench in a horizontal position.

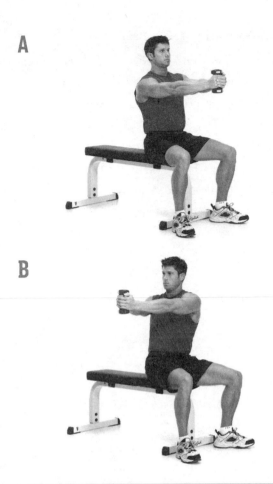

A

B

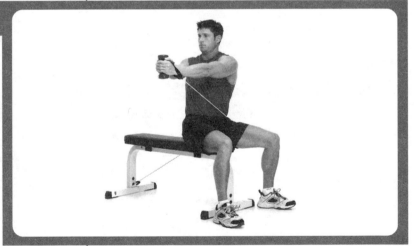

VERTICAL LEG CRUNCH

This movement isolates the upper abs, the first step to obtaining that coveted six-pack. To reduce difficulty, this move can also be done with your lower legs resting on a chair or weight bench.

A Lie on your back and extend your legs straight up, feet crossed at the ankles, knees slightly bent. Put your hands loosely behind your head.

B Contract your abdominals and slowly raise your head, shoulders, and upper back at about a 30-degree angle. Pause, then slowly return to the starting position.

MAKE IT EASIER

- Bend your knees.
- Cross your arms on your chest

DO IT HARDER

- Hold tubing or a cable handle for more resistance.
- Hold a small dumbbell between your feet.

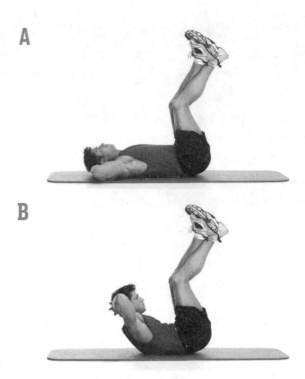

WEIGHTED CURLUP

This movement will strengthen both the upper and lower abdominal muscles. It's a superb exercise for preventing lower back problems—and may decrease back pain that already exists.

A Lie flat on your back with one knee bent at about a 45-degree angle about 6 inches from your butt and the other leg straight. Hold a weight plate behind your head, with your elbows pointed out.

B Curl your upper torso in toward your knees, pressing your lower back to the floor and raising your shoulder blades as high off the floor as you can get them. Keep your knees in line with your feet, and don't use your hands to pull your head up. Concentrate on contracting your abdominal muscles. Hold for a second, then slowly return to the starting position.

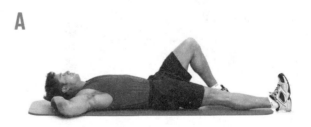

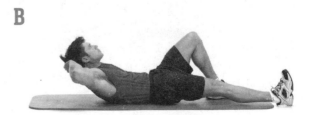

MAKE IT EASIER

- Place the weight on your chest.
- Hold the weight in front of your head.

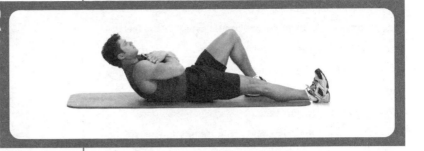

DO IT HARDER

- Hold the weight plate farther away from your body and move your arms, shoulders, and spine as if they were in a straight line.
- Hold your legs up off the ground; don't let your feet touch the floor.

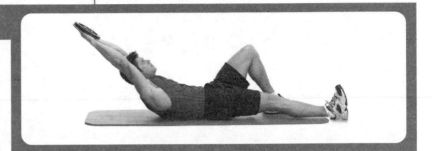

BREATHING LESSONS

Situps can be safe or dangerous. It all depends on how you do them.

Men who hold their breath while doing situps essentially perform an involuntary Valsalva maneuver: forcing the epiglottis against the glottis and jacking up blood pressure in the brain. There have been reports of healthy young men suffering stroke or spinal epidural hematoma when doing situps improperly. For older men, the risks are even greater.

Make sure you brush up on proper breathing techniques—exhaling on the exertion phase, inhaling during the relaxation phase—if situps are part of your workout.

WOOD CHOP

This exercise works all of the abdominals; you should feel the effects all the way across your midsection.

A Stand between two pulley stacks, as though doing cable crossovers. Grab a single high handle with both hands, keeping your arms overhead.

B Pull the handle diagonally across your body toward the opposite foot. Imagine that you're swinging an ax. Slowly return to the starting position, then repeat to finish the set. Repeat on the other side.

MAKE IT EASIER

- Stand close to the stack so that the weight is resting when you start.
- Keep your hands close to your head.

DO IT HARDER

- Stand farther away from the stack so that the weight is not resting when you start.
- Keep your hands away from your head.

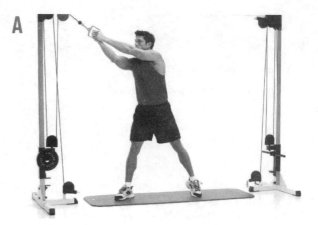

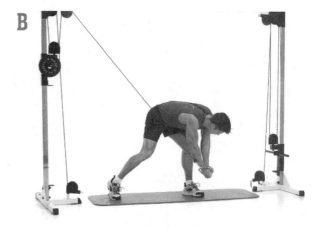

IS THERE A DIFFERENCE BETWEEN UPPER AND LOWER AB WORKOUTS?

Lifters talk about upper and lower abdominal training. Researchers make it more complicated by talking about supra- and infra-umbilical abdominal training. The idea underlying these discussions is that, in theory, you can target different areas of the rectus abdominis muscle to make that six-pack pop.

The rectus abdominis is a single muscle that runs from the pubic bone to the rib cage. Since it is only one muscle, some argue, it's physiologically impossible to contract only the upper or lower portion. This is true, but only up to a point.

Muscles are made up of individual muscle fibers (cells). Individual fibers are connected in series; the end of one connects to the next one in line. These serial fibers run parallel to other serial fibers. They don't all contract simultaneously. When you do a particular exercise, some muscle fibers fatigue first. When that happens, others jump in to help out. Now, suppose you do a different exercise. The fibers that were latecomers the first time around will start off the action, and the initial starters will come into play second.

Some exercises, such as the reverse curl, place more stress on muscle fibers at the muscle origin, near your pubic bone. Other exercises, such as trunk rotation with a cable, place more stress on the muscle insertion, on your rib cage. For complete abdominal development, do a variety of ab workouts. That guarantees that you'll emphasize both areas.

LEVEL 1 (FOCUS ON SIZE)

- Do the complete exercise program 3 days a week. Allow at least 1 day of rest between workouts.

- Choose any one of the workouts we've provided. You can do one of the workouts three times a week. Or you can do different workouts on different days.

- Start out by doing 1 set of 10 repetitions for each exercise. Perform all exercises in a row without resting in between. Take a 1-minute rest after the last exercise, then repeat for a second circuit. Then, for each workout, add 1 repetition to each set. Keep going until you reach 20 reps. Then increase the resistance and return to 10 reps.

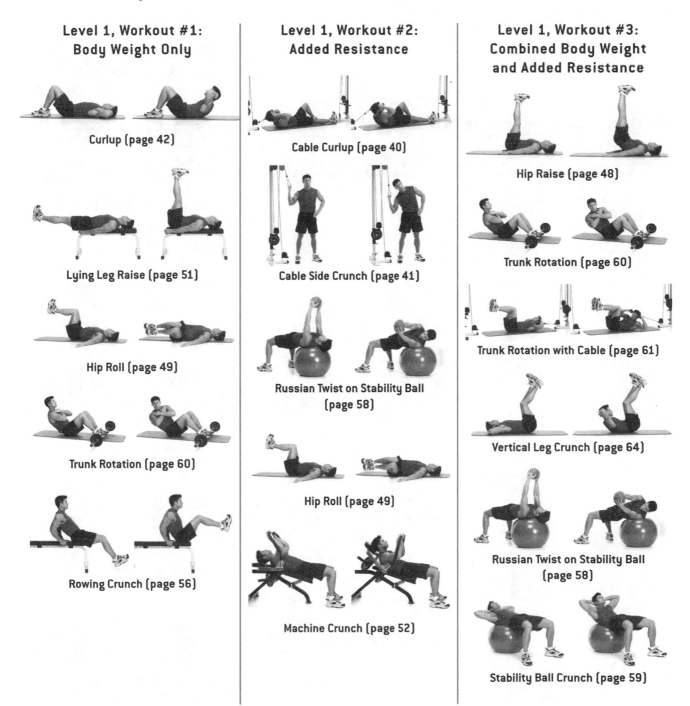

Level 1, Workout #1: Body Weight Only

Curlup (page 42)

Lying Leg Raise (page 51)

Hip Roll (page 49)

Trunk Rotation (page 60)

Rowing Crunch (page 56)

Level 1, Workout #2: Added Resistance

Cable Curlup (page 40)

Cable Side Crunch (page 41)

Russian Twist on Stability Ball (page 58)

Hip Roll (page 49)

Machine Crunch (page 52)

Level 1, Workout #3: Combined Body Weight and Added Resistance

Hip Raise (page 48)

Trunk Rotation (page 60)

Trunk Rotation with Cable (page 61)

Vertical Leg Crunch (page 64)

Russian Twist on Stability Ball (page 58)

Stability Ball Crunch (page 59)

LEVEL 2 (FOCUS ON STRENGTH)

- Do the complete exercise program 3 days per week. Allow at least 1 day of rest between workouts.

- Choose one of the workouts below. You can do only one of them three times per week or you can do all of them in an alternating fashion.

- Start out by doing 2 to 3 sets of 10 repetitions for each exercise. Perform all exercises in a row without resting in between. Take a 1-minute rest after the last exercise, then repeat for a second circuit. Every time you work out, add 1 repetition to each set. Keep going until you reach 20 reps. Then increase the resistance and return to 10 reps.

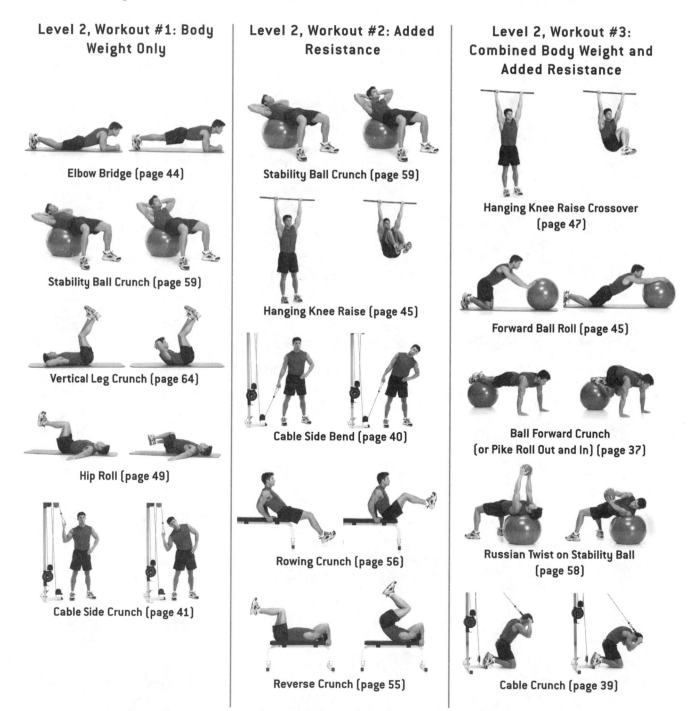

Level 2, Workout #1: Body Weight Only

Elbow Bridge (page 44)

Stability Ball Crunch (page 59)

Vertical Leg Crunch (page 64)

Hip Roll (page 49)

Cable Side Crunch (page 41)

Level 2, Workout #2: Added Resistance

Stability Ball Crunch (page 59)

Hanging Knee Raise (page 45)

Cable Side Bend (page 40)

Rowing Crunch (page 56)

Reverse Crunch (page 55)

Level 2, Workout #3: Combined Body Weight and Added Resistance

Hanging Knee Raise Crossover (page 47)

Forward Ball Roll (page 45)

Ball Forward Crunch (or Pike Roll Out and In) (page 37)

Russian Twist on Stability Ball (page 58)

Cable Crunch (page 39)

LEVEL 3 (HYBRID TRAINING—FOCUS ON SIZE AND STRENGTH)

- Do the complete exercise program 3 days per week. Allow at least 1 day of rest between workouts.

- Choose any one of the workouts we've provided. You can do one of the workouts three times a week. Or you can do different workouts on different days.

- Start out by doing 1 set of 10 repetitions for each exercise. Perform all exercises in a row without resting in between. Take a 1-minute rest after the last exercise, then repeat for a second circuit. Then, for each workout, add 1 to 2 repetitions to each set. Keep going until you reach 20 reps. Then increase the resistance and return to 10 reps.

- After warming up, take all sets to positive failure.

- As you get in better shape, progress to 2 to 3 circuits of the 5 exercises.

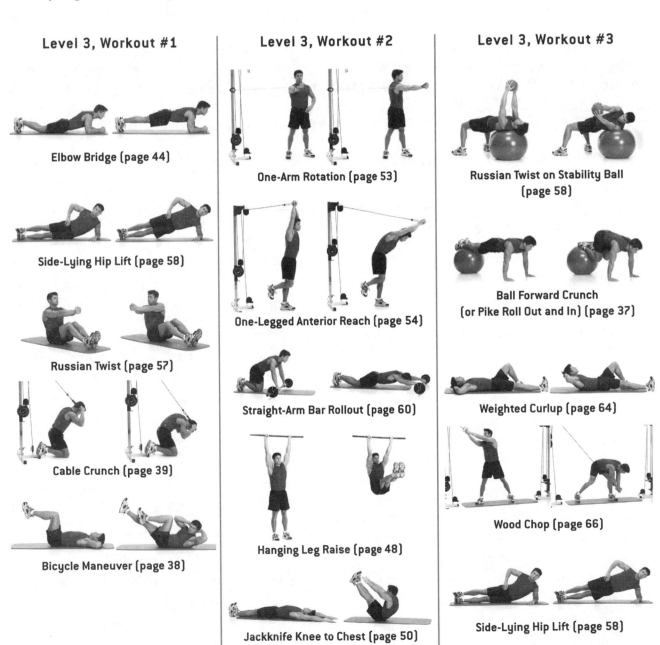

Level 3, Workout #1

Elbow Bridge (page 44)

Side-Lying Hip Lift (page 58)

Russian Twist (page 57)

Cable Crunch (page 39)

Bicycle Maneuver (page 38)

Level 3, Workout #2

One-Arm Rotation (page 53)

One-Legged Anterior Reach (page 54)

Straight-Arm Bar Rollout (page 60)

Hanging Leg Raise (page 48)

Jackknife Knee to Chest (page 50)

Level 3, Workout #3

Russian Twist on Stability Ball (page 58)

Ball Forward Crunch (or Pike Roll Out and In) (page 37)

Weighted Curlup (page 64)

Wood Chop (page 66)

Side-Lying Hip Lift (page 58)

7
BIGGER ARMS

What do you see when you stand in front of the mirror? The first thing men notice, for better or worse, is their midsection. After that, they look at the biceps, shoulders, and chest. Which explains why most men spend a disproportionate amount of their workouts working the upper body, particularly the upper arms.

Looks aside, there are good, practical reasons to develop strong arms. Think gripping. Pulling. Pressing. Lifting. Just about everything you do, including your daily workouts, requires good arm strength. Strong arms *last*. They won't give out when you're doing the heavy training involved in building the chest, back, and shoulders.

ARMS EXPLAINED

It doesn't make a lot of sense to talk about "arm exercises" because the upper and lower arms have different functions and muscle groups. Let's start with the muscles in the upper arm. Their basic function is to flex the elbow joint, bringing the forearm closer to the upper arm, or extend the elbow joint, moving the forearm away from the upper arm.

- The primary upper arm elbow flexors are the biceps brachii and brachialis. The biceps are probably the most widely recognized muscle group—the ones that pop when you "make a muscle." The brachialis, a smaller muscle, is located on the outer part of the upper arm.

- The triceps brachii is the major upper arm muscle involved in elbow extension. Located on the back of the upper arm, it is divided into three sections, or "heads": the lateral (outer) head, the medial (middle) head, and the long (inner) head.

The lower arms, or forearms, are an often neglected muscle group. A well-muscled forearm isn't as eye-catching as big biceps, but you need that strength, especially if you're doing serious lifting and need to maximize grip strength.

The lower arms have several muscle groups that move the wrist: supinators, pronators, flexors, and extensors.

- Wrist supinators turn the hand from a palms-down to a palms-up position.

- Wrist pronators turn the hand from a palms-up to a palms-down position.

- Wrist flexors bring your hand toward your forearm.
- Wrist extensors pull your hand away from your forearm.

Some of the lower arm muscles get a decent workout during upper arm exercises. But if you really want to make them pop, you need to train them more directly with dedicated exercises.

THE TOTAL ARM WORKOUT

A mistake that a lot of men make is overworking the biceps at the expense of the triceps or forearm. The body is precisely balanced; working one muscle and neglecting its counterpart almost guarantees soreness as well as injuries. It also makes the arms look disproportionately large or small in places. You have to train the arms as a whole, not as a series of unrelated parts.

To get the most out of your arm workouts, here are some points to keep in mind.

Stand or sit with your back against a wall when doing curls. It holds your body stable and concentrates more of the stress on the upper arms.

Change hand positions. A neutral grip (palms facing each other) when doing curls gives the most power, but you can subtly shift the angle of attack with supinated (underhand) and pronated (overhand) grips. While you're at it, try different handle attachments—straight or angled bars, for example. They work the muscles from different angles and force them into greater growth.

Keep your back straight. Take a look at that guy curling massive weights. If he's rocking back and forth like he's training for the limbo, you know that his ego is dominating his common sense. The idea is to work the biceps. All of that arching and jerking creates momentum that makes the exercise easier—the opposite of what you want. If you can't lift a weight without arching or rocking, drop down to a lighter weight.

Keep the wrists and forearms parallel. And check to make sure that your elbows are close to your body. These positions evenly distribute the stress between arms when doing curls, and also exert the most stress where you want it.

Train your forearms last. If you work the lower arms too hard initially, you won't have the grip strength to finish your upper arm workout. The exception to this rule is if your grip strength isn't what it should be. In that case, work the forearms first.

Move through the full range of motion. This is true of all exercises, but particularly those involving the lower arms. The muscles in the forearms fatigue more quickly than the bigger muscles in the upper arms. It's easy to get tired and inadvertently shorten the range of motion to make the exercises easier. Don't do it. Maximum range of motion means more muscle size and more functional wrist and hand strength.

Keep the elbows fixed while doing lower arm exercises. Moving the elbows will rob your forearms of their ability to do the lifting. At the same time, keep the hands horizontal when doing wrist flexion or extension movements.

Don't neglect the triceps. A lot of men do, if only because triceps exercises are usually more difficult than working the biceps. Here's something to keep you motivated: The triceps stay big even when they aren't contracting. In other words, building the triceps will make your arms look bigger even when you're standing still.

Lead with the "big three." When you want to really blast your biceps to growth, the best workouts are the barbell preacher curl (page 86), alternating incline dumbbell curl (page 84), and narrow-grip standing barbell curl. For triceps, the best are the barbell decline lying triceps extension (page 95), angled bar pushdown (page 102), and dips (page 91).

BICEPS CURL WITH STRAIGHT BAR

If you want to develop massive, well-defined arms, this exercise is a must. It exerts a lot of tension on the biceps, the large muscle group located mainly in the upper arm.

A Stand with your feet shoulder width apart, knees slightly flexed. Hold the barbell with your palms facing up, spaced slightly more than shoulder width apart. Your arms should be fully extended, with the bar resting lightly on your upper thighs.

B Keeping your upper arms close to your sides, curl the barbell toward your collarbone. Pause for a second at the top of the curl, then lower the bar to the starting position.

MAKE IT EASIER

- Lean forward and take advantage of mild back extension to complete the movements.
- Use a narrower grip.

DO IT HARDER

- Use a wider grip to reduce biceps activation and recruit more synergistic muscles.

BICEPS CURL WITH EZ BAR

Besides increasing the size of your biceps, this move will also strengthen your elbow flexors.

A Stand straight with your knees slightly bent. Hold the EZ barbell underhanded (palms up), with your hands about shoulder width apart. Your arms should be extended, and the barbell should be at thigh level.

A
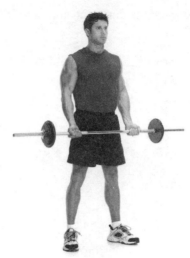

B
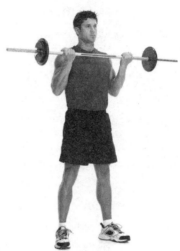

A
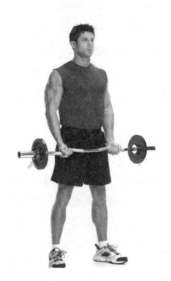

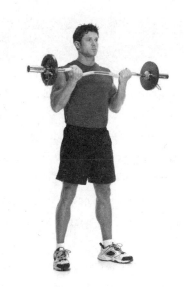

B Keeping your elbows close to your body, use your biceps to curl the bar slowly up toward your chin. Keep your wrists straight throughout the curl; don't sway or rock your body for momentum. Hold for a second, then lower the barbell slowly to the starting position.

MAKE IT EASIER

- Use a narrower grip.
- Lean forward and take advantage of mild back extension to complete the movements.

DO IT HARDER

- Use a wider grip to reduce biceps activation and recruit more synergistic muscles.

ALTERNATING SEATED BICEPS CURL WITH TUBING

This exercise uses resistance rather than weights to work the biceps, the large muscle group at the front of the upper arm.

A Sit on the end of a bench or chair, your feet flat on the floor. Place the tubing under both feet and step on it firmly. Grip each end of the tubing, keeping your fists at waist level; there shouldn't be any slack in the tubing. Lean forward slightly at the hips so that the tubing doesn't rub against the bench or chair.

B Raise one fist up to your shoulder, then slowly lower it back to waist level. Repeat on the other side. If you don't feel significant resistance on the exertion phase, adjust the tubing to take up any slack.

MAKE IT EASIER

- Use a lower tension tubing. Most are color-coded to indicate their level of tension.

DO IT HARDER

- Use a higher tension tubing. Most are color-coded to indicate their level of tension.
- Double the tubing for more resistance.

A

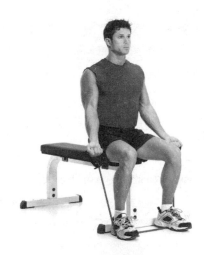

B

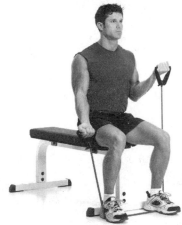

DOUBLE SEATED BICEPS CURL WITH TUBING

This movement works the biceps, the large muscle group at the front of the upper arm. The seated position makes it easier on the back.

A Sit at the end of a bench or chair, your feet flat on the floor. Place the tubing under both feet and step on it firmly. Hold each end of the tubing, keeping your fists at waist level. The tubing should be taut, with no slack. Lean forward slightly at the hips so that the tubing doesn't rub against the bench or chair.

B Raise your fists up to your shoulders, then slowly lower them back to waist level. If you don't feel significant resistance on the exertion phase, adjust the tubing to take up any slack.

MAKE IT EASIER
- Bend your knees more or move your feet closer together to reduce the tension in the band.
- Use a lower tension tubing. Most are color-coded to indicate their level of tension.

DO IT HARDER
- Set up farther away from the far end of the band to increase tension and stress on the biceps.
- Use a higher tension tubing. Most are color-coded to indicate their level of tension.
- Double the tubing for more resistance.

ALTERNATING STANDING BICEPS CURL WITH TUBING

This exercise works the biceps as well as the elbow flexor muscles.

A Stand with your feet shoulder width apart. Hook the tubing under each foot, gripping the handles. Your arms should be fully extended.

B With your arms at your sides and your palms facing forward, slowly curl your left arm up, keeping your left elbow near your side. Continue to curl until your hand reaches shoulder height. Slowly lower your arm and return to the starting position. Finish the set, then switch arms.

A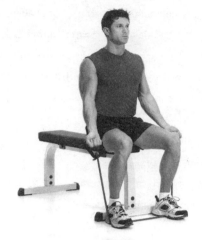

B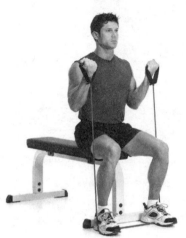

A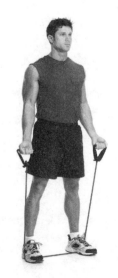

MAKE IT EASIER

- Move your feet closer together to reduce the tension in the band.
- Use a lower tension tubing. Most are color-coded to indicate their level of tension.

DO IT HARDER

- Move your feet farther away from the far end of the band to increase the tension on the band.
- Use a higher tension tubing. Most are color-coded to indicate their level of tension.
- Double the tubing for more resistance.

CABLE CURL WITH STRAIGHT BAR

This exercise works all of the biceps muscle groups: the biceps brachii (front of upper arm), the brachialis (outside of upper arm), and the brachioradialis (upper forearm). You need a low pulley on a multistation weight machine.

A Stand facing the pulley; there should be a bar handle on the cable. Place your feet shoulder width apart, about $1\frac{1}{2}$ feet from the pulley post. Keep your knees bent and your back straight. Using an underhand grip, hold the bar with both hands, keeping your arms fully extended. Your shoulders should lean back slightly.

B Keeping your upper arms tight against your body and perpendicular to the floor, slowly curl the bar toward your chest. Pause for a second at the top, then slowly lower the bar to the starting position.

MAKE IT EASIER

- Stand closer to the pulley so that the weight can rest on the stack between reps.
- Lean forward and use some mild back extension to assist with the movement.

DO IT HARDER

- Use a wider grip to minimize biceps activation and recruit more synergistic muscles.

B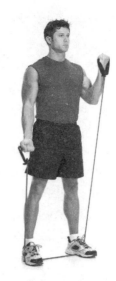

A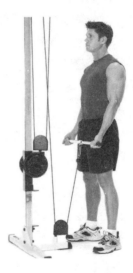

B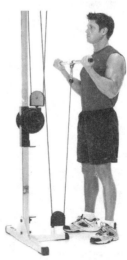

CABLE CURL WITH EZ BAR

This exercise works all of the biceps muscle groups: the biceps brachii (front of upper arm), the brachialis (outside of upper arm), and the brachioradialis (upper forearm). You need a low pulley on a multistation weight machine.

A Stand facing the pulley. There should be an EZ bar handle on the cable. Place your feet shoulder width apart, about 1¹/₂ feet from the pulley post. Keep your knees slightly bent and your back straight. Using an underhand grip, hold the bar with both hands, keeping your arms fully extended. Your shoulders should lean back slightly.

B Keeping your upper arms tight against your body and perpendicular to the floor, slowly curl the bar toward your chest. Pause for a second at the top, then slowly lower the bar to the starting position.

MAKE IT EASIER

- Set up closer to the pulley so that the weight can rest on the stack between reps.
- Lean forward and use some mild back extension to assist with the movement.

DO IT HARDER

- Use a wider grip to minimize biceps activation and recruit more synergistic muscles.

A
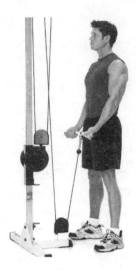

B
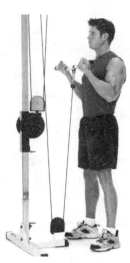

THE "CURL-PLUS"

Even though you get the most bang for your exercise buck when you keep the upper arms motionless when doing curls, it's not the perfect approach to getting big arms. The biceps crosses the shoulder and the elbow joints, which means you want movements that train the biceps at the elbow as well as at the shoulder.

Try this. When you do a barbell curl and reach the top of the movement, raise your elbows forward and up until your upper arms are horizontal to the floor. This motion flexes the shoulder joint and cause a stronger contraction in the biceps at the elbow and at the shoulder.

CABLE CONCENTRATION CURL

Besides concentrating on the biceps, this exercise also strengthens your elbow flexors.

A Position a weight bench so one end is close to a multi-station weight machine; there should be a D-handle low pulley cable. Sit on the end of the bench with your feet a little more than shoulder width apart. Hold the handle in your right hand, with your palm facing up and your arm fully extended. Rest your right elbow on your inner right thigh. With your left hand on your left thigh, bend forward slightly, keeping your back straight.

B Slowly curl the handle up toward your shoulder, keeping your upper arm perpendicular to the floor. Hold for a second, then slowly return to the starting position. Finish the set, then switch arms.

MAKE IT EASIER

- Set up closer to the pulley so that the weight can rest on the stack between reps.
- Lean forward and use some mild back extension to assist with the movement.

DO IT HARDER

- Use a wider grip to minimize biceps activation and recruit more synergistic muscles.

A

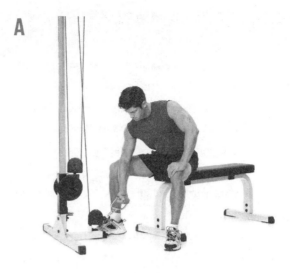

B

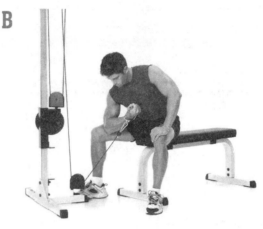

DUMBBELL CONCENTRATION CURL

Because this exercise involves little extraneous body movement, it's very effective at isolating the biceps.

A Sit on a chair or the end of a weight bench, with your feet a little more than shoulder width apart. Hold a dumbbell in your right hand, your palm facing up and your arm fully extended. Rest your right elbow on your inner right thigh. With your left hand on your left thigh, bend forward slightly, keeping your back straight.

B Slowly curl the dumbbell up toward your shoulder, keeping your upper arm perpendicular to the floor. Hold for a second, then lower the dumbbell slowly with a controlled motion to the starting position. Finish the set, then switch arms.

MAKE IT EASIER

- Use your free hand to assist your loaded hand.
- Shorten the range of motion. You can increase the range of motion as your strength increases.

DO IT HARDER

- Pause at the bottom and the top to emphasize stronger muscle contractions.

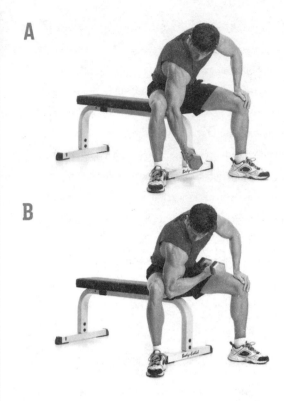

A

B

TUBING CONCENTRATION CURL

This movement uses resistance rather than weight to isolate and strengthen the biceps.

A Sit comfortably on a bench, with your feet slightly wider than shoulder width apart. Keeping your back straight, lean forward so that your right elbow can be placed on the inside of your right thigh, just behind the knee. Secure the exercise tubing with your right foot and hold the handle with your palm facing up, wrist straight.

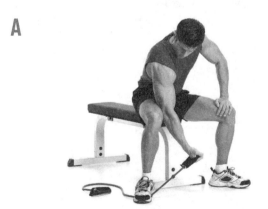

A

B Keeping your elbow on your leg and your wrist locked, exhale as you curl your arm up toward your upper right chest; contract the biceps at the top of the movement. Pause for a moment, then slowly lower your arm back to the starting position.

MAKE IT EASIER

- Set up closer to the far end of the band to reduce tension and stress on the biceps.
- Use a lower tension tubing. Most are color-coded to indicate their level of tension.

DO IT HARDER

- Set up farther away from the far end of the band to reduce tension and stress on the biceps.
- Use a higher tension tubing. Most are color-coded to indicate their level of tension.
- Double the tubing for more resistance.

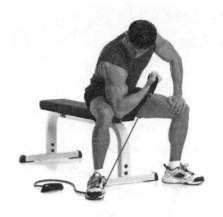

ALTERNATING SEATED DUMBBELL CURL

Alternating curls allows you to concentrate on one set of muscles at a time, maximizing the workout of each arm.

A Sit at the edge of a weight bench, with your feet shoulder width apart. Hold a dumbbell in each hand, with your arms at your sides and your palms facing forward.

B Slowly curl the left dumbbell up toward your collarbone. Hold for a second at the top of the lift, then lower the weight slowly with a controlled motion to the starting position. Repeat with your right arm.

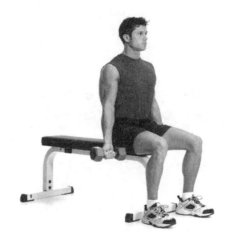

MAKE IT EASIER

- Lean back a little to make the movement easier to complete.
- Shorten the range of motion. You can increase the range of motion as your strength increases.

DO IT HARDER

- Pause at the bottom and the top to emphasize stronger muscle contractions.

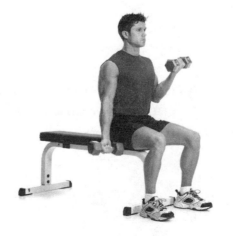

DOUBLE SEATED DUMBBELL CURL

Sitting rather than standing decreases the difficulty of this exercise, putting less strain on the back.

A Sit on the edge of a weight bench, with your feet shoulder width apart. Hold a dumbbell in each hand using an underhand grip, with your arms at your sides.

B Slowly curl the dumbbells up toward your collarbone. Hold for a second at the top of the lift, then lower the weights slowly with a controlled motion to the starting position.

MAKE IT EASIER

- Lean back a little to help assist you in completing a rep when the going gets tough.
- Shorten the range of motion so that you are only lifting the weight where you feel comfortable. You can increase the range of motion as your strength increases.

DO IT HARDER

- Pause at the bottom and the top to emphasize stronger muscle contractions.

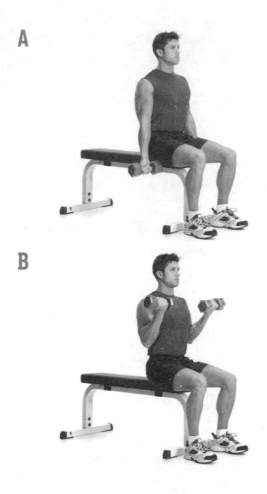

ALTERNATING STANDING DUMBBELL CURL

A Stand straight, with your feet shoulder width apart and your knees slightly bent. Hold a dumbbell in each hand using an underhand grip, with your arms at your sides.

B Slowly curl the left dumbbell up toward your collarbone. Hold for a second at the top of the lift, then lower the weight slowly with a controlled motion to the starting position. Repeat with your right arm.

MAKE IT EASIER

- Lean back a little to make the movement easier to complete.
- Shorten the range of motion. You can increase the range of motion as your strength increases.

DO IT HARDER

- Pause at the bottom and the top to emphasize stronger muscle contractions.

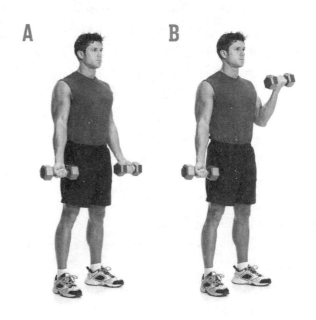

DOUBLE STANDING DUMBBELL CURL

A Stand straight, with your feet shoulder width apart and your knees slightly bent. Hold a dumbbell in each hand using an underhand grip, with your arms at your sides and your palms facing forward.

B Slowly curl the dumbbells up toward your collarbone. Hold for a second at the top of the lift, then lower the weights slowly with a controlled motion to the starting position.

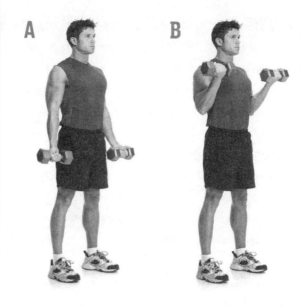

MAKE IT EASIER

- Lean back a little to make the movement easier to complete.
- Shorten the range of motion. You can increase the range of motion as your strength increases.

DO IT HARDER

- Pause at the bottom and the top to emphasize stronger muscle contractions.

ALTERNATING SEATED HAMMER CURL

In addition to working the biceps, this exercise works the elbow flexor muscles on the front of your arms.

A Sit at the end of the bench, with your knees bent and your feet shoulder width apart. Hold the dumbbells so that your palms are facing your body.

B Curl one weight up toward your shoulder, as though you're lifting a hammer to drive a nail. Alternate sides, curling first with one arm, then with the other. Don't rotate your wrist. Keep your shoulders back and your back straight.

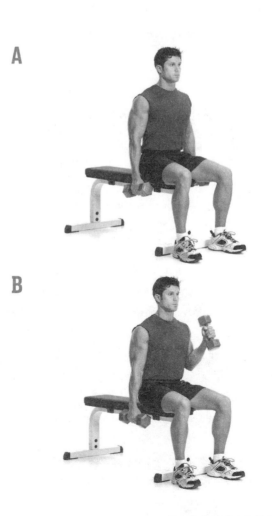

MAKE IT EASIER

- Lean back a little to make the movement easier to complete.
- Shorten the range of motion. You can increase the range of motion as your strength increases.

DO IT HARDER

- Pause at the bottom and the top to emphasize stronger muscle contractions.

DOUBLE SEATED HAMMER CURL

To achieve the greatest benefit from this exercise, keep constant tension on your arms throughout the movements.

A Sit on the end of the bench. Hold a pair of dumbbells, with your arms hanging straight down from your shoulders, your palms facing in.

B Without moving your upper arms, bend your elbows to lift the weights toward your shoulders, keeping your palms facing inward. Stop when you've lifted the weights as high as you can without moving your upper arms. Pause, then slowly lower the weights to the starting position.

MAKE IT EASIER

- Lean back a little to make the movement easier to complete.
- Shorten the range of motion. You can increase the range of motion as your strength increases.

DO IT HARDER

- Pause at the bottom and the top to emphasize stronger muscle contractions.

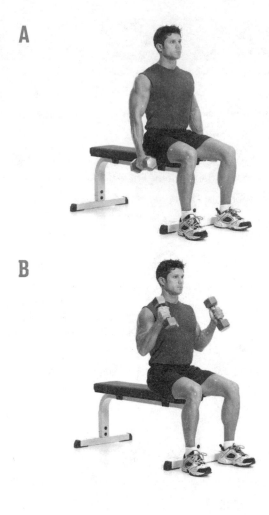

ALTERNATING STANDING HAMMER CURL

This exercise is particularly good for isolating and building the biceps (front of upper arm) muscles.

A Stand straight, with your feet shoulder width apart and your knees slightly bent. Hold a dumbbell in each hand, with your palms facing in and your arms fully extended.

B Slowly curl one dumbbell until the end touches your shoulder. Don't rotate your wrist while curling; keep the hand neutral and upper arm stationary. Hold for a second at the top, then lower the dumbbell slowly with a controlled motion to the starting position. Repeat with the other arm.

MAKE IT EASIER

- Lean back a little to make the movement easier to complete.
- Shorten the range of motion. You can increase the range of motion as your strength increases.

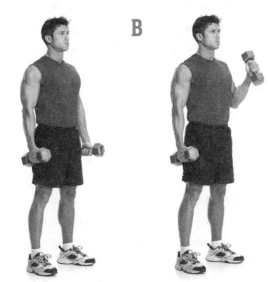

DO IT HARDER

- Pause at the bottom and the top to emphasize stronger muscle contractions.

DOUBLE STANDING HAMMER CURL

This exercise will work the biceps (front of upper arm) muscles as well as the elbow flexors at the front of your arm. Performing this movement while standing increases the level of difficulty.

A Stand straight with your feet shoulder width apart and your knees slightly bent. Hold a dumbbell in each hand, with your palms facing in and your arms fully extended.

B Keeping your upper arms stationary, bend your elbows to lift the weights toward your shoulders, keeping your palms facing inward. Stop when you've lifted the weights as high as you can. Pause, then slowly lower the weights to the starting position. Repeat.

MAKE IT EASIER

- Lean back a little to make the movement easier to complete.
- Shorten the range of motion. You can increase the range of motion as your strength increases.

DO IT HARDER

- Pause at the bottom and the top to emphasize stronger muscle contractions.

A

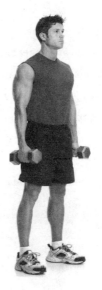

B

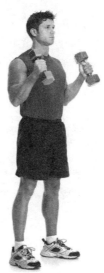

ALTERNATING INCLINE DUMBBELL CURL

Performing these curls on an incline bench provides good back support. Keeping your head in constant contact with the bench will help prevent neck strain.

A Holding a dumbbell in each hand, sit on an incline bench, keeping your head and upper body in full contact with the bench. Let your arms hang down, fully extended and perpendicular to the floor, palms facing forward. Keep your wrists straight throughout the exercise.

B Contracting the biceps muscles, bend one arm at the elbow, stopping when the weight is just short of touching your shoulder. Contract the muscle tightly in this position for a 2-second count. Slowly return to the starting position, stopping just short of the elbow fully extending. Repeat with the other arm, then alternate sides.

MAKE IT EASIER

- Use a higher incline, one that's greater than 60 degrees.
- Shorten the range of motion. You can increase the range of motion as your strength increases.

DO IT HARDER

- Use a lower incline, one that's less than 60 degrees.
- Pause at the bottom and the top to emphasize stronger muscle contractions.

DOUBLE INCLINE DUMBBELL CURL

The reclining position puts a lot of stress on the biceps and the supinator muscles near the elbows, giving your arms a great workout.

A Holding a dumbbell in each hand, sit on an incline bench, keeping your head and upper body in full contact with the bench. Let your arms hang down, fully extended and perpendicular to the floor, palms facing out.

A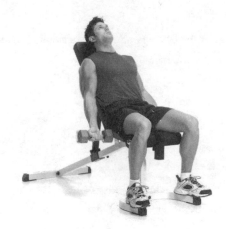

B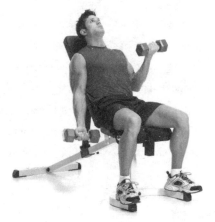

A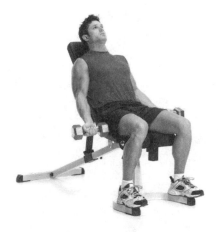

B Slowly curl the dumbbells up to your shoulders, keeping your upper arms stationary and your elbows pointed down. Hold for a second, then slowly lower your arms with a controlled motion to the starting position.

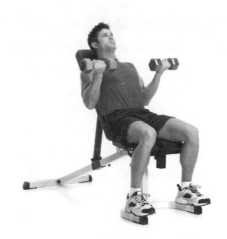

MAKE IT EASIER

- Use an incline greater than 60 degrees.
- Shorten the range of motion. You can increase the range of motion as your strength increases.

DO IT HARDER

- Use an incline less than 60 degrees.
- Rotate your wrists at the top of the lift so that the palms face outward.

TUBING INCLINE CURL

This movement works the elbow flexor, the muscles on the front of your arms. Various thicknesses of tubing create various levels of resistance.

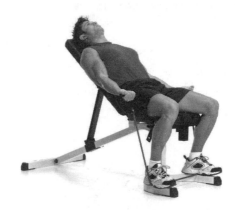

A Sit on the incline bench, hook the exercise tubing under each foot, and grip the handles with your arms fully extended.

B With your arms at your sides and your palms facing out, slowly curl your arms up, keeping your elbows against your sides. Curl until your hands reach shoulder height. Slowly lower your arms to the starting position.

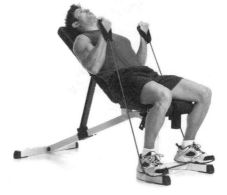

MAKE IT EASIER

- Move your feet closer to the far end of the band to reduce the tension on the band.
- Use a lower tension tubing. Most are color-coded to indicate their level of tension.

DO IT HARDER

- Move your feet farther away from the far end of the band to increase the tension on the band.
- Use a higher tension tubing. Most are color-coded to indicate their level of tension.
- Double the tubing for more resistance.

BARBELL PREACHER CURL

This movement is one of the best exercises for working the biceps. Because it's done in a seated position, it is easier on your back than standing curls.

A Sit on a bench, with your arms hanging over a platform. Your elbows should be low on the platform, with your armpits almost touching the pad. Hold the barbell with your palms facing up, your hands closer than shoulder width apart.

B Slowly curl the bar toward your chin, keeping your upper arms in contact with the pad. Hold for a second, then lower slowly with a controlled motion to the starting position.

MAKE IT EASIER

- Use an incline greater than 60 degrees.
- Shorten the range of motion. You can increase the range of motion as your strength increases.

DO IT HARDER

- Use an incline less than 60 degrees.
- Pause at the bottom and the top to emphasize stronger muscle contractions.

A

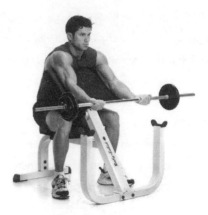

B

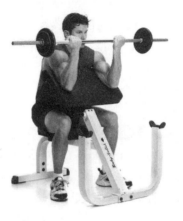

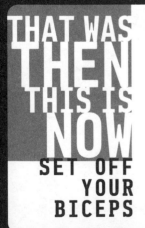

THAT WAS THEN THIS IS NOW
SET OFF YOUR BICEPS

Pity the lifters of yesteryear. They'd do 50, 60, even 70 sets for a single biceps workout. Some workouts even had guys doing additional sets of curls every hour throughout the day. It was thought that the biceps needed that kind of training to reach their maximum size. The science has changed—and so, thankfully, has the workload. As long as you lift to the point of muscle failure, you can get the same biceps blast with 12 or fewer sets.

ALTERNATING DUMBBELL PREACHER CURL

Using free weights allows you to use an increased range of motion, increasing overall strength and stability.

A Sit on a bench, with your arms hanging over a platform. Your elbows should be low on the platform, with your armpits almost touching the pad. Hold a dumbbell in each hand, with your palms facing up and your hands spaced closer than shoulder width apart.

B Keeping your upper arms in contact with the pad, slowly curl the left dumbbell up until your arm is at about a 90-degree angle. Hold for a second, then lower with a controlled motion to the starting position. Repeat on the right side.

MAKE IT EASIER

- Use an incline greater than 60 degrees.
- Shorten the range of motion. You can increase the range of motion as your strength increases.

DO IT HARDER

- Use an incline less than 60 degrees.
- Pause at the bottom and the top to emphasize stronger muscle contractions.

A

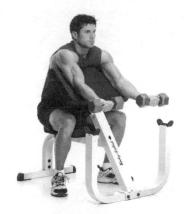

B

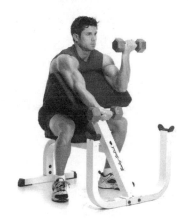

DOUBLE DUMBBELL PREACHER CURL

Those who are new to weight training may recognize a natural strength discrepancy between their right and left arms. To balance arm strength, it's important to raise and lower both dumbbells at the same speed and in the same range of motion.

A Sit on a bench, with your arms hanging over a platform. Your elbows should be low on the platform, with your armpits almost touching the pad. Hold a dumbbell in each hand, with your palms facing up and your hands spaced closer than shoulder width apart.

B Keeping your upper arms in contact with the pad, slowly curl the dumbbells up until your arms are at about a 90-degree angle. Hold for a second, then lower with a controlled motion to the starting position.

MAKE IT EASIER

- Use an incline greater than 60 degrees.
- Shorten the range of motion. You can increase the range of motion as your strength increases.

DO IT HARDER

- Use an incline less than 60 degrees.
- Pause at the bottom and the top to emphasize stronger muscle contractions.

EZ BAR PREACHER CURL

This movement works the biceps. Stabilizing the upper arm maximizes stress and makes each repetition more efficient.

A Sit on a bench, with your arms hanging over a platform. Your elbows should be low on the platform, with your armpits almost touching the pad. Hold the EZ bar with your palms facing up, your hands spaced closer than shoulder width apart.

A
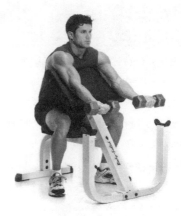

B
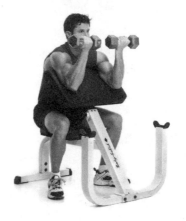

A
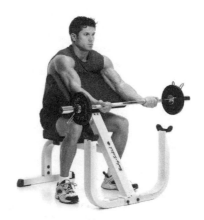

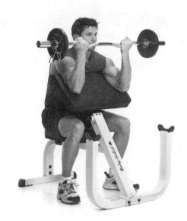

B Slowly curl the bar toward your chin, keeping your upper arms in contact with the pad. Hold for a second, then lower slowly with a controlled motion to the starting position.

MAKE IT EASIER

- Use an incline greater than 60 degrees.
- Shorten the range of motion. You can increase the range of motion as your strength increases.

DO IT HARDER

- Use an incline less than 60 degrees.
- Pause at the bottom and the top to emphasize stronger muscle contractions.

BARBELL REVERSE-GRIP CURL

Changing the hand position from the traditional underhand grip stresses the biceps from a slightly different angle, resulting in greater strength and balance.

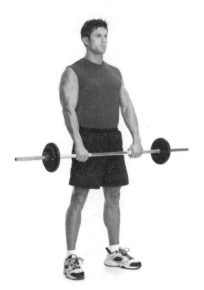

A Stand with your feet shoulder width apart, your knees slightly bent. Hold the barbell with an overhand grip, your hands spaced shoulder width apart. Your arms should be fully extended, with the bar resting against your upper thighs. Keep your elbows close to your sides.

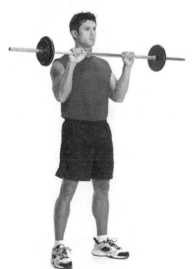

B Curl the bar toward your collarbone. Pause for a second, then slowly lower to the starting position.

MAKE IT EASIER

- Use a narrow grip.
- Use dumbbells instead of a bar.
- Use an EZ bar to reduce strain on your wrists.
- Lean forward and use some mild back extension to assist with the movement.

DO IT HARDER

- Use a wider grip to minimize biceps activation and recruit more synergistic muscles.

CABLE REVERSE-GRIP CURL

This movement works smaller muscles that cross the elbow joint and your forearms. Use less weight for this than you would for a regular cable curl.

A Stand with your feet slightly more than shoulder width apart and hold a bar-handle low pulley cable palms down, with your hands no more than shoulder width apart. Keep your arms fully extended.

B Curl the bar in a semicircular motion toward your body as far as you can. Hold for a second at the top of the curl, then lower down to the starting position.

MAKE IT EASIER

- Set up closer to the pulley so that the weight can rest on the stack between reps.
- Lean forward and use some mild back extension to assist with the movement.

DO IT HARDER

- Use a wider grip to minimize biceps activation and recruit more synergistic muscles.

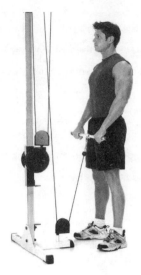

A

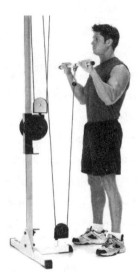

B

CLOSE-GRIP BENCH PRESS

This movement works the triceps (back of upper arm) muscles and helps to balance and develop strength equally on both sides of the elbow joint.

A Lie on a weight bench with your knees bent, feet on the floor. Unrack a barbell, with your hands slightly less than shoulder width apart. Extend both arms directly over your chest.

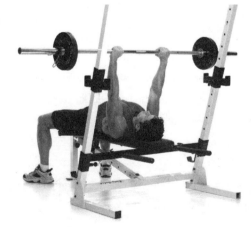

A

B Lower the bar straight down toward your chest. Bring your elbows past your sides and lightly touch the bar against the lower part of your chest. Then press back to the starting position.

MAKE IT EASIER

- Make the grip a little wider, but keep the elbows moving down along your sides.
- Use an EZ bar to reduce strain on your wrists.

DO IT HARDER

- Pause the weight on your chest before pressing up.
- Let your elbows flare out to the sides while pressing and lowering.

DIPS

Dips are an excellent exercise for developing the upper body. Descending in the dip with your arms close to your sides and your elbows moving back places more stress on the triceps and works all three of the triceps heads.

A On a set of parallel bars, assume a neutral grip (palms facing each other). Start with a straight-arm supported position. Keep your legs straight and head up; minimize the amount of forward lean.

B Take a deep breath, bend your elbows, and lower yourself until you feel a mild stretch in your shoulder. The depth of your dip will depend on your flexibility and strength level. At the bottom position, breathe out and push up by extending your arms.

MAKE IT EASIER

- Let your elbows flare out to bring in more chest fibers to assist in the movement.
- Use bands or an assistance machine if you can't lift your body weight initially.

B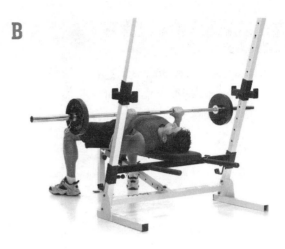

A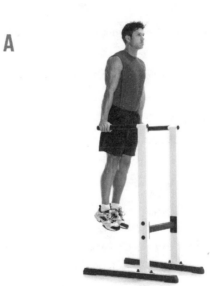

B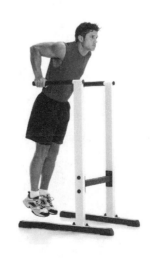

DO IT HARDER

- Pause at the bottom before pushing up.
- Add extra weight by holding a dumbbell between your legs. Or use a dip belt, as shown.

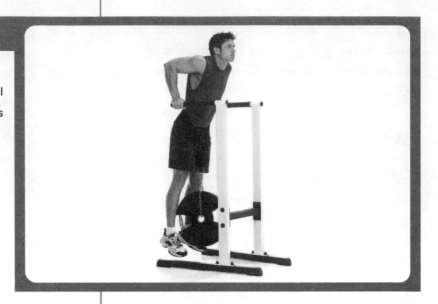

CABLE KICKBACK

Kickbacks are a great exercise for working the back head of the triceps. Maintaining good form and control throughout this movement is difficult; make the effort. The use of a cable provides equal resistance through the entire range of motion.

A Attach a handle to a floor cable. Grab the pulley in your left hand. Stand up and take one step forward with your right foot and one step backward with your left foot. Bend at the waist, and support your torso with your right hand on your right knee. With your left palm facedown, keep your elbow in and raise the upper arm so that it is slightly above parallel.

B With your left hand perpendicular to the floor, slowly straighten your arm, keeping your upper arm stationary. Return to the starting position in a slow, controlled motion.

MAKE IT EASIER

- Use a rope handle to put less strain on your wrists.
- Raise your torso to place less strain on your elbow.

DO IT HARDER

- Pause the weight at the top to put extra tension on the triceps.
- Use a thicker handle to increase grip strength while working the triceps.

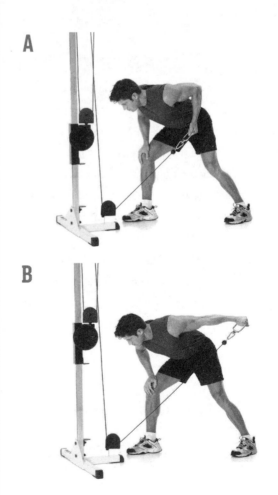

A

B

SINGLE-ARM DUMBBELL KICKBACK

This exercise isolates the triceps. Because you don't get much help from the surrounding muscles, it can be difficult to maintain good form and control.

A Hold a dumbbell in your right hand. Place your left knee and left arm on a weight bench, with your right foot on the floor. Keep your back straight and parallel to the floor. Your right arm should be bent 90 degrees.

B Slowly straighten your right arm and extend the weight behind your body, keeping your upper arm parallel to the floor. You should feel your right arm's triceps fully contract. Then, slowly bend your right arm again, bringing the weight back to the starting position. Finish the set and switch arms.

MAKE IT EASIER

- Raise your shoulders during the movement.
- Raise your torso to place less strain on your elbow.

A

B

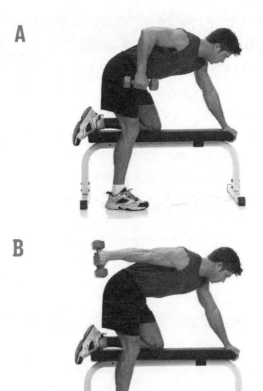

DO IT HARDER

- Pause the weight at the top to put extra tension on the triceps.
- Keep your back parallel to the ground.
- Use tubing instead of a dumbbell.

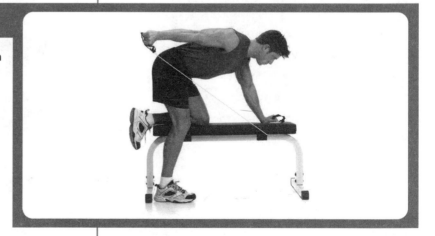

SINGLE-ARM DUMBBELL LYING CROSS-SHOULDER TRICEPS EXTENSION

This across-the-body movement resembles a military salute. It's strenuous and difficult to control. Start out using a relatively light weight until you get the hang of it.

A Lie on a bench with your knees bent. Hold a dumbbell in your right hand, with your right arm extended straight up from your body, your palm facing your feet.

B Keeping your upper arm and elbow stationary, slowly lower the dumbbell across your upper chest until the end touches your left shoulder. Then slowly extend your arm back to the starting position. Finish the set, then switch arms.

MAKE IT EASIER

- Lower the weight as usual, but press it up on the return motion.
- Use your free hand to assist your loaded arm.

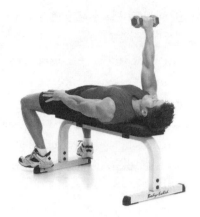

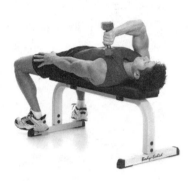

DO IT HARDER

- Use a heavier dumbbell that requires the assistance of your free hand during the exertion phase. Let go with your free hand and do a negative on the way down.
- Pause at the top and contract the triceps.
- Use tubing instead of a dumbbell.

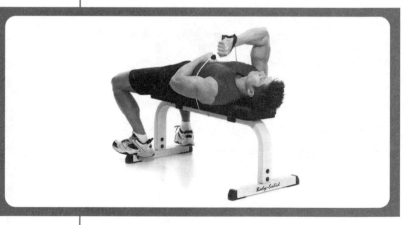

BARBELL DECLINE LYING TRICEPS EXTENSION

Performing this exercise on a decline bench increases the demand on your triceps muscles.

A Lie on your back on a decline bench. Hold a curl bar over your chest with your arms extended, palms facing up and away from you. Your hands should be in a narrow grip, 4 to 6 inches apart.

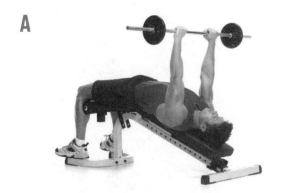

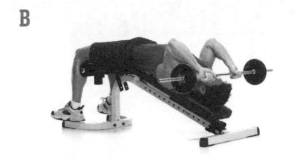

B Keeping your upper arms stationary, slowly bend your elbows, lowering the weight toward the top of your head. Hold for a second, then slowly return to the starting position.

MAKE IT EASIER

- Lower the weight as usual, but press it up on the return motion.
- Don't come down all the way.

DO IT HARDER

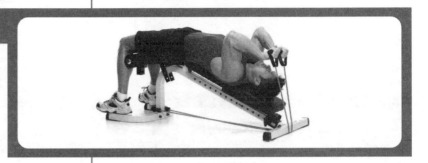

- Lower the weight behind your head.
- Pause at the top and contract the triceps.
- Use tubing instead of a dumbbell.

BARBELL INCLINE LYING TRICEPS EXTENSION

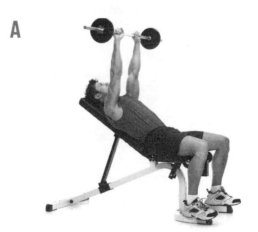

This exercise works the biggest and strongest part of the triceps muscle, covering the inside and back of your upper arm.

A Lie on an incline bench, with the back of your head on the upper corner of the bench. Hold a curl bar over your head with your arms fully extended, palms facing up and away from you. Your hands should be in a narrow grip, 4 to 6 inches apart.

B Keeping your upper arms stationary, bend your elbows, lowering the barbell toward your head. Hold for a second, then slowly return to the starting position.

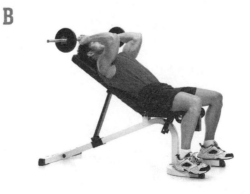

MAKE IT EASIER

- Lower the weight as usual, but press it up on the return motion.
- Don't come down all the way.

DO IT HARDER

- Lower the weight behind your head.
- Pause at the top and contract the triceps.
- Use tubing instead of a barbell.

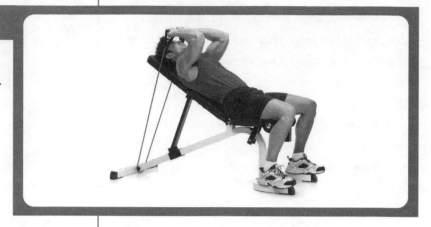

BARBELL LYING TRICEPS EXTENSION

This exercise should be practiced with good control because overhead lifts can be dangerous if the weight slips. Begin by using lighter weights—and a spotter.

A Lie on your back on a weight bench. Hold a curl bar over your chest with your arms fully extended, palms facing up and away from you. Your hands should be about shoulder width apart.

B Keeping your upper arms stationary, slowly bend your elbows, lowering the weight toward the top of your head. Hold for a second, then slowly return to the starting position.

MAKE IT EASIER

- Lower the weight as usual, but press it up on the return motion.
- Don't come down all the way.
- Use an EZ bar to reduce strain on your wrists.

DO IT HARDER

- Lower the weight behind your head.
- Pause at the top and contract the triceps.

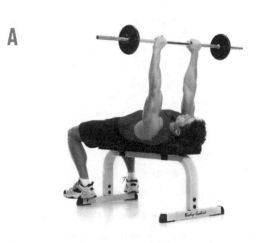

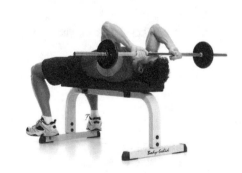

A

B

CABLE LYING TRICEPS EXTENSION

This exercise, sometimes referred to as the French Cable Curl, develops the three heads of the triceps muscles.

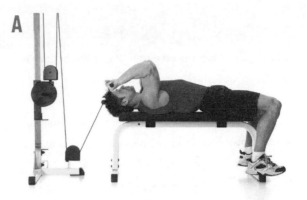

A Position a weight bench so that one end is about a foot from a multistation weight machine with a bar-handle low pulley cable. Grip the bar while standing, then lie on your back on the bench, with your head pointed toward the machine. Grip the bar with your palms facing up and away from you. Space your hands 4 to 6 inches apart. Your elbows should be bent 90 degrees, with the bar just over the top of your head, your upper arms perpendicular to the floor.

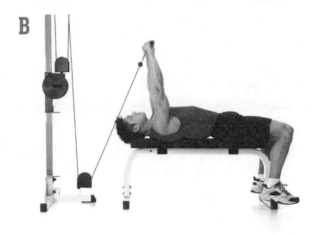

B Slowly unbend your elbows until your arms extend directly out from your shoulders. Hold for a second, then slowly return to the starting position.

MAKE IT EASIER

- Lower the weight as usual, but press it up on the return motion.
- Don't come all the way down.

DO IT HARDER

- Lower the weight behind your head.
- Pause at the top and contract the triceps.

DOUBLE DUMBBELL LYING TRICEPS EXTENSION

This exercise will increase the overall stability of the elbow joint, and because it requires more coordination, it brings more supporting muscles into play.

A Lie on your back on a weight bench. Hold a dumbbell in each hand, over your chest, with your palms facing up and away from you and your arms fully extended.

B Keeping your upper arms stationary, in a slow, controlled motion, bend your elbows, lowering the dumbbells toward the top of your head. Hold for a second, then slowly return to the starting position.

MAKE IT EASIER

- Lower the weight as usual, but press it up on the return motion.
- Don't come all the way down.

DO IT HARDER

- Lower the weight behind your head.
- Pause at the top and contract the triceps.

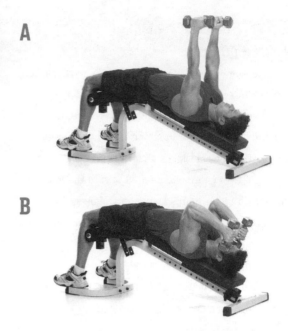

SEATED ONE-ARM DUMBBELL TRICEPS EXTENSION

Performing this exercise while seated stabilizes the back and reduces the risk of injury.

A While sitting on a weight bench, hold a moderately heavy dumbbell with your right hand, using a palm-down grip. Hold the dumbbell over your head, with your thumb around the handle and the weight resting on your palms. Start with your arm fully extended, your shoulder relaxed, and your elbow close to your head.

B Lower the dumbbell behind your head as far as it will go. Hold for a second, then raise to the fully extended position. Complete a set, then repeat with the other arm.

MAKE IT EASIER

- Lower the weight as usual, but press it up on the return motion.
- Don't come all the way down.

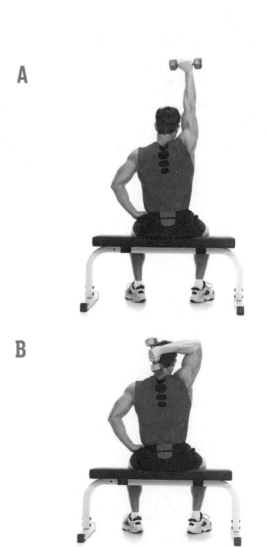

DO IT HARDER

- Don't lock your arms at the top; keep constant tension on the triceps.
- Pause at the top and contract the triceps.
- Use tubing instead of a dumbbell.

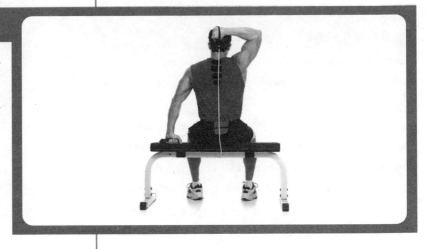

TUBING LYING TRICEPS EXTENSION

This exercise works your triceps and strengthens elbow extensors. Using exercise tubing utilizes resistance rather than weight and eliminates the need for a spotter.

A Run a length of tubing underneath the long bar that connects the feet of a weight bench. Lie on your back on the bench. Hold the tubing's handles over your head, with your elbows bent and your palms facing away from you. Your hands should be 4 to 6 inches apart and there should be no slack in the tubing.

B Keeping your upper arms stationary, slowly uncurl your arms over your chest until they are fully extended. Hold for a second, then slowly return to the starting position.

MAKE IT EASIER

- Lower your hands as usual, but press them up on the return movement.
- Don't come down all the way.

DO IT HARDER

- Pause your hands at head level.
- Pause at the top and contract the triceps.

A

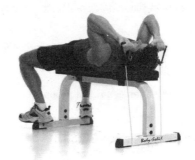

B

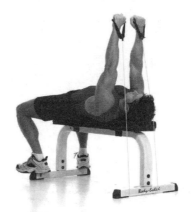

ONE-ARM CABLE TRICEPS EXTENSION

This exercise works the entire triceps, but it is especially good for strengthening the lateral head on the outer back part of your upper arm.

A Attach a D-handle to the low pulley of a cable machine. Grip the handle with one hand, your palm facing up and away from you. Place the hand with the cable behind your neck, your palm facing your neck, and your elbow positioned upward. Keep your upper arm perpendicular to the floor and your shoulder stationary as you bring the weight down behind your head.

B Slowly unbend your elbow until your arm is extended directly out from your shoulder. Hold for a second, then slowly return to the starting position. Complete a set, then switch to the other arm.

MAKE IT EASIER
- Lower the weight as usual, but press it up on the return movement.
- Don't come down all the way.

DO IT HARDER
- Pause the weight behind your head.
- Pause at the top and contract the triceps.

A

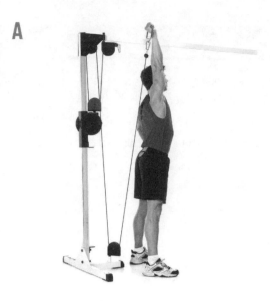

B

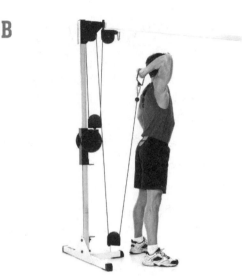

BARBELL SEATED OVERHEAD TRICEPS EXTENSION

This exercise develops the three heads of the triceps muscles.

A With your hands slightly narrower than shoulder width apart, hold a barbell with a full, overhand grip. Straddle a weight bench and hold the bar over your head with your arms straight, your elbows unlocked. Your upper arms should be just outside your ears.

A

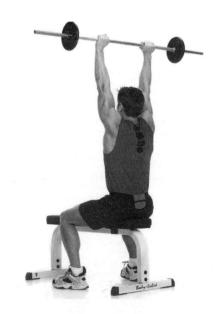

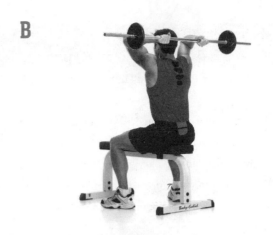

B Bend your elbows back and slowly lower the bar toward the back of your neck. Stop when your forearms are just past parallel to the floor. Pause, then press back up to the starting position. Keep your upper arms stationary throughout the exercise.

MAKE IT EASIER

- Use tubing instead.
- Don't come down all the way.

DO IT HARDER

- Pause the weight behind your head.
- Pause at the top and contract the triceps.
- Use tubing instead of a barbell.

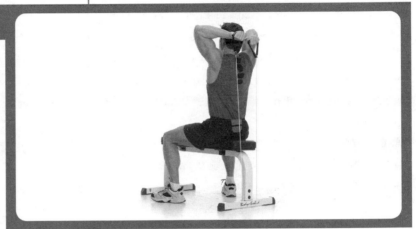

DUMBBELL SEATED OVERHEAD TRICEPS EXTENSION

Performing this exercise while seated stabilizes the back and reduces the risk of strain.

A Grip the end of a moderately heavy dumbbell with both hands and sit on a weight bench. Hold the dumbbell over your head, with your thumbs around the bar and the weight resting on your palms. Start with your arms fully extended, your shoulders relaxed, and your elbows close to your head.

B Lower the dumbbell behind your head as far as it will go. Hold for a second, then raise to the fully extended position.

MAKE IT EASIER

- Use tubing instead.
- Don't come down all the way.

DO IT HARDER

- Pause the weight behind your head.
- Pause at the top and contract the triceps.

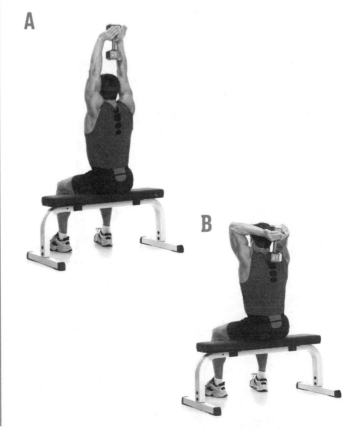

CABLE PUSHDOWN (OR ANGLED BAR PUSHDOWN)

This is a great exercise that works all three heads of the triceps muscle.

A Stand facing an overhead pulley with a bar handle on the cable. Your legs should be shoulder width apart, your knees slightly bent. Hold the bar with both hands palms down, in a narrow grip. Your forearms should be at a 45-degree angle to the floor, your upper arms and elbows close to your body.

B Keeping your wrists locked and straight, slowly and smoothly straighten your arms, pressing the bar down as far as you can without locking your elbows. Hold for a second at the fully straightened position, then slowly allow the bar to rise to the starting position.

MAKE IT EASIER

- Lower the weight as usual, but press it down.
- Push the arms until they are straight; don't come all the way back up.

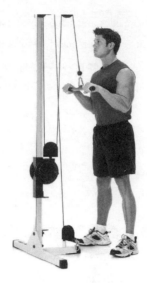

A

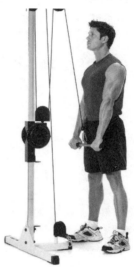

B

DO IT HARDER

- Keep the elbows along your sides, and the weight in front of your body. As you push down, do not let your elbows drift back.
- Use a Y-shaped rope handle, pause at the bottom, and pull the hands apart.

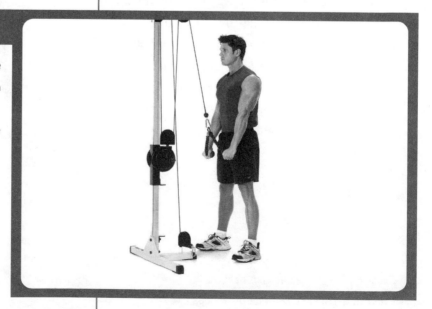

REVERSE-GRIP CABLE PUSHDOWN

While this exercise works the entire triceps, it is especially good for strengthening the lateral head, the outer back part of your upper arm.

Stand facing an overhead pulley with a bar handle on the cable. Your legs should be shoulder width apart, your knees slightly bent. Hold the bar with your palms up, using a narrow hand spacing. Keep your upper arm vertical, with your elbows bent at 45 to 90 degrees.

Keep your wrists straight as you smoothly push the weight down and straighten your arms. Hold for a second, then slowly return to the starting position.

A

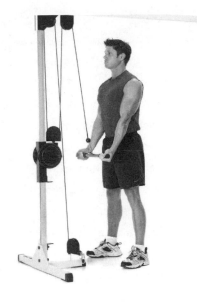

MAKE IT EASIER

- Lower the weight as usual, but lean forward to push it down.
- Push the arms until they are straight; don't come all the way back up.

DO IT HARDER

- Keep the elbows along your sides and the weight in front of your body. As you push down, do not let your elbows drift back.
- Perform the movement as described above with a rope handle, but pause at the bottom and pull the rope taut by pushing your hands apart laterally.

REVERSE DIP

Also known as bench dips or desk dips, this exercise works all three heads of the triceps. Note: Don't do this exercise if you have wrist problems.

A Place two exercise benches, or two heavy chairs, side by side, 3 to 4 feet apart. Sit on one end of a bench and hold on to the edge of the bench with your arms shoulder width apart. Plant your heels firmly on the facing bench, about 6 inches in from the edge. Your butt should be suspended slightly in front of your hands.

B Slowly bend your arms and lower your body toward the floor. Go as low as you can without touching the floor. Then slowly extend your arms, raising yourself back to the starting position.

MAKE IT EASIER

- Don't lower yourself all the way down.
- Keep one foot on the floor to help push your body back up.

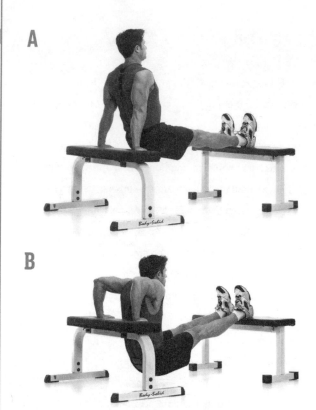

A

B

DO IT HARDER

- Keep the elbows close to your sides.
- Place a dumbbell or weight plates on your lap.

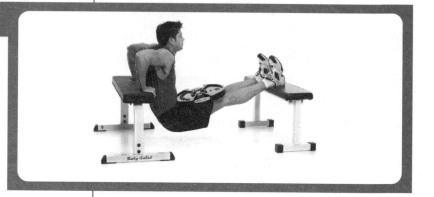

BARBELL FOREARM CURL

This exercise strengthens the wrist flexors (underside of forearm), hand abductors (inside of forearm), and the hand adductors (outside of forearm).

A Sit on a weight bench, with your legs a little more than hip width apart. Hold a barbell or EZ bar with an underhand grip and lean your forearms on your thighs. For maximal mobility, the backs of your wrists should be just slightly over your knees. Lower the weight toward the floor, stopping when you've gone as far as you can without moving your forearms.

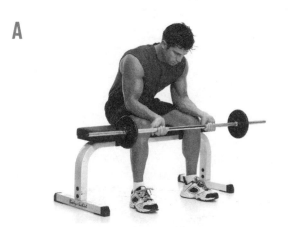

A

B Slowly lift the weight as high as you can toward your body. Pause for a second, then return to the starting position.

MAKE IT EASIER

- Use a narrow grip.
- Attach tubing to a stationary object and perform the curl against the resistance provided by the tubing (see Tubing Forearm Curl on page 106). Or use no weight at all if the unloaded barbell is too heavy.

DO IT HARDER

- Use a wide grip.
- Pause at the top and bottom of the movements.

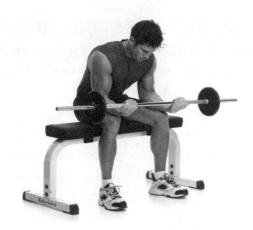

CABLE FOREARM CURL

Working the muscles of the forearm increases hand strength and stability. This exercise is more efficient than gripping exercises alone.

A Position a weight bench about a foot from a bar-handle low pulley cable. Sit on the bench, with your feet slightly wider than shoulder width apart. Hold the bar with your palms up, hands positioned no more than shoulder width apart. Your wrists should be over your knees so you can bend them through the full range of motion. The tops of your forearms should rest on the back of your thighs, and your body should remain as upright as possible.

B Curl the bar in a semicircular motion toward your body as far as you can without letting your forearms rise off your thighs. At the top of the curl, pause for a second, then return to the starting position.

MAKE IT EASIER

- Use a narrow grip.
- Set up close to the pulley so that you can do partial reps.

DO IT HARDER

- Use a wide grip.
- Set up farther away from the pulley and pause at the top and bottom of the movements.

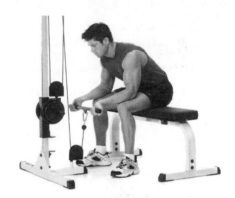

A

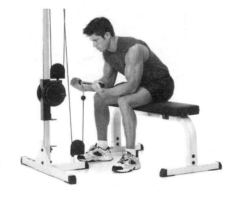

B

DUMBBELL FOREARM CURL

Similar to the barbell forearm curl, this exercise works both wrists at one time, strengthening the muscles of the forearms, wrists, and hands.

A Sit on a weight bench, with your legs a little more than hip width apart. With your palms up, hold a dumbbell in each hand. Lean your forearms on your thighs. For maximal mobility, the backs of your wrists should be just slightly over your knees. Keep your body upright. Allow your wrists to bend back naturally as the weight pulls them down.

B Keeping your arms stationary and using only your wrists, curl the dumbbells toward your body as far as they will go. Hold for a second, then return to the starting position.

MAKE IT EASIER

- Allow the dumbbells to touch each other to reduce muscle strain involved in balance.
- Attach tubing to a stationary object and perform the curl against the resistance provided by the tubing (see Tubing Forearm Curl, below).

DO IT HARDER

- Keep the dumbbells farther apart.
- Pause at the top and bottom of the movements.

A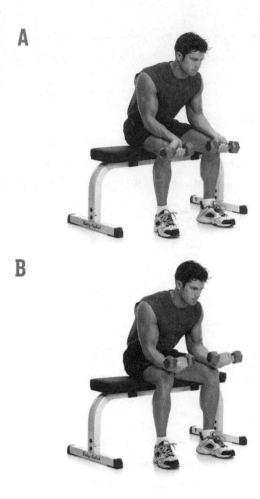

B

TUBING FOREARM CURL

Utilizing the power of resistance rather than weights, this exercise builds strength in the wrist flexors (front of the forearms).

A Sit on a bench, with your feet slightly more than hip width apart. Secure a length of exercise tubing under both feet. Hold the handles with your palms up and your wrists slightly over your knees so you can bend them through their full range of motion. The tops of your forearms should rest against your thighs. Keep your upper body upright, though you may lean into your legs for comfort.

A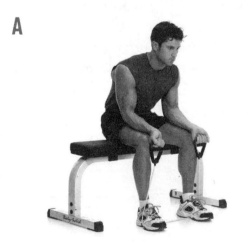

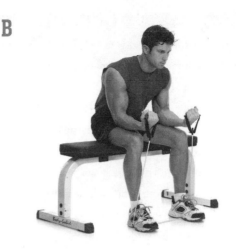

B Slowly curl the tubing handles in a semicircular motion up toward your body as far as you can, without letting your forearms rise off your thighs. Pause at the top of the curl, then lower the handles to the starting position.

MAKE IT EASIER

- Use a narrow grip.
- Set up closer to the anchored end of tubing so that there is less resistance.

DO IT HARDER

- Use a wide grip.
- Double the tubing and pause at the top and bottom of the movements.

BARBELL REVERSE FOREARM CURL

This exercise works the muscles on the outside of the forearm.

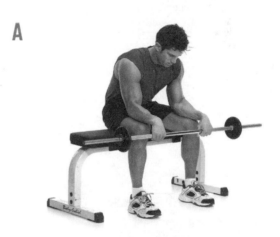

A Sit on a weight bench, with your legs a little more than hip width apart. With your palms up, hold a barbell with an overhand grip and lean your forearms on your thighs. For maximal mobility, the backs of your wrists should be just slightly over your knees.

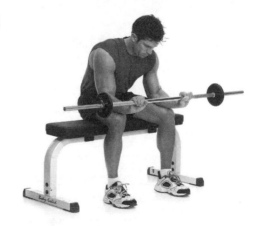

B Curl your palms toward your biceps. Pause, then reverse the motion.

MAKE IT EASIER

- Use a narrow grip.
- Attach tubing to a stationary object and perform the curl against the resistance provided by the tubing (see Tubing Reverse Forearm Curl on page 109). Use no weight at all if the unloaded barbell is too heavy.

DO IT HARDER

- Use a wide grip.
- Pause at the top and bottom of the movements.

CABLE REVERSE FOREARM CURL

This exercise works the wrist extensors, the muscles located on the back of the forearm. As a complement to forearm curls, it develops strength and flexibility.

A Position a weight bench about a foot from a multi-station weight machine with a bar-handle low pulley cable. Sit on the bench, with your legs slightly more than shoulder width apart. Hold the bar with a palms-down grip. Your hands should be about shoulder width apart. Your wrists should be slightly over your knees, so you can bend them through their full range of motion. Let your forearms rest against your thighs. Keep your body as upright as possible, slightly leaning on your legs for comfort.

B Curl the bar in a semicircular motion up toward your body as far as you can without letting your forearms rise off your thighs. Hold for a second at the top of the curl, then return to the starting position.

MAKE IT EASIER

- Use a narrow grip.
- Set up close to the pulley so that you can do partial reps.

DO IT HARDER

- Use a wide grip.
- Set up farther away from the pulley and pause at the top and bottom of the movements.

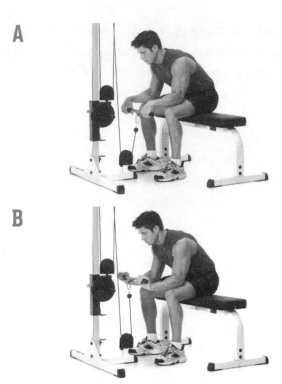

A

B

DUMBBELL REVERSE FOREARM CURL

This exercise works the muscles on the outside of the forearm, providing a stronger backhand for sports like tennis and racquetball. Use a lighter weight than you would for the forearm curl.

A Sit on a weight bench, with your legs a little more than hip width apart. Using a palm-down grip, hold a dumbbell in each hand. Lean your forearms on your knees, with your wrists positioned just over your knees so you can bend them through their full range of motion. Keep your body upright. Allow your wrists to bend naturally as the weight pulls them.

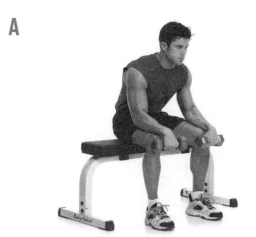

A

B Using the wrists only and keeping the rest of your arms stationary, curl the dumbbells as far as you can. Hold for a second, then return to the starting position.

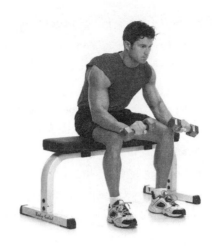

MAKE IT EASIER

- Allow the dumbbells to touch each other.
- Attach tubing to a stationary object and perform the curl against the resistance provided by the tubing (see Tubing Reverse Forearm Curl, below).

DO IT HARDER

- Keep the dumbbells farther apart.
- Pause at the top and bottom of the movements.

TUBING REVERSE FOREARM CURL

This exercise builds your wrist extensors.

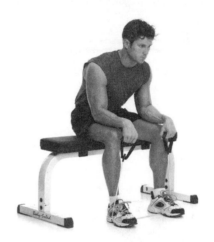

A Sit on a bench, with your feet slightly more than hip width apart. Secure a length of exercise tubing under both feet. Hold one handle in each hand, palms down. Drape your wrists slightly over your knees so you can flex and extend them through their full range of motion. The meaty part of your forearms should rest against your thighs. Your upper body should be fairly upright, though you may lean into your legs for comfort.

B Slowly curl the tubing handles in a semicircular motion up toward your body as far as you can without letting your forearms rise off your thighs. Pause at the top of the curl, then return to the starting position.

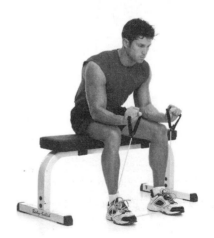

MAKE IT EASIER

- Use a narrow grip.
- Set up closer to the anchored end of tubing so that there is less resistance.

DO IT HARDER

- Use a wide grip.
- Double the tubing and pause at the top and bottom of the movements.

REVERSE WRIST RAISE

This movement, also known as ulnar deviation, works the muscles and tendons around the ulna, one of two forearm bones. Strengthening the wrist and forearms increases elbow strength and helps prevent injuries, such as tennis elbow.

A Stand with your right arm at your side, holding a hammer or dumbbell with a weight on one end only. The weighted end should be behind your hand.

B Slowly raise and lower the weight through a comfortable range of motion. Don't move your elbow or shoulder. Finish the set, then switch arms.

MAKE IT EASIER

• Grip the handle closer to the weighted end.

DO IT HARDER

• Grip the handle farther away from the weighted end.
• Pause at the top and bottom of the movements.

A

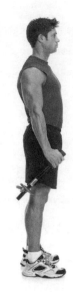

B

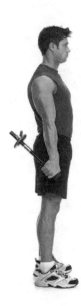

WRIST RAISE

The muscles that control forearm, wrist, and hand movement actually originate near the elbow joint. This exercise, sometimes known as radial deviation, works the muscles and tendons around your radius bone (forearm) and strengthens nearly all the muscles that support the wrist joint.

A Stand with your right arm at your side. Hold a hammer or dumbbell with a weight on one end only. The weighted end should be in front of your hand.

A

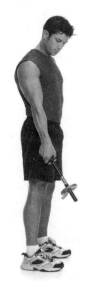

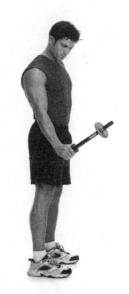

B Slowly raise and lower the weight through a comfortable range of motion. Don't move your elbow or shoulder; focus all the exertion in the wrist. Finish the set, then switch arms.

MAKE IT EASIER

- Grip the handle closer to the weighted end.
- For less resistance, use tubing to perform the exercise by standing on one end and holding the other end in your hand.

DO IT HARDER

- Grip the handle farther away from the weighted end.
- Pause at the top and bottom of the movements.

WRIST ROLLER

This move builds strength in the muscles in your wrists, fingers, and the outer forearm. If you're only going to do one wrist exercise, this should be the one.

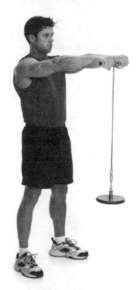

A Stand straight with your feet about shoulder width apart. Hold the wrist roller in both hands, palms facing down, and arms extended in front of you and parallel to the floor. The weight should be dangling in front of you.

B Slowly roll the weight up with your wrists, using long, exaggerated, up-and-down movements. Keep the rest of your body stationary; don't sway your body or drop your arms. When the weight reaches the top, slowly lower it using the same motion.

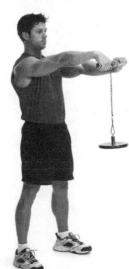

MAKE IT EASIER

- Use a narrow grip.
- Set up closer to the floor, by kneeling or sitting, so that the weight travels less distance.

DO IT HARDER

- Use a wide grip.
- Stand on a bench so that the weight travels more distance.

LEVEL 1 (FOCUS ON SIZE)

- Do the complete exercise program 3 days a week. Allow at least 1 day of rest between workouts.

- Choose any one of the workouts we've provided. You can do one of the workouts three times a week. Or you can do different workouts on different days.

- Start out by doing 2 sets of 5 repetitions for each exercise. Do 1 set of 5 reps without stopping. Rest 1 minute, then repeat.

- For each workout, add 1 to 2 repetitions. Keep going until you reach 10 reps. Then increase the resistance and return to 5 reps.

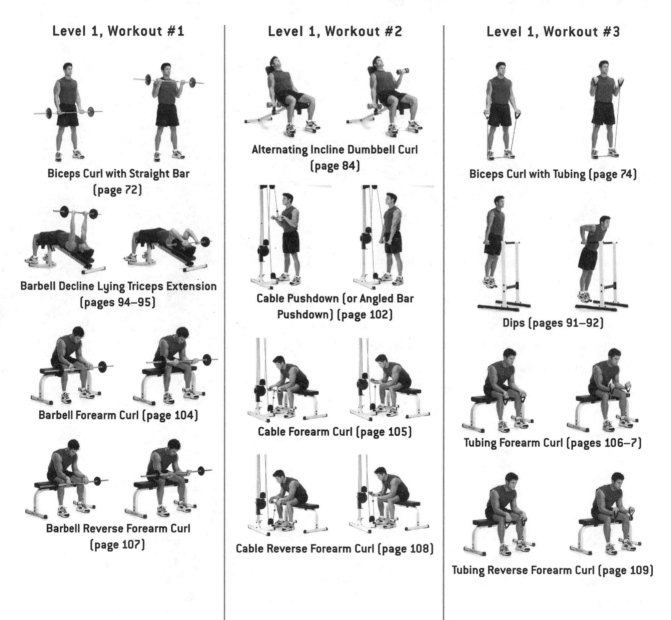

Level 1, Workout #1

Biceps Curl with Straight Bar
(page 72)

Barbell Decline Lying Triceps Extension
(pages 94–95)

Barbell Forearm Curl (page 104)

Barbell Reverse Forearm Curl
(page 107)

Level 1, Workout #2

Alternating Incline Dumbbell Curl
(page 84)

Cable Pushdown (or Angled Bar
Pushdown) (page 102)

Cable Forearm Curl (page 105)

Cable Reverse Forearm Curl (page 108)

Level 1, Workout #3

Biceps Curl with Tubing (page 74)

Dips (pages 91–92)

Tubing Forearm Curl (pages 106–7)

Tubing Reverse Forearm Curl (page 109)

LEVEL 2 (FOCUS ON STRENGTH)

- Do the complete exercise program 3 days a week. Allow at least 1 day of rest between workouts.

- Do one of the workouts three times a week. Or do different workouts on different days.

- Start out by doing 2 sets of 5 repetitions for each exercise. Do 1 set of 5 reps without stopping. Rest 1 minute, then repeat.

- For each workout, add 1 to 2 repetitions until you reach 10 reps. Increase the resistance and return to 5 reps.

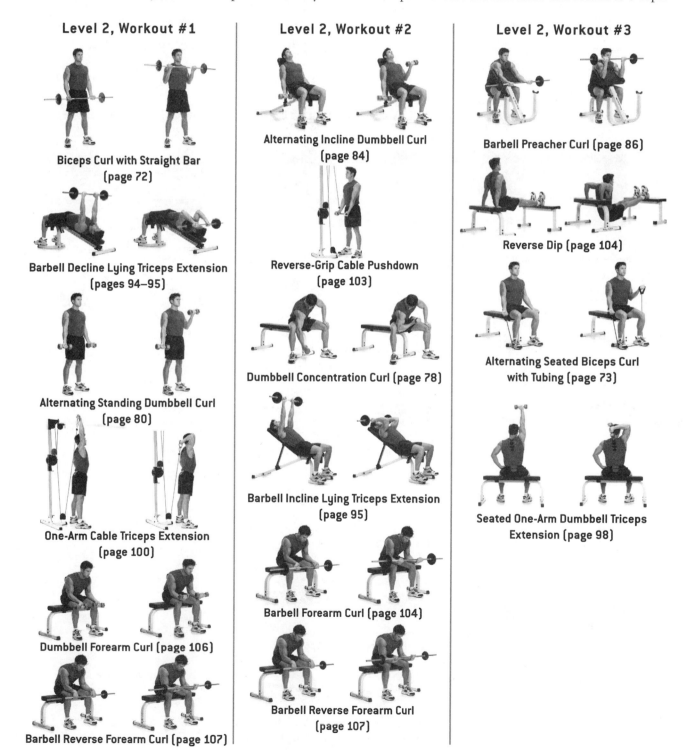

Level 2, Workout #1

Biceps Curl with Straight Bar (page 72)

Barbell Decline Lying Triceps Extension (pages 94–95)

Alternating Standing Dumbbell Curl (page 80)

One-Arm Cable Triceps Extension (page 100)

Dumbbell Forearm Curl (page 106)

Barbell Reverse Forearm Curl (page 107)

Level 2, Workout #2

Alternating Incline Dumbbell Curl (page 84)

Reverse-Grip Cable Pushdown (page 103)

Dumbbell Concentration Curl (page 78)

Barbell Incline Lying Triceps Extension (page 95)

Barbell Forearm Curl (page 104)

Barbell Reverse Forearm Curl (page 107)

Level 2, Workout #3

Barbell Preacher Curl (page 86)

Reverse Dip (page 104)

Alternating Seated Biceps Curl with Tubing (page 73)

Seated One-Arm Dumbbell Triceps Extension (page 98)

LEVEL 3 (HYBRID TRAINING—SIZE AND STRENGTH)

- Do the complete exercise program 3 days a week. Allow at least 1 day of rest between workouts.

- Do one of the workouts three times a week. Or do different workouts on different days.

- Start out by doing 2 sets of 5 repetitions for each exercise. Do 1 set of 5 reps without stopping. Rest 1 minute, then repeat.

- For each workout, add 1 to 2 repetitions. Keep going until you reach 10 reps. Then increase the resistance and return to 5 reps.

- Slightly higher reps (for example, 8 to 12) and volume (three exercises, with 3 sets of each) is best for increasing biceps size.

- Build basic mass first. Start with exercises such as barbell and dumbbell curls. Then move on to "shaping" movements—exercises that utilize cables and machines.

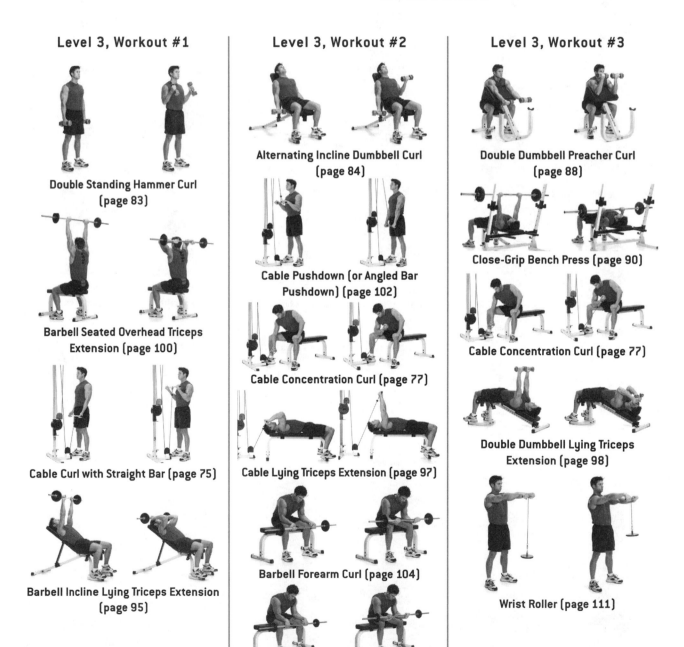

Level 3, Workout #1

Double Standing Hammer Curl (page 83)

Barbell Seated Overhead Triceps Extension (page 100)

Cable Curl with Straight Bar (page 75)

Barbell Incline Lying Triceps Extension (page 95)

Level 3, Workout #2

Alternating Incline Dumbbell Curl (page 84)

Cable Pushdown (or Angled Bar Pushdown) (page 102)

Cable Concentration Curl (page 77)

Cable Lying Triceps Extension (page 97)

Barbell Forearm Curl (page 104)

Barbell Reverse Forearm Curl (page 107)

Level 3, Workout #3

Double Dumbbell Preacher Curl (page 88)

Close-Grip Bench Press (page 90)

Cable Concentration Curl (page 77)

Double Dumbbell Lying Triceps Extension (page 98)

Wrist Roller (page 111)

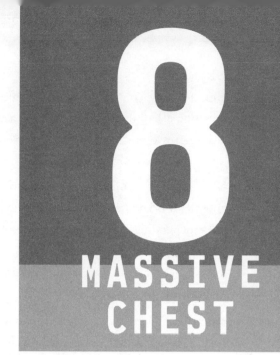

8

MASSIVE CHEST

Men with a powerful look to them invariably have big, well-developed chests. A strong upper body in general, and a strong chest in particular, are what get a man noticed. Feeling good about how you look can vastly improve self-confidence, a must in today's competitive world. Even if you don't sport a bodybuilder's physique, a large chest makes your waist appear smaller. That's an optical illusion most of us can appreciate.

Here's another reason to work your chest more. If you have good upper body strength, you'll be less likely to spend weeks inspecting ceiling tiles due to

muscle, tendon, or ligament injuries. A strong chest can also save your back. No matter how many times doctors advise men to lift heavy objects carefully, no one does it consistently. A strong chest will help you circumvent those lapses by compensating for the extra muscular strain.

Most men spend a disproportionate amount of gym time working their chests, shoulders, and arms. Yet relatively few guys have decent chest development. This is mainly because they don't really understand what the chest muscles are or what they do. They don't utilize the workouts that can generate impressive increases in size and strength, often in as little as 8 to 12 weeks.

THE CHEST EXPLAINED

The chest is made up primarily of two muscles: the pectoralis major and the pectoralis minor. The pec

major is the large superficial chest muscle that pops when you wear a tight T-shirt. The pectoralis minor is a smaller muscle that lies underneath the pec major.

That's the simple version—too simple, really, because men tend to focus their attention on the obvious, the pectoralis major. Unless you hit the different *parts* of this muscle, and also work the pec minor, you'll never get any serious kind of chest development. So let's break things down a little more.

- The pectoralis major spreads out like a fan and covers the rib cage like an armor plate. Its main job is to pull the arm and shoulder across the front of the body. It consists of two parts: the clavicular (upper) portion and the sternal (lower) portion. The upper part is attached to the clavicle (collarbone). At the lower end, it attaches to the sternum (breastbone) and the cartilage of several ribs. The pectoralis major muscle lets you perform such motions as pitching a ball underhanded, doing a wide-grip bench press, twisting off a bottle cap, swimming the crawl stroke, and doing dips.

- The pectoralis minor is also an upper chest muscle. It originates on the third, fourth, or fifth ribs (depending on the man), and inserts on the scapula. Its main job is to lift the ribs. When you take a deep breath and your chest rises, that's the pec minor at work.

Together, these muscles consist of an enormous number of fibers that fan out across the chest. To develop any kind of size, you need to include a *lot* of exercises in your workout.

THE TOTAL CHEST WORKOUT

The great thing about bench and dumbbell presses is that they quickly improve the appearance of the chest, making it broader and more rounded. But concentrating mainly on these exercises actually works a very small percentage of the chest muscles. They'll get bigger, sure, but won't come anywhere near their full potential.

Just as it's important to work different and opposing muscle groups as part of a well-balanced workout, you want to achieve balance in your chest workouts, as well. That means hitting muscles in the upper, lower, inner, and outer chest.

Incline to work the upper part. Exercises that are performed on an incline, such as dumbbell bench presses, barbell bench presses, and dumbbell flies, exert more tension on the upper chest.

Lie flat or on a decline to work the lower and outer chest. The best way to build muscles near the sternum at the lower part of the chest is to do workouts on either a flat surface or a decline. Examples include decline dumbbell or barbell presses, flat barbell bench presses, or cable crossovers.

Contract to work the inner chest. Just about any chest exercise exerts some strain on muscle fibers on the inner chest. To really work these muscles, though, you need to contract the muscles strongly at the top of the movement. Good inner-chest exercises include machine flies, flat dumbbell flies, or cable crossovers.

Build the back to build the chest. The chest and back muscles work together. Your chest will never reach its full potential size unless you also take the time to really work the back, particularly the latissimus dorsi muscles in the upper back. (See "The Middle Back" on page 163.)

Recruit more muscle fibers. When you're getting ready to lift heavy weights in barbell movements, such as a bench press, unrack the weight, position the bar at arm's length, and pause for a moment to let your body *feel* the weight before you start to lower the bar. This will help your body recruit more muscle fibers and get comfortable with the movement.

Bring the triceps into play. When gripping a barbell, use an overhand grip with the thumbs wrapped around the bar. This grip allows you to squeeze the bar when the weight starts to feel heavy. This activates more of the triceps and allows you to lift heavier weights or increase your reps.

Don't use a *false grip,* with all of your fingers on the same side of the bar. This grip takes the triceps out of play—and is also dangerous because it doesn't let you grip the bar securely.

Balance your chest with a balanced grip. When using dumbbells, always grip them in the center of the handle, and make sure that they're both at the same height and in the same position. You'll see a lot of men simply grab a pair of dumbbells and hoist them up, without paying attention to this all-important detail. Dumbbells that are uneven at the initial, starting position will follow different movement paths. The result: lopsided chest development. If you want your right and left pecs to resemble each other, always lift both dumbbells in the same trajectory, keeping the same beginning and end points.

Keep the weight off your chest. Unless you're a competitive power lifter, don't rest the weighted bar on your chest in between movements. You want to maximize chest muscle fiber involvement, and that requires lowering the weight under full control, letting the bar lightly touch your chest, then quickly changing direction and pressing upward with a little more speed. This movement increases the number of muscle fibers you overload, causing faster gains in size and strength.

Strengthen your chest by strengthening everything else. Many chest exercises involve pressing—bench presses, dumbbell presses, and so on. These movements work a lot of muscles, such as the triceps, anterior deltoid (front of the shoulder), and serratus anterior (area under the armpits). So if you're having trouble doing presses, don't assume that your chest is to blame. Any one of these other muscles could be the weak link. That's why we rec-ommend training every major muscle group each week. Strengthening these other muscles will allow you to optimize your chest workouts at the same time.

Warm up tight muscles. Arm swings are a great chest warmup. Also perform the dynamic stretching routine on page 285.

Shrug off chest pain. If you ever notice that you're aching in the area where your chest and shoulder connect, the first thing to suspect is impingement. It's an inflammation of the rotator cuff that often occurs when men overwork their chests and underwork their backs. You can prevent it by increasing exercises (or sets of any particular exercise) that work the upper back. A good example is horizontal shrugs. Strengthening the rhomboids in the upper back will help prevent the shoulder joint from being pulled forward during your chest workouts.

CABLE CROSSOVER

This works a huge number of muscle groups, including the pectoralis major and minor (chest) muscles, serratus anterior (upper and outer rib cage), deltoids (shoulder), and coracobrachialis (inner upper arm).

A Stand between two overhead pulleys with D-handles on the cables. Position your feet shoulder width apart. Grip the handles using an overhand grip. Bend at the waist so that your upper body is at a 45-degree angle to the floor. Keeping your elbows slightly bent and your wrists straight, pull the handles down until they are in line with your shoulders. This is the starting position.

B Slowly pull the handles down and in until they meet in front of your knees. Pause for a second, then slowly return to the starting position.

MAKE IT EASIER

- Bend elbows more to make it easier to pull the handles together.
- Lean forward to increase leverage.

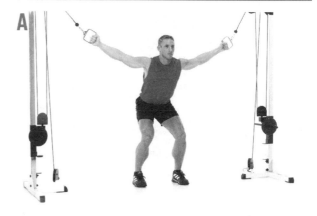

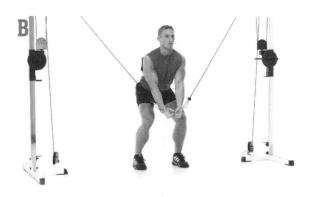

DO IT HARDER

- Use a thicker handle to increase the workload.
- Use a bench with a back support and do the exercise while seated.
- Press the weight forward, but lower it slowly with straight arms.
- Use tubing at chest height on either side so that it stretches as you draw your hands together.

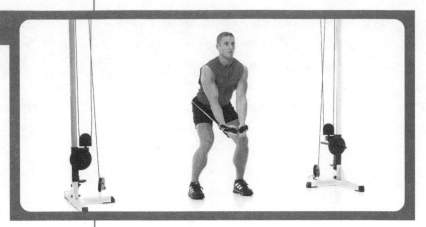

DECLINE BARBELL BENCH PRESS

The declined position of this exercise puts a lot of tension on the lower chest. It's a difficult and potentially dangerous move, so use lighter-than-usual weights—and a spotter if you can. This form of benching puts the body in the strongest mechanical position for the chest to press big weights.

A Lie on a decline bench, with your head under the barbell rack and your knees over the far end of the bench. Hook your feet under the support pads. With your arms shoulder width apart, hold the bar with an overhand grip, palms facing your feet. Lift the bar off the rack and hold it straight over your chest.

B Bend your elbows and lower the bar under control to slightly below your nipple line, keeping your elbows pointed at 45 to 60 degrees from your sides. Lightly touch your chest with the bar, then quickly reverse direction and press the bar back to the starting position.

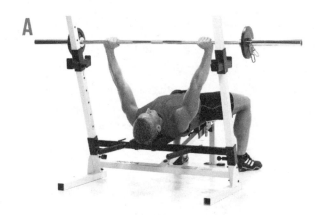

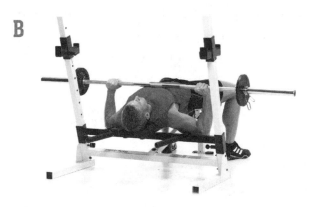

MAKE IT EASIER

- Use a wider grip.

DO IT HARDER

- Use a closer grip.
- Add bands or chains to each side of the bar.

THE SECRET TO A BIG BENCH PRESS

A big bench press is a head-turner in any gym. To lift those kinds of weights, you have to be blessed with certain genetic advantages—and you also have to know how to lift. The following tips will help you lift weights so heavy that it will make all the other guys wish they could be you.

- Take a deep breath and hold it. You need maximum stability to move maximum weights. By holding a deep breath, you stabilize internal pressures, which allows you to exert more force. Warning: Don't use this technique if you've been diagnosed with high blood pressure.

- Push your feet into the floor so that you "drive" through the legs. Your knees should be bent at about 90 degrees. This allows you to lift your lower body slightly and shift the load from the weighted barbell onto your upper back and traps.

- Squeeze your shoulder blades together. Hold them there before unracking the weight. This draws your shoulders downward and reduces the distance the bar has to travel.

- Lower the bar to your lower chest or lower ribs, depending on your body dimensions.

- Keep your elbows under the bar. This allows you to transfer more force to lifting. If the elbows flare out to the sides, more force goes into working the chest as opposed to lifting the bar.

- Push the bar in a straight line. It shortens the distance it has to travel. That means less work—and more weight.

DECLINE DUMBBELL BENCH PRESS

The decline position of this exercise works the lower chest muscle. The advantage of using dumbbells instead of a bar is that they reduce the tendency of stronger muscle groups to compensate for weaker ones. This is a difficult and potentially dangerous move; use lighter-than-usual weights—and a spotter if you can.

A Lie on a decline bench with your knees over the far end of the bench, feet on the floor. With your arms shoulder width apart, hold a dumbbell in each hand, palms facing your feet. The dumbbells should extend straight over your chest at arm's length.

A

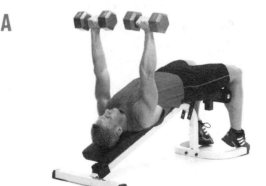

B Lower the dumbbells under control to your nipple line. Your elbows should point down and flare at 45 to 60 degrees from your sides. Lightly touch your chest, then quickly reverse direction and press the dumbbells back to the starting position. Hold for a second, then repeat.

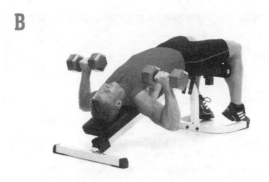

MAKE IT EASIER

• Use a wider hand-spacing between the dumbbells.

DO IT HARDER

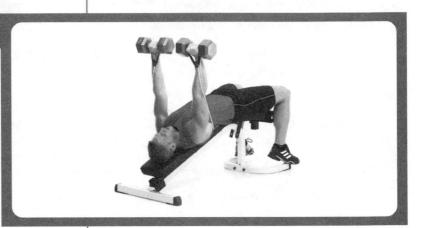

• Perform the exercise in an alternating fashion, or on a small stability ball.
• Add bands or chains to each dumbbell.
• Hold the dumbbells so that your palms face each other throughout the movement.

DECLINE TUBING FLY

This exercise works the lower chest as well as the shoulders.

A Grab the ends of a length of exercise tubing in each hand and position it so that when you lie down on a decline bench it crosses your shoulder blades. Your arms should be extended above you, palms facing each other.

B Lower your arms out and away from each other in a semi-circular motion to chest level. Keep your wrists locked, your elbows bent at roughly 90 degrees, and your back straight. Hold for a second, then slowly return to the starting position.

MAKE IT EASIER

• Keep the elbows slightly bent.
• Use dumbbells instead of tubing.

DO IT HARDER

• Keep your elbows nearly straight, but not locked.
• Add bands or chains to each dumbbell.
• Hold the dumbbells so that your palms face your feet throughout the movement.

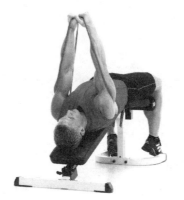

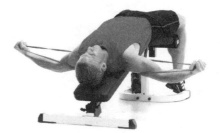

DIPS

Dips are an excellent exercise for developing the upper body. Descending in the dip with your arms close to your sides and your elbows moving back places more stress on the triceps and works all three of the triceps heads.

A On a set of parallel bars, assume a neutral grip (palms facing each other). Start with a straight-arm supported position. Keep your head up and bend your knees; minimize the amount of forward lean.

B Take a deep breath, bend your elbows, and lower yourself until you feel a mild stretch in your shoulder. The depth of your dip will depend on your flexibility and strength level. At the bottom position, breathe out and push up by extending your arms.

MAKE IT EASIER

• Use a dip machine with a counterweight.
• Use a closer hand-spacing between the handles.

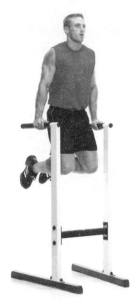

A

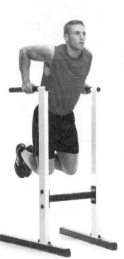

B

DO IT HARDER

• Use a wider hand-spacing between the handles.
• Use a dip belt to add extra weight or hold a dumbbell between your legs.
• Loop bands over the handle and rest your knees on top of the band.
• Hold your legs out in front of you, at a 90-degree angle to the hips.

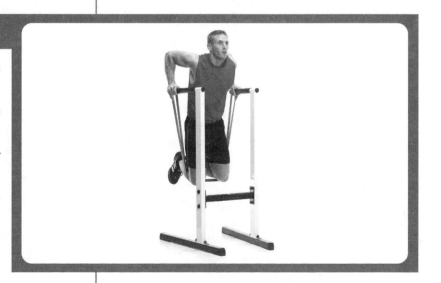

FLAT BARBELL BENCH PRESS

Bench presses are probably the most popular exercise in the weight room. They give a superb workout to the chest, shoulders, and triceps.

A Lie on a bench, with your head under the barbell rack, your feet flat on the floor. Grip the barbell with an overhand grip. Your hands should be at or slightly more than shoulder width apart. Press the barbell off the rack. Hold it extended at arm's length above your chest. Keep your back straight and against the bench.

B Bend your elbows and lower the bar under control to your nipple line, keeping your elbows pointed at 45 to 60 degrees from your sides. Lightly touch your chest with the bar, then quickly reverse direction and press the barbell back to the starting position. Hold for a second, then repeat.

MAKE IT EASIER

• Use a wider grip.

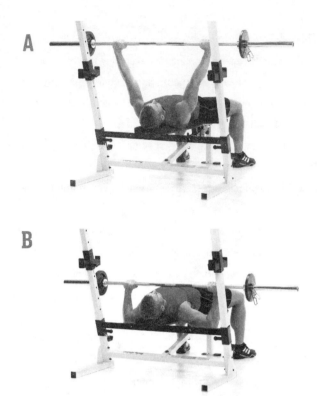

DO IT HARDER

• Use a closer grip.
• Add bands or chains to each side of the bar.

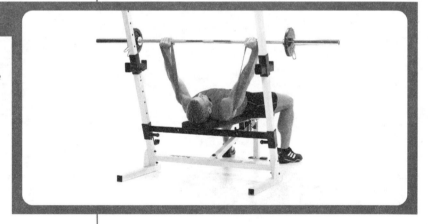

FLAT DUMBBELL BENCH PRESS

This exercise is nearly identical to the barbell bench press. However, using dumbbells makes it more difficult because you have to support and balance two separate weights.

A Lie on a weight bench, with a dumbbell in each hand and your arms fully extended and perpendicular to the floor. The ends of the dumbbells should almost touch. Keep your feet flat on the floor, your palms facing out. Keep your head and body in full contact with the bench.

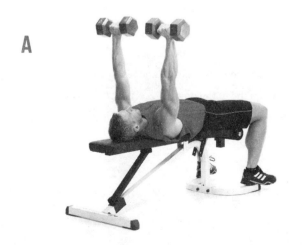

B Lower the dumbbells under control to your nipple line. Your elbows should point down and flare at 45 to 60 degrees from your sides. Lightly touch your chest, then quickly reverse direction and press the dumbbells back to the starting position. Hold for a second, then repeat.

MAKE IT EASIER

- Use a wider hand-spacing between the dumbbells to place more stress on your chest.

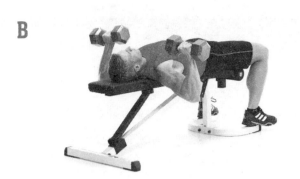

DO IT HARDER

- Perform the exercise in an alternating fashion, or on a stability ball.
- Add bands or chains to each dumbbell.
- Hold the dumbbells so that your palms face each other throughout the movement.

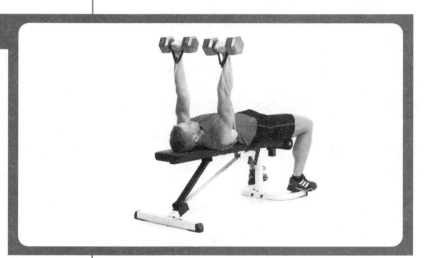

FLAT TUBING FLY

This movement works the shoulder adductors as well as the chest.

A Grab the ends of a length of exercise tubing in each hand and position it so that when you lie down on a weight bench it crosses your shoulder blades. Lie on your back with your legs parted and your feet firmly on the floor. Your arms should be extended above you, palms facing each other. Your back should be straight and firm against the bench. Don't lock your elbows.

B Lower your arms out and away from each other in a semicircular motion to chest level. Keep your wrists locked, your elbows slightly bent, and your back straight. Hold for a second, then slowly return to the starting position.

MAKE IT EASIER

- Bend the elbows more.

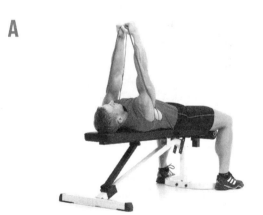

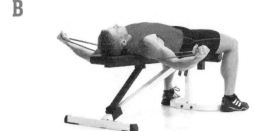

DO IT HARDER

- Keep your elbows almost straight, but not locked.
- Perform this exercise using dumbbells.
- Hold the dumbbells so that your palms face your feet throughout the movement.

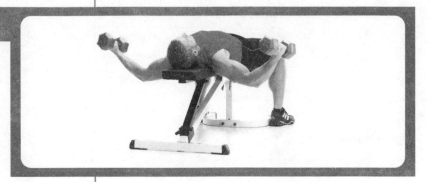

INCLINE BARBELL BENCH PRESS

This exercise helps build the upper and outer pectoralis (chest) muscles and shoulders. It also works the serratus anterior (located around the upper and outer rib cage) muscles.

A Lie on a 45-degree incline bench. Grip the barbell, with your hands shoulder width apart and palms facing your feet. Keep your back flat against the bench and your feet flat on the floor. Press the weight off the barbell rack. Completely extend your arms until they are perpendicular to the floor.

B Bend your elbows and lower the bar to your upper chest, keeping your elbows pointed at 45 to 60 degrees from your sides. Lightly touch your chest, then quickly reverse direction and press the barbell back to the starting position. Hold for a second, then repeat.

MAKE IT EASIER

- Use a wider grip to place more stress on your chest.

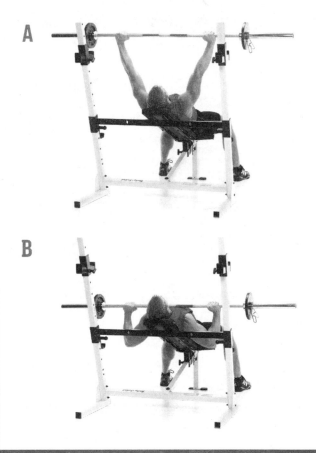

DO IT HARDER

- Use a closer grip to place more stress on your triceps.
- Add bands or chains to each side of the bar.

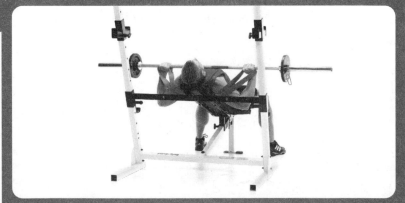

SHOULDERING THE BURDEN OF CHEST PRESSES

Chest training and shoulder pain seem to happen to everyone at some point. The reason is that many of the presses used to build the chest put a lot of stress on the rotator cuff—the muscles and tendons in the shoulder that hold the "ball" of the upper arm bone firmly in the shoulder socket.

As you get older, your risk of a rotator cuff injury increases. Mild cases can be treated with self-care measures or exercise therapy. More advanced cases require steroid injections and surgery. A minor injury can heal on its own if you take good care of it. Try these steps.

Rest. This doesn't mean finishing your workout even though your shoulder is killing you. It means stop—*now*. Limit heavy lifting or overhead activity until your shoulder starts to feel better. This usually takes about a week.

Apply ice and heat. Putting ice on your shoulder helps reduce inflammation and pain. Use a cold pack, a bag of frozen vegetables, or a towel filled with ice cubes. Apply cold for 15 to 20 minutes, and repeat every few hours for the first day or two. After that, switch to heat. Again, limit applications to about 20 minutes.

Take pain relievers. Aspirin, ibuprofen, and similar drugs are all equally effective. Acetaminophen is good for pain, but won't reduce inflammation as well as the other drugs.

Stay limber. After a couple of days, do some gentle exercises to keep your shoulder muscles limber. Total inactivity causes stiff, painful joints. It also increases the risk of "frozen shoulder," which basically means the joint gets so stiff that you can't move it. Keep the shoulder moving—and once it's healed, get serious about daily shoulder stretches and a balanced shoulder-strengthening program to prevent future injuries.

INCLINE DUMBBELL BENCH PRESS

This movement works the triceps as well as the chest.

A Lie on a 45-degree incline bench. Hold a dumbbell in each hand, using an overhand grip, your palms facing your feet. Hold the dumbbells shoulder width apart, with your arms fully extended and perpendicular to the floor. Keep your back pressed against the bench, your feet flat on the floor.

B Lower the dumbbells to your nipple line. Your elbows should point down and flare at 45 to 60 degrees from your sides. Lightly touch your chest, then quickly reverse direction and press the dumbbells back to the starting position. Hold for a second, then repeat.

MAKE IT EASIER

- Use a wider hand-spacing between the dumbbells to place more stress on your chest.

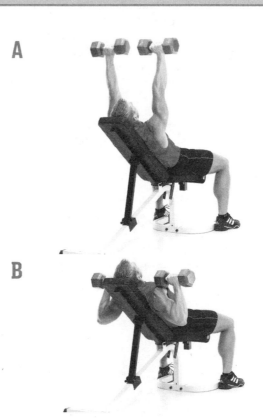

A

B

DO IT HARDER

- Perform the exercise in an alternating fashion, or on a large stability ball.
- Add bands or chains to each dumbbell.
- Hold the dumbbells so that your palms face each other throughout the movement.

INCLINE TUBING FLY

The key to this movement is keeping your chest tensed throughout. The more slowly you move your hands, particularly as you lower them, the more you will feel your chest working.

A Grab the ends of a length of exercise tubing in each hand and position it so that when you lie down on a bench, it crosses your shoulder blades. Lie on a 45-degree incline bench. Keep your back pressed against the bench and your feet flat on the floor. Your arms should be extended above you, palms facing each other. Don't lock your elbows.

B Slowly lower your arms out and away from each other in a semicircular motion to chest level. Keep your wrists locked, your elbows slightly bent, and your back straight. Hold for a second, then slowly return to the starting position.

MAKE IT EASIER

- Bend the elbows more.

A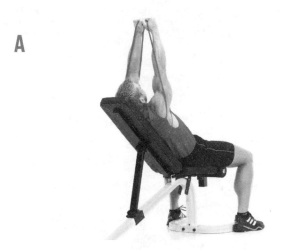

B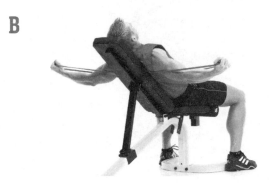

DO IT HARDER

- Keep your elbows straighter, but not locked.
- Use dumbbells as well as tubing.

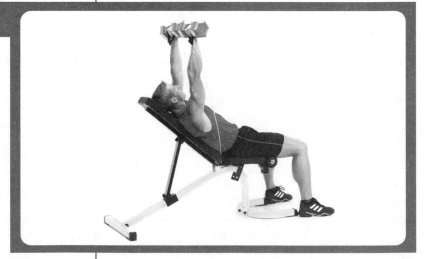

FLOOR PUSHUP

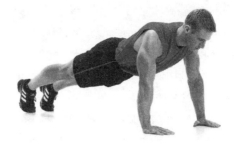

A   Lie facedown on the floor with hands spaced wider than your shoulders, positioned under your chest, with your thumbs pointing toward each other and middle fingers pointing straight ahead. Your feet shoulld be about hip width apart with legs straight. Don't let your hips sag down. Extend your arms until they are straight and your upper body is at about a 45-degree angle to the floor.

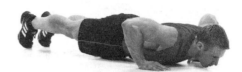

B   Lower your body until your chin or chest touches the floor. Pause for a second and press up. Maintain a straight line between your feet, hips, and head as you move up and down. Repeat.

MAKE IT EASIER

• Bend your knees so they rest on the floor.
Don't lower yourself all the way to the floor.

DO IT HARDER

• Try the one-hand version on page 128.
• Try the T Pushup on page 130.

HOW TO DO MORE PUSHUPS

The average 35-year-old man can only do about 30 pushups before crashing to the floor. That's not too impressive, especially when you consider that there are middle-school girls who can do them with ease.

Pushups are great for upper-body strength—and it's not that hard to push your count into the "wow" zone.

• Do them at your own pace. Men can do more pushups when they self-pace than they can using the traditional (and arbitrary) two-up, four-down count.

• Never use an internally rotated hand position, in which the fingers point inward. It puts too much stress on the elbows. Keep your hands and fingers pointed straight ahead, or slightly pointed outward.

• Train with one-arm pushups to build strength quickly—and make two-arm pushups to feel a lot easier later on.

• Do pushups on wobble boards, medicine balls, or barbells to make them more challenging, and also to develop better stabilization muscles. Then, when you go back to regular pushups, you should be able to do a lot more.

• Train progressively. In the first week, do as many pushups as you can in 5 seconds. Rest for 1 minute, then do another 5-second set. Rest for 1 minute, then do the final 5-second set. Do this two to three times a week. Each week, add 5 seconds to your pushup time. Reduce your rest time by 5 seconds. At the end of 13 weeks, you'll be doing pushups for 180 straight seconds! That's enough to win any bar bet.

ONE-HAND PUSHUP

This pushup variation works one side of the body at a time. One-hand pushups aren't for beginners. You need very strong arms and shoulders, and good balance, to avoid serious injury when doing them.

A Set up as though you're about to do a two-hand floor pushup. Spread your feet apart wider than your shoulders. Move your left hand so it is directly under your head or neck. Your body should form a triangle on the floor. Put your right hand on your right hip or hamstring.

B Lower yourself with your left hand. Go down until you touch the floor, then quickly push yourself back to the start position using only your left hand. Complete your reps, then switch sides.

MAKE IT EASIER

- Do the movement with your knees touching the ground.
- Perform the exercise using tubing.
- Use your free hand to assist you by lightly pushing up with it just enough to help your other arm do the movement.

DO IT HARDER

- Bring your feet closer together.
- Do this with your hand on a medicine ball, dumbbell, or stability ball.
- Do this with only one hand and the opposite foot in contact with the ground.

A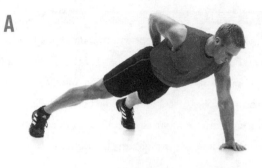

B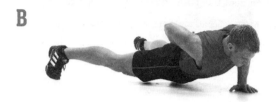

STABILITY BALL PUSHUP

This classic exercise works to strengthen the chest, shoulders, arms, wrists, and upper back. Because the exercise ball forces you to concentrate on balance, you build core body stabilization as well.

A In a facedown position, place your toes on an exercise ball. Put your palms on the floor, hands aligned under your shoulders.

B Lower your chest toward the floor, keeping your upper arms and elbows close to your rib cage as your arms bend. Then return to the starting position, and repeat.

MAKE IT EASIER

- Do the movement with your knees on the ball.
- Use a smaller ball to reduce the amount of force needed to push up.

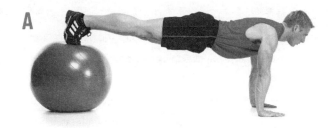

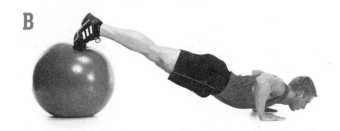

DO IT HARDER

- Add tubing around your arms and shoulders.
- Put only one foot on the ball and hold the other one in the air.
- Do this with your hands on medicine balls, dumbbells, or wobble boards.
- Do this with only one hand on the ground, and both feet on the ball.
- Do this with your hands on the stability ball and feet on the ground.

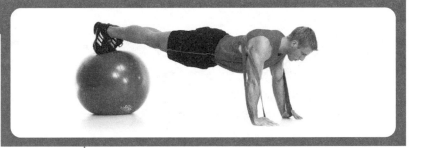

T PUSHUP

This nontraditional pushup works the chest, shoulders, arms, and wrists, while also developing core body strength and balance.

A   Lie facedown on the floor. Balance your weight on the balls of your feet and the palms of your hands. With your hands shoulder width apart, extend your arms until your body is at a 45-degree angle to the floor. Your legs should be together and fully extended.

B   Roll onto the outside edge of the left foot while rotating your body 180 degrees, lifting your right arm toward the ceiling and perpendicular to the floor. Be sure to keep the left shoulder blade rolled in and down, to prevent shoulder injuries. Rotate back until the right arm is once again on the floor. From this position, perform a traditional pushup. Return to the "up" position, and repeat, this time balancing on the right hand and rotating the left arm and torso.

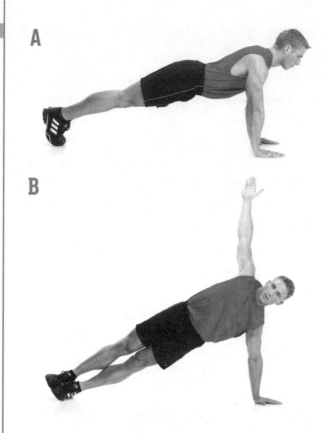

A

B

MAKE IT EASIER

- Spread your feet farther apart.
- Roll on both feet instead of just one foot.

DO IT HARDER

- Bring your feet closer together.
- Do this with your hands on medicine balls or dumbbells.
- Use only one hand.

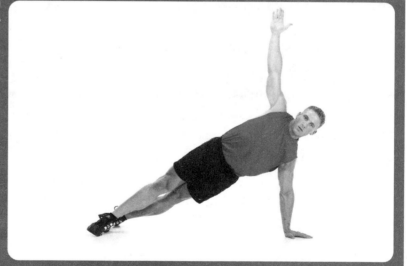

HOW USEFUL IS "PRE-EXHAUST" TRAINING?

The usual training strategy is to start workouts with compound movements that work multiple muscle groups, such as a bench press, then progress to isolation exercises, such as flies. Some bodybuilders, however, insist that they get better results by turning this around. They do the isolation exercises first to *pre-exhaust* the chest, then follow up with pressing movements. The idea is that this stimulates more muscle growth.

Not true. If anything, this is a pretty poor approach to training. If your chest is fatigued, you'll lift less on the pressing movements. That means less overload, and less of the stimulation needed to achieve maximal size and strength. This reverse strategy may be helpful for men with some types of injuries. It can also help increase muscular endurance. But if you're trying to get big, stick to the traditional approach.

LEVEL 1 (FOCUS ON SIZE)

- Do the complete exercise program 3 days a week. Allow at least 1 day of rest between workouts.

- Choose any one of the workouts we've provided. You can do one of the workouts three times a week. Or you can do different workouts on different days.

- For the first exercise, start with 1 to 2 sets using relatively light weights to warm up. Perform all sets for one exercise before moving to the next exercise. Take 1 to 2 minutes' rest between each set or exercise.

LEVEL 1 WORKOUTS

We've provided three different workouts for Level 1. Workout variations mean more strength and size—and less boredom.

One option is to do all three workouts weekly. For example, do Workout #1 on Monday, Workout #2 on Wednesday, and Workout #3 on Friday. If you choose this option, do 2 warmup sets for the first exercise, followed by 3 sets of 6 repetitions using "real" weight. Next, do 3 sets of 10 reps for the second exercise, followed by 3 sets of 14 reps for the third exercise. Do only 1 set of the last exercise, going for maximum reps.

Another option is to do just one of the workouts, three times a week. Vary the rep count daily. On Monday, for example, do 3 sets of 6 reps for the first three exercises; on Wednesday, do 3 sets of 10 reps for the first three exercises; and on Friday, do 3 sets of 14 reps for the first three exercises. Always start with two warmup sets for the first exercise (these don't go toward the final "count"). Do only 1 set of the last exercise, going for maximum reps.

Level 1, Workout #1

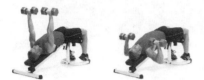

Decline Dumbbell Bench Press (page 119)

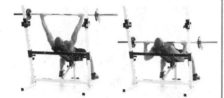

Flat Barbell Bench Press (page 122)

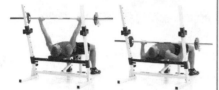

Incline Barbell Bench Press (page 124)

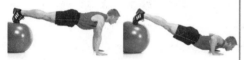

Stability Ball Pushup (page 129)

Level 1, Workout #2

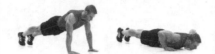

Floor Pushup (page 127)

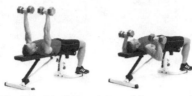

Flat Dumbbell Bench Press (page 122)

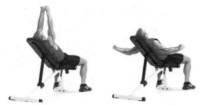

Incline Tubing Fly (page 126)

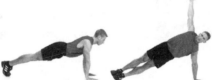

T Pushup (page 130)

Level 1, Workout #3

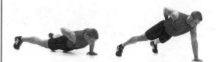

One-Hand Pushup (page 128)

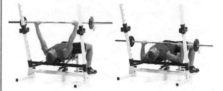

Decline Barbell Bench Press (page 118)

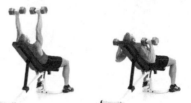

Incline Dumbbell Bench Press (page 125)

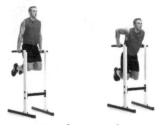

Dips (page 121)

LEVEL 2 (FOCUS ON STRENGTH)

- Do the complete exercise program 3 days a week (except for Workout 1). Allow at least 1 day of rest between workouts.

- Choose any one of the workouts we've provided. You can do one of the workouts three times a week. Or you can do different workouts on different days.

- For the first exercise, start with 1 to 2 sets using relatively light weights to warm up. Perform all sets for one exercise before moving to the next exercise. Take 1 to 2 minutes' rest between each set or exercise.

Level 2, Workout #1
MAX BENCH PRESS ROUTINE

It's possible to increase your bench weight by more than 50 pounds in less than 12 weeks by following this routine. You only have to do it twice a week—a "light" day and a "heavy" day. First, determine your 1 repetition maximum (1RM) for the bench press. (See page 14.) Then use the chart below to determine your flat bench press weight and reps for a given workout. Round the weights to the nearest 5 pounds.

To stay limber (and safe), start each workout with two 5-rep warmup sets, using 50 percent and 70 percent of your 1RM. After you've done all sets and reps of your bench press, complete the workout with the additional exercises on the following page.

Level 2, Workout 1, Bench Press Cycle

WEEK	DAY	% 1RM	#SETS	#REPS
1	1	80	6	2
1	2	80	6	3
2	1	80	6	2
2	2	80	6	4
3	1	80	6	2
3	2	80	6	5
4	1	80	6	2
4	2	80	6	6
5	1	80	6	2
5	2	85	5	5
6	1	80	6	2
6	2	90	4	4
7	1	80	6	2
7	2	95	3	3
8	1	80	6	2
8	2	100	2	2
9	1	80	6	2
9	2	105	2	1*

*AFTER THE 2 SETS AT TOP WEIGHT, KEEP DOING SINGLES, WITH 2 MINUTES' REST BETWEEN SETS. INCREASE THE WEIGHT 5 TO 10 POUNDS EACH TIME UNTIL YOU FIND YOUR NEW 1RM.

ADDITIONAL EXERCISES FOR WORKOUT #1

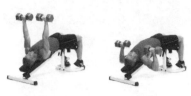

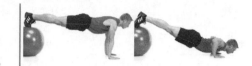

Decline Dumbbell Bench Press (page 119)

On Day 1, do 2 to 3 sets, 8 to 10 reps each; on Day 2, do the same number of sets, but only 4 to 6 reps.

Incline Dumbbell Bench Press (page 125)

On Day 1, do 2 to 3 sets, 8 to 10 reps each; on Day 2, do the same number of sets, but only 4 to 6 reps.

Stability Ball Pushup (page 129)

On both days, do 1 set, maximum reps.

Level 2, Workout #2

Do this workout three times a week. Perform 2 warmup sets for each exercise. Vary the rep count on successive days. For example, do 1 set of 3 reps on Monday, 1 set of 11 reps on Wednesday, and 1 set of 7 reps on Friday.

Each week, add 1 set to each exercise until you're up to 5 sets.

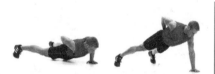

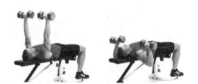

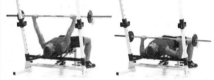

One-Hand Pushup (page 128)

Flat Dumbbell Bench Press (page 122)

Decline Barbell Bench Press (page 118)

Level 2, Workout #3

Do this workout three times a week. Perform 2 warmup sets for each exercise.

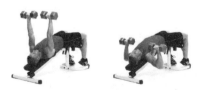

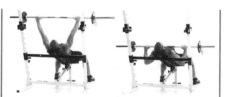

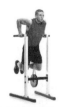

Decline Dumbbell Bench Press (page 119)

Do 2 to 3 sets of 3 reps.

Incline Barbell Bench Press (page 124)

Do 2 to 3 sets of 7 reps.

Dips with Weight (page 121)

Use a dip belt to add the weight or hold a dumbbell between your legs. Do 2 to 3 sets of 11 reps.

LEVEL 3 (HYBRID TRAINING—FOCUS ON SIZE AND STRENGTH)

We've provided three different programs for the Level 3 chest workouts. You can stick to one program throughout the week. Or shake things up and do different programs on different days. Always allow at least 1 day of rest between workouts. The number of sets and repetitions you'll do in each workout depends on the approach you take. Here are the two main options.

Option A

- Perform all three workouts in a single week. For example, do Workout #1 on Monday, Workout #2 on Wednesday, and Workout #3 on Friday.

- After a general warmup, do 2 warmup sets for the first exercise, lifting lighter-than-usual weights.

- Do 5 sets of 2 reps for the first exercise.

- Next, do 2 sets of 6 reps for the second exercise.

- Do 2 sets of 12 reps for the third exercise.

Option B

- Pick one of the workouts and stick with it all week.

- After a general warmup, do 2 warmup sets for the first exercise, lifting lighter-than-usual weights.

- Vary the rep count on each day. For example, do 3 sets of 2 reps for the first three exercises on Monday. On Wednesday, do 3 sets of 6 reps for the first three exercises. On Friday, do 3 sets of 12 reps for the first three exercises.

Level 3, Workout #1

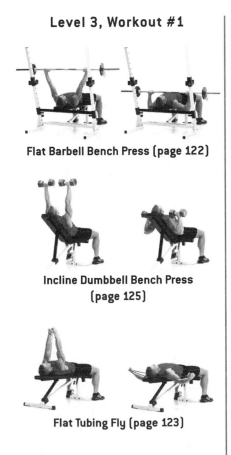

Flat Barbell Bench Press (page 122)

Incline Dumbbell Bench Press (page 125)

Flat Tubing Fly (page 123)

Level 3, Workout #2

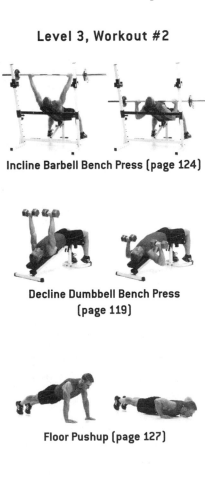

Incline Barbell Bench Press (page 124)

Decline Dumbbell Bench Press (page 119)

Floor Pushup (page 127)

Level 3, Workout #3

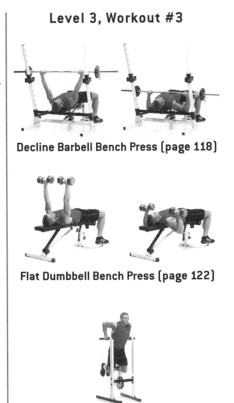

Decline Barbell Bench Press (page 118)

Flat Dumbbell Bench Press (page 122)

Dips with Weight (page 121)

Use a dip belt to add the weight or hold a dumbbell between your legs.

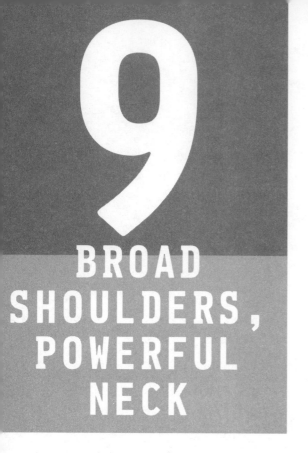

9

BROAD SHOULDERS, POWERFUL NECK

When you build up the large shoulder muscles, the deltoids, you'll have the look that most men only wish for. Large deltoids help create the wide, V-shaped, tapered look that makes the waist look smaller and projects a strong, powerful, and healthy appearance. The shoulders are an incredibly complex network of joints, bones, nerves, and muscles. The stronger you make those muscles, the less likely you are to spend a week in bed—or a few hours in the operating room—after hammering your shoulders with more force than they were meant to handle. Shoulder injuries are so common, and

potentially so serious, that trainers sometimes call shoulder workouts prehabilitation—exercises that dramatically reduce the risk of damage.

Different parts of the deltoids come into play when you do chest exercises (pushing movements) or back exercises (pulling movements). In fact, it's hard to think of any upper-body movement—everything from loading weight plates onto a bar to raising your arm—that doesn't bring these muscles into play.

The other main muscle, the trapezius, is responsible for raising your shoulder, rotating the shoulder blades, and turning your head. It also makes the neck look larger, and gives a powerful appearance when viewed from either the front or the back. These muscle groups are so closely related that a lot of the same exercises work for both, at least to some extent. A well-rounded workout, of course, includes exercises that are specific to either the delts or the traps.

DELTOIDS EXPLAINED

The shoulder is categorized as a ball-and-socket joint, similar in design to the hip. The anatomy of the shoulder gives it the greatest range of motion of any joint in the body. At the same time, the complexity of this joint makes it highly prone to injuries, such as nerve impingement or shoulder dislocation.

Every joint is supported by opposing muscles. When one muscle pulls in a given direction, an opposing muscle also contracts. This is what keeps the joint stable. This interplay is much more pronounced in the shoulder. Unlike, say, the elbow joint, which only moves back and forth, the shoulder's multidirectional range of motion means that a great number of muscles come into play. A workout that hits all of the muscles—and different parts of the same muscles—is essential. Imbalances in strength between opposing muscles is a common cause of injuries.

The main shoulder muscle, the deltoids, is divided into three areas, or heads.

- The anterior (front) deltoid is involved in shoulder abduction (moving the arm away from the body), flexion (moving the arm upward to the front), transverse flexion (moving the arm across the chest), and internal rotation (turning the arm inward).

- The lateral (side) deltoid is involved in many of the same movements as the anterior deltoid: abduction, flexion, and transverse flexion.

- The posterior (rear) deltoid is involved in shoulder extension (moving the upper arm down to the rear), transverse extension (moving the arm away from the chest with the elbows out to the sides), transverse abduction (moving the arm away from the chest with the elbows down), and external rotation (turning the upper arm outward).

THE TOTAL DELTOID WORKOUT

For the most part, it's better to work the deltoids with free weights rather than cables, tubing, or machines. You recruit more muscle fibers when using free weights. The other workouts are fine for variety, but spend most of your time using dumbbells, barbells, and plates.

Balance the shoulders and chest. A lot of men attempt to balance their workouts by doing the same number of back and chest exercises. This is *wrong*. What they should be doing is the same number of upper-back exercises and sets as they do for the chest *plus* the shoulders. This is the only way to balance the pulling and pushing movements across the joint.

If you haven't been doing this in the past, you might want to develop a 12-week program in which you perform more back work relative to the chest and shoulder exercises you do.

Listen to your body. If your shoulder joint is tight and you can't externally rotate the joint without feeling as though something's about to pop, you're better off avoiding some exercises than trying to push your muscles to a point they aren't prepared to go. For example, you might be too stiff to lower a barbell behind your head, the key move in behind-the-neck presses. Rather than forcing it, switch to dumbbells and work the rotator cuff for a while. In a few weeks, you'll probably be loose enough to try the exercise again.

Don't bounce. It's always tempting to bounce dumbbells or barbells at the bottom of pressing movements. Bouncing makes exercises easier. Don't do it. Dropping weights too fast almost guarantees you'll have to deal with painful inflammation at some point. Always lower weights slowly, and with full control, rather than bouncing them off your shoulder, clavicle, or—yikes!—neck.

Pay attention to arm position. You want your arms to be perpendicular to the floor through most of the pressing movements involved in shoulder workouts. This allows you to transfer more force into the movement and lift heavier weights.

Order counts. Do compound movements, such as presses and upright rows, before doing isolation movements, such as laterals or side raises. Doing your workouts in this order will allow you to lift heavier weights and stimulate more muscle fibers—the shortcut to getting bigger.

Balance your right and left hands. A lot of shoulder exercises utilize dumbbells. Be sure to grip them in the center of the handles, and move the right and left arms at the same rate and through the same range of motion. If you don't pay attention to this little detail, you're setting yourself up for lopsided shoulder development.

Warm up tight muscles. Perform the dynamic stretching routine on page 285.

ANTERIOR (FRONT) SHOULDER EXERCISES

BARBELL SHOULDER PRESS

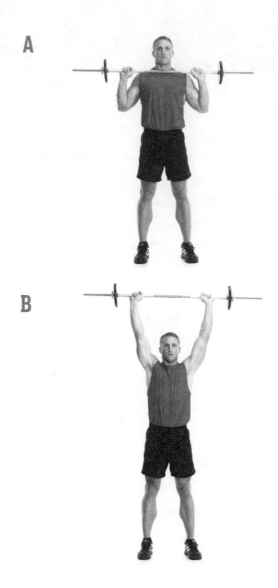

Sometimes referred to as a military press, this movement works the front and side deltoid (shoulder) muscles.

A Stand with your back straight, your feet shoulder width apart, and your knees slightly bent. Hold a barbell with an overhand grip, with your hands shoulder width or slightly farther apart. Bend your elbows and raise the bar to shoulder level. Keep your elbows pointing down, and your chest high.

B Press the barbell straight over your head, using total control. Hold for a second, slowly lower it to chest level, and repeat.

MAKE IT EASIER

- Lower the bar in front of your head only to chin level. Or do partial presses in a power rack.
- Do the exercise while seated, with good back support.
- Use a Smith machine.

DO IT HARDER

- Clean the weight into position to make this exercise more of a total body movement.
- Use bands or tubing.
- Use your legs to help drive the weight up, then lower it slowly. The negatives will stimulate shoulder size and strength.

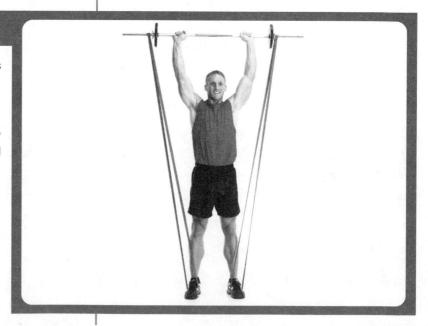

SEATED FRONT DUMBBELL SHOULDER PRESS

This exercise works the front and side deltoid (shoulder) muscles, the triceps (back of upper arm), and the trapezius (upper back and neck) muscles. It's a must for building massive shoulders.

A Sit on the end of a bench with your back straight. Hold a dumbbell in each hand, with your palms facing forward at shoulder height.

B Press both dumbbells overhead until they almost touch. Extend your arms fully. Pause for a second, then slowly return to the starting position.

MAKE IT EASIER

- Press only one dumbbell at a time, using the other hand for support.
- Lower the dumbbells at the side of your head, going only to ear level.
- Press the dumbbells overhead with a neutral hand position, palms facing your ears.

A

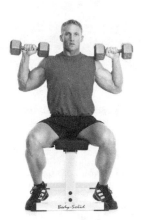

B

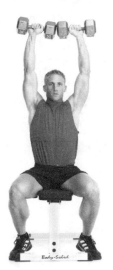

DO IT HARDER

- Use bands or tubing instead of dumbbells.
- Clean the dumbbells into position. This exerts more tension in the initial stages of the movement.
- Do the exercise while standing.
- Press the dumbbells in an alternating fashion. While pressing one dumbbell, hold the other dumbbell over your head.

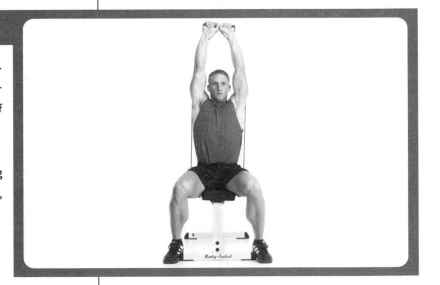

LATERAL (SIDE) SHOULDER EXERCISES

CABLE SIDE DELTOID RAISE

This exercise works the deltoids as well as the trapezius (upper back and neck) and rhomboid (between the spine and shoulder blades) muscles.

A Stand sideways in front of a low pulley with a D-handle on the cable. Your right shoulder should be closest to the machine. Stand with your legs shoulder width apart. Bend your knees slightly, keeping your back straight. Grip the handle with your left hand, with your arms hanging down and your palms facing your body.

B Raise the left hand in an arc away from the body until it goes just above shoulder level. Don't jerk the weight at the start of the movement. Keep your left elbow pointed outward, keeping the cable close to your body. Hold for a second, then slowly return to the starting position. Finish the set, then turn around and switch arms.

MAKE IT EASIER

- Use tubing or stretch bands and perform the exercise as described (see Tubing Side Deltoid Raise on page 142).
- Use dumbbells.
- Do the exercise while seated, with good back support.

DO IT HARDER

- Change to thicker handles with a 2-inch diameter to make it harder to grip. Or use thick-handled dumbbells, or wrap towels around the dumbbells.
- Train both sides simultaneously by standing in the middle of two pulleys. The cables will cross in front of you diagonally.
- Press the weight up, but lower it as a negative raise.

A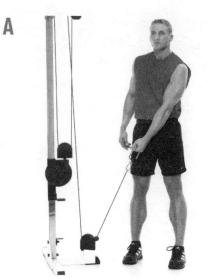

B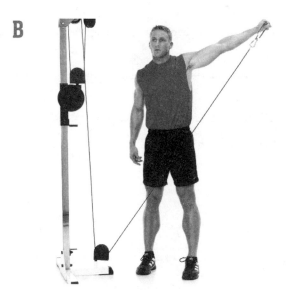

DUMBBELL SIDE DELTOID RAISE

This very effective exercise works the deltoid (shoulder) muscles.

A Stand straight, with your feet shoulder width apart and your knees slightly bent. Hold a dumbbell in each hand, with your arms hanging at your sides. Your palms should face your upper thighs. Lean forward slightly at the waist, keeping your shoulders back and your back straight.

B With your elbows slightly bent, raise your arms up and out to the sides until they reach slightly above shoulder level. Your palms should be facing the floor. Hold for a second, then slowly return to the starting position.

MAKE IT EASIER

- Use tubing or stretch bands and perform the exercise as described (see Tubing Side Deltoid Raise on page 142).
- Do the exercise while seated, with good back support.

DO IT HARDER

- Use thick-handled dumbbells or wrap a towel around the dumbbells to make them harder to grasp.
- Press the weight up, but lower it as a negative raise.

A

B

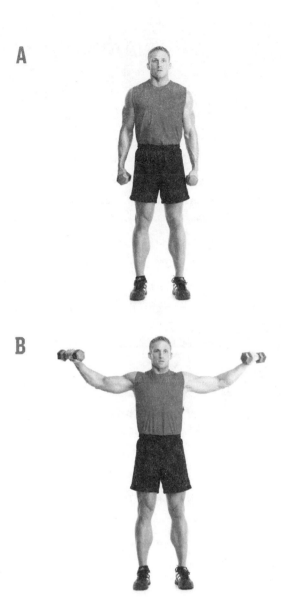

INCLINE SIDE DELTOID RAISE

The incline position of this exercise isolates the deltoid (shoulder) muscles, which makes the movement more rigorous. Because it's done on a bench, the lower back is supported, reducing the risk of injury.

A Sit facing an incline bench, with your chest leaning against the incline. Your legs should be shoulder width apart, your feet on the floor, and your chin just above the top of the bench. Hook tubing under the bench and hold one end in each hand, with your arms dangling below the bench. Keep your elbows slightly bent, and your palms facing each other.

B Keeping your elbows relaxed, raise your arms to the sides until they are slightly higher than the shoulders. Hold for a second, then slowly lower to the starting position.

MAKE IT EASIER

- Perform this exercise with dumbbells.
- Change the incline of the bench to target different areas of the deltoid.

DO IT HARDER

- Raise the arms in an alternating fashion. Raise one arm and hold at the top position, then raise the other arm and hold while lowering the first arm.
- Press the handles up, then lower them as a negative raise.

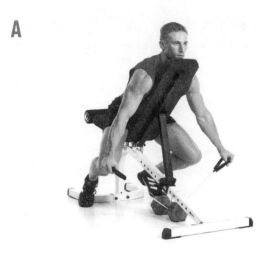

A

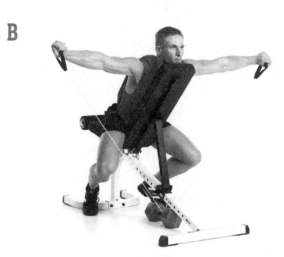

B

TUBING SIDE DELTOID RAISE

This very effective exercise works the side deltoid (shoulder) muscles.

A Stand straight, with your feet shoulder width apart and your knees slightly bent. Hold a tubing or stretch band handle in one hand, with your arm hanging at your sides. Your palm should face your upper thighs. Lean forward slightly at the waist, keeping your shoulders back and your back straight.

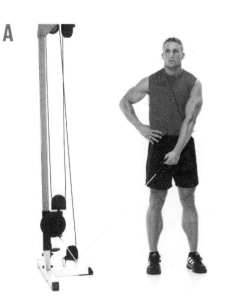

A

B With your elbow slightly bent, raise your arm up and out to the side until it's slightly above shoulder level. Your palm should be facing the floor. Hold for a second, then slowly return to the starting position. Finish the set, then repeat on the other side.

MAKE IT EASIER

- Stand closer to the base of the tubing for less tension.
- Do the exercise while seated, with good back support.

DO IT HARDER

- Face away from the tubing to put more stress at the start of the movement.
- Press the weight up, but lower it as a negative raise.

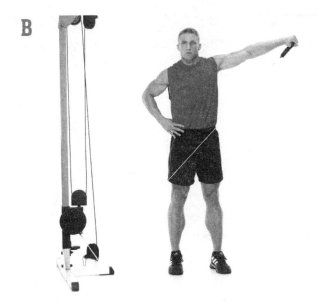

HOW TO HOIST BEFORE YOU LIFT

Dumbbells are one of the best workout tools ever devised, but they have a major drawback. If you've gotten to the point where you're lifting major weight, just getting them into position can be a challenge.

If you're lucky enough to own a private gym, definitely invest in a special cradle that allows you to unrack dumbbells that are already in the proper position. Failing that, you have a couple of options:

- Have a workout partner hand you one or both dumbbells when you're in the start-up position.

- Take advantage of momentum and swing them into the start-up position.

- When doing seated exercises, rest the dumbbells on your knees, then pop them into position, one at a time, by raising your knees.

- If you're already pretty strong, you can probably clean them into position. Don't try this unless you're in good shape and already know how to do a dumbbell clean. Resorting to a deadlift and arching your back isn't a clean—and it can hurt you in ways you won't soon forget.

Cleaning a weight, incidentally, is the move used to initiate the first half of the clean and jerk. You set up as though you're preparing to do a deadlift. Get a good grip on the weight, then rise up and pull the weight up along the body into position.

BARBELL UPRIGHT ROW

This exercise works the side deltoid (shoulder) and trapezius (upper back and neck) muscles, as well as the chest and forearm muscles.

A Hold a barbell in both hands, with your palms shoulder width apart. Your arms should be fully extended in front of you, with the barbell at your upper thighs. Allow your shoulders to relax slightly, but keep your back straight.

B Pull the barbell straight up and tuck it under your chin. Your elbows should be pointing up and out. Hold briefly, then slowly lower the weight.

MAKE IT EASIER

- Stand on tubing or stretch bands and perform the exercise as described above.
- Use an EZ bar to reduce stress on your wrists.
- If you have an injury, shorten the range of motion and train the shoulder at specific angles where there is no pain.

DO IT HARDER

- Pause at three different positions on the way down. Hold each position for a count of 3.
- Use your legs to get the weight into the top position, and then slowly lower the bar.
- Use a staggered, or asymmetrical, grip to place more stress on one side of the body. Alternate hand positions in each set so that the total stress on each side is the same.

A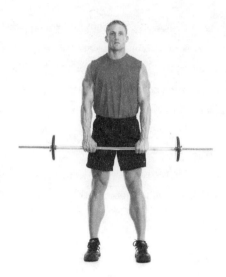

B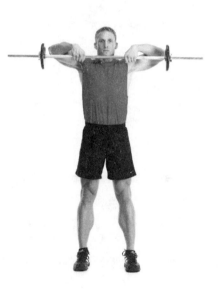

CABLE UPRIGHT ROW

This exercise works the shoulders as well as the chest, biceps, and forearms.

A Stand in front of a low pulley with a T-handle on the cable. Keep your back straight, your feet shoulder width apart, and your knees slightly bent. Grip the handle overhand, with your hands 4 to 6 inches apart. Extend your arms so that the bar touches your upper thighs. Allow your shoulders to relax slightly, but don't slouch.

B Pull the bar straight up and tuck it under your chin. Your elbows should point up and out. Hold briefly, then lower the weight to the starting position.

MAKE IT EASIER

- Stand on tubing or stretch bands and perform the exercise as described above.
- Use an EZ bar to reduce stress on your wrists.

DO IT HARDER

- Pause at three different positions on the way down. Hold each position for a count of 3.
- Use your legs to get the weight into the top position, then slowly lower the bar.
- Use a staggered, or asymmetrical, grip to place more stress on one side of the body. Alternate hand positions each set so that the total stress on each side is the same.

A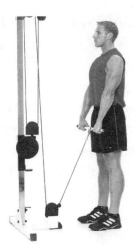

B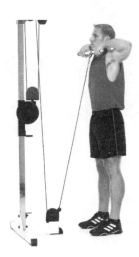

DUMBBELL UPRIGHT ROW

Performing this exercise with dumbbells instead of a barbell increases the level of difficulty. This movement will strengthen your shoulders, chest, biceps, and forearms.

A Stand with your feet shoulder width apart, and your knees slightly bent. Hold a dumbbell in each hand, with your arms extended so that the dumbbells touch your upper thighs. Allow your shoulders to relax slightly, but don't slouch.

B Pull the dumbbells straight up toward your shoulders. Your elbows should point up and out. Hold briefly, then lower the weights to the starting position.

MAKE IT EASIER

- Stand on tubing or stretch bands and perform the exercise as described above.
- If you have an injury, shorten the range of motion and train the shoulder at specific angles where there is no pain.

DO IT HARDER

- Pause at three different positions on the way down. Hold each position for a count of 3.
- Use your legs to get the weight into the top position, then slowly lower.
- Alternate dumbbells by lifting and holding first one and then the other. Hold one dumbbell at the top until the other reaches the top position.

A

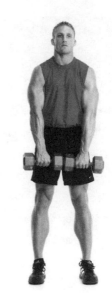

B

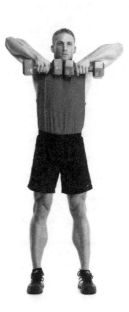

POSTERIOR (BACK) SHOULDER EXERCISES

SEATED DUMBBELL BENT LATERALS

This exercise works the deltoid (shoulder) muscles. Specifically, it works the middle and posterior deltoids (shoulder), the trapezius (upper back and neck), rhomboid (upper back), teres minor (outside of shoulder blade), and infraspinatus (shoulder blade) muscles. During the movement, keep the arms moving backward in the same plane. Don't let the dumbbells break the plane and drift toward your hips.

A Sit at the end of a weight bench, with a dumbbell in each hand. Lean forward from your waist and bring the dumbbells together behind your calves. Your palms should face each other.

B Keeping your body still, raise the weights out to your sides, turning your wrists so that the rear of each dumbbell is higher than the front. Don't swing your body; let your shoulders lift the weight. With your arms just slightly bent, raise the dumbbells a bit lower than your head. Hold for a second, then slowly return to the starting position.

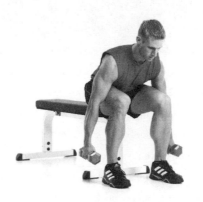

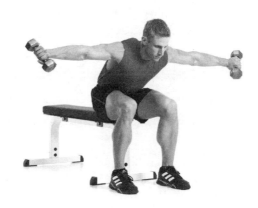

MAKE IT EASIER

- Hook tubing or stretch bands under your feet and perform the exercise as described above.
- Keep the dumbbells parallel throughout the range of motion.
- If you have an injury, shorten the range of motion and train the shoulder at specific angles where there is no pain.

DO IT HARDER

- Pause at three different positions on the way down. Hold each position for a count of 3.
- Change the angle of your torso so that you can stress different muscle fibers.
- Alternate dumbbells by lifting and holding first one and then the other. Hold one dumbbell at the top until the other dumbbell reaches the top position.

STANDING CABLE BENT-OVER LATERAL RAISE

This exercise looks similar to the standing dumbbell bent-over lateral raise, but it uses cables instead. Specifically, this movement works the middle and posterior deltoids (shoulder), the trapezius (upper back and neck), rhomboid (upper back), teres minor (outside of shoulder blade), and infraspinatus (shoulder blade) muscles.

A Stand between two low pulleys, with your feet shoulder width apart and your knees slightly bent. With both hands, reach across your body to grip the pulley handles. Allow your arms to hang down, with your elbows slightly bent and your forearms crossed. Bend forward at the waist, keeping your back slightly arched, until your upper body is parallel with the floor.

B Raise your arms outward and upward as high as you can. Hold for a second, then slowly lower to the starting position.

MAKE IT EASIER

- Stand on tubing or stretch bands and perform the exercise (see Standing Bent-Over Lateral Raise with Tubing on opposite page).
- Keep the torso parallel throughout the range of motion.

DO IT HARDER

- Pause at three different positions on the way down. Hold each position for a count of 3.
- Change the angle of your torso so that you stress different muscle fibers.
- Alternate handles by lifting and holding first one and then the other. Hold one handle at the top until the other handle reaches the top position.

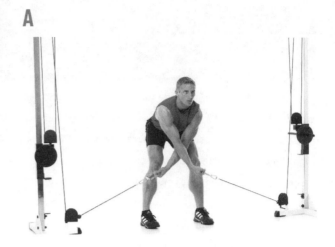

A

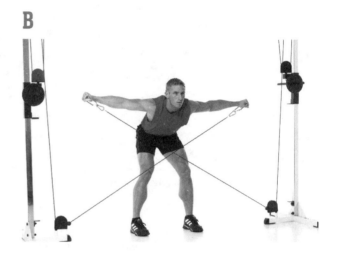

B

STANDING BENT-OVER LATERAL RAISE WITH TUBING

This exercise emphasizes the back deltoid (shoulder) muscles. Specifically, it works the middle and posterior deltoids (shoulder), the trapezius (upper back and neck), rhomboid (upper back), teres minor (outside of shoulder blade), and infraspinatus (shoulder blade) muscles.

A Bend over at the waist with a handle in each hand, with your arms in front of you and your elbows slightly bent. Your palms should face each other. Place your feet a little more than shoulder width apart, keeping your back straight and roughly parallel to the floor.

B Raise your arms until they're parallel to the floor, keeping your back straight. Hold for a second, then slowly return to the starting position.

A

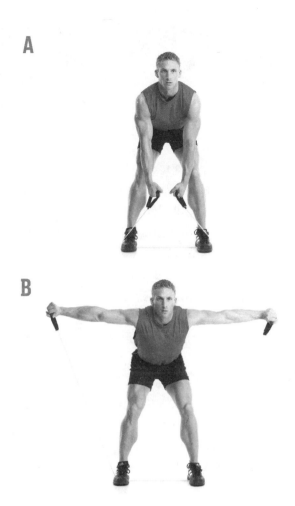

B

MAKE IT EASIER

- Use dumbbells instead of tubing.
- If you have an injury, shorten the range of motion and train the shoulder at specific angles where there is no pain.

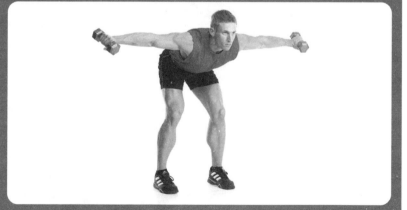

DO IT HARDER

- Change the angle of your torso so that you stress different muscle fibers.
- Alternate handles by lifting and holding first one and then the other. Hold one handle at the top until the other reaches the top position.

TRAPS EXPLAINED

The trapezius is a large muscle on both sides of the spine between the shoulder joint and the neck. The trapezius is, in effect, one large, diamond-shaped muscle. It attaches at the top of the neck, spreads to the shoulder attachment along the clavicle bone, travels all the way down to the middle of the back, and ties in the shoulders and lats.

The traps are actually larger than the abdominals. If more men understood this, they might put a lot more work into trap training, though in all honesty, there isn't a lot you can do. Only a few exercises directly target the traps. The muscle isn't one that "pops," which probably explains why it tends to get neglected in most workouts.

Because the trapezius supports many different muscle groups, and because you need it for moving furniture and other lifting activities, it's worth giving it more attention.

The traps are divided into upper, middle, and lower muscle fibers.

- The upper fibers move the scapula up, move the spine back, and allow the neck to move away from the chest. They also allow the head to move sideways toward the shoulders and to pivot to both sides.

- The middle fibers allow the scapula to move back toward the spine as well as upward and to the sides.

- The lower fibers move the scapula laterally and upward, as well as down. They also control spinal extension, in which the spine shifts backward.

THE TOTAL TRAP WORKOUT

There are only a handful of exercises that directly target the traps. As always, good technique is critical to making them as strong as possible.

Shrug off bad habits. The best exercises for training the trapezius are shrugs. When performing shrugs of any type, don't stick your head forward and downward. Most guys get into the bad habit of leaning their head forward when they shrug. This can set you up for injury—and it also prevents the traps from achieving optimal development.

When doing shrugs, keep your head neutral—look straight ahead into a mirror. Check to be sure that your head and neck are in alignment with the rest of your spine.

Train the traps second. For most men, the ideal workout order is to train the shoulders first, followed by the traps. If you are one of those rare men who already have awesome shoulder development, but you have relatively weak-looking traps, you can reverse the order and train the traps first.

Use wrist straps. The traps are strong muscles that can handle quite a bit of work. If you are doing dumbbell or barbell shrugs and your grip gives out before the traps do, you'll seriously short-change your workout. Get in the habit of using wrist straps. They'll help you train past the point when your grip gives out.

Train heavy. The traps need heavy weights to develop any kind of size. A lot of men can easily shrug 400 to 500 pounds. You won't be starting at that point, of course, but plan on moving serious weight. It's the only way to stimulate new muscle growth.

TRAPEZIUS EXERCISES
BARBELL SHRUG

This movement works the deltoid and trapezius muscles. More specifically, it strengthens your trapezius (shoulder), levator scapulae (beneath the trapezius), and rhomboid (upper back) muscles. This is an exercise where you can really pile on the weight for maximum gains.

A Stand with your back straight, your feet shoulder width apart, and your knees slightly bent. Hold a barbell with an overhand grip with your hands shoulder width or slightly farther apart. The barbell should rest against the front of your upper thighs.

B Shrug your shoulders straight up toward your ears, keeping your arms straight and your head still. Pause when your shoulders are as high as they can go. Then slowly return to the starting position.

MAKE IT EASIER

- Stand on tubing or stretch bands and perform the exercise as described above.
- Use an EZ bar.
- If you have an injury, shorten the range of motion and train the shoulder at specific angles where there is no pain.

DO IT HARDER

- Pause at three different positions on the way down. Hold each position for a count of 3.
- Change the angle of your torso so that you can stress different muscle fibers.

A

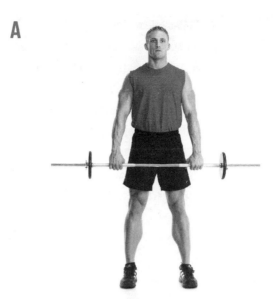

B

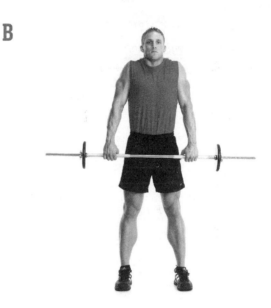

CABLE SHRUG

The cable creates continuous resistance so that you can maintain tension on your trapezius (shoulder) muscles.

A Stand straight, with your feet shoulder width apart and your knees slightly bent. Grip a bar that is attached to a low cable pulley. Using an overhand grip, hold it at arm's length in front of you.

B Shrug your shoulders as high as possible; try to touch your ears with your shoulders. Hold for a second, then slowly return to the starting position.

MAKE IT EASIER

- Stand on tubing or stretch bands and perform the exercise as described above.
- Use an EZ bar.
- If you have an injury, shorten the range of motion and train the shoulder at specific angles where there is no pain.

DO IT HARDER

- Pause at three different positions on the way down. Hold each position for a count of 3.
- Change the angle of your torso so that you stress different muscle fibers. Use two separate handles and alternate sides by lifting and holding first one and then the other. Hold one handle at the top until the other handle reaches the top position.

A

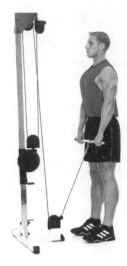

B

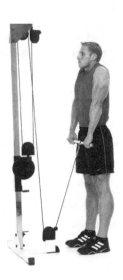

DUMBBELL SHRUG

Dumbbells provide more variety in hand positioning. This exercise strengthens your trapezius (shoulder), levator scapulae (beneath the trapezius), and rhomboid (upper back) muscles.

A Stand straight, with your feet shoulder width apart and your knees slightly bent. Hold a dumbbell in each hand, letting your arms hang alongside your body. Your palms should face your body. Make sure your shoulders are back and relaxed.

B Shrug your shoulders as high as they'll go, keeping your head still and your chin slightly tucked. Hold for a second, then slowly return to the starting position.

MAKE IT EASIER

- Stand on tubing or stretch bands and perform the exercise as described above.
- Keep the dumbbells touching throughout the range of motion.
- If you have an injury, shorten the range of motion and train the shoulder at specific angles where there is no pain.

DO IT HARDER

- Pause at three different positions on the way down. Hold each position for a count of 3.
- Use your legs to get the weight into the top position, then slowly lower the dumbbells.
- Alternate dumbbells by lifting and holding first one and then the other. Hold one dumbbell at the top until the other dumbbell reaches the top position.

A

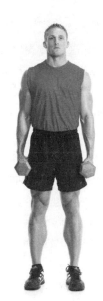

B

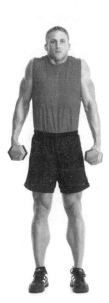

NECK EXERCISES
CABLE NECK FLEXION

This movement involves the use of a head-strap attachment or rope handle. It works all the muscles of the neck that bring the chin toward the chest (neck flexors).

A Sit on a weight bench facing away from the pulley on the weight stack. Place your neck in the harness cable attachment. Hold on to the bench for support.

B Move your head away from the pulley by bending your neck forward until your chin touches the upper chest. Return your head to the initial position by hyperextending the neck.

MAKE IT EASIER

- Use tubing or stretch bands. Loop tubing securely around head so that it does not slide off and hold other end of tubing in hands behind back. Adjust tension by pulling down more or less on tubing.
- If you have any neck pain, shorten the range of motion. Train the neck at specific angles where there is no pain.

DO IT HARDER

- Pause at three different positions on the way back. Hold each position for a count of 3.
- Use your hands to assist the movement, then lower the weight slowly.

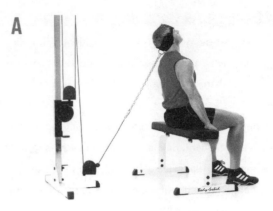

A

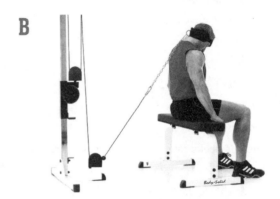

B

WEIGHTED NECK FLEXION

This movement involves the use of a weight plate. It works the muscles of the neck that bring the chin toward the chest (neck flexors).

A Place a folded towel on a weight plate. Place the weight and towel on your forehead. Support and balance the weight with both hands throughout the movement.

B Move your head up by flexing the neck until your chin touches the upper chest. Return by hyperextending the neck, and repeat.

MAKE IT EASIER

- Use tubing or stretch bands. Loop tubing securely around head and hold other end of tubing in hands behind back. Adjust tension by pulling down more or less on tubing.
- If you have any neck pain, shorten the range of motion.

DO IT HARDER

- Pause at three different positions on the way back. Hold each position for a count of 3.
- Use your hands to assist the movement, and lower the weight slowly.

A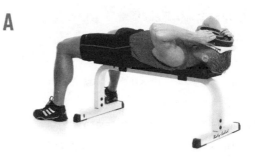

B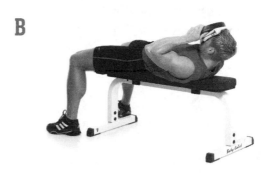

NO KIDDING?

CAN YOU TRAIN THE ROTATOR CUFF?

The shoulder joint is supported by the rotator cuff, a series of four muscles that both rotate the shoulder and support (cuff) the joint. When you throw a baseball, the movement essentially throws your arm away from your body. The ball flies away because you release your grip. The only reason that your arm and shoulder don't follow after it is because the rotator cuff holds your upper arm bone in place.

The ironic thing is that the structure designed in part to protect the shoulder is itself so prone to injury. Keeping the rotator cuff strong can save you a lot of grief. But because the small, internal muscles that make up the rotator cuff are out of sight, a lot of men never give them a second thought. Until the day when their shoulder gives out while they're lifting something heavy.

Strengthening the rotator cuff muscles is straightforward. Moves that rotate the joint through its full range of motion, which are usually done with light weights while lying on your side, are all that's needed to keep the rotator cuff— and, by extension, the shoulder—strong.

WEIGHTED NECK LATERAL FLEXION

This movement involves the use of a dumbbell It works all the muscles of the neck that bring the ear toward the shoulder (lateral neck flexors).

A Place a folded towel on a dumbbell. Lie on a mat on your side, with your knees and hips bent. Position the weight and towel on the side of your upper head. Hold the weight against the side of your head. Place the hand on your lower arm on the floor for support.

B Move your head up and to the side by laterally flexing the neck. Lower your head to the opposite side, and repeat. Finish a set, then switch sides.

MAKE IT EASIER

- Use tubing or stretch bands. Loop tubing securely around head and hold other end of tubing in right hand in order to provide resistance as you flex the neck to the left. Adjust tension by pulling down more or less on tubing. Complete all reps then switch sides.
- If you have any neck pain, shorten the range of motion.

DO IT HARDER

- Pause at three different positions on the way back. Hold each position for a count of 3.
- Use your hands to assist you, then lower the weight slowly.

CABLE NECK EXTENSION

This movement involves the use of a head-strap attachment or rope handle. It works all the muscles of the neck that bring the head back, or the chin away from the chest (neck extensors).

A Sit on a bench facing a pulley. Place your neck in the harness cable attachmentand grip the edge of the bench with both hands.

B Move your head away from the pulley by hyperextending your neck. Return by bending the neck forward until your chin touches your upper chest.

A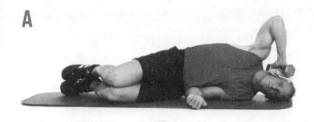

B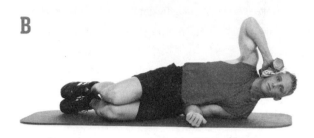

A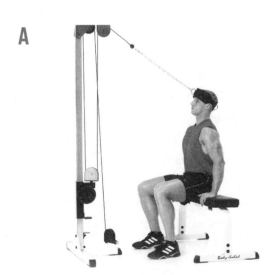

MAKE IT EASIER

- Use tubing or stretch bands. Loop tubing securely around head and hold other end of tubing in hands in front of chest. Adjust tension by pulling down more or less on tubing.
- If you have any neck pain, shorten the range of motion until it's more comfortable.

DO IT HARDER

- Pause at three different positions on the way back. Hold each position for a count of 3.
- Use your hands to assist you and then lower the weight slowly.

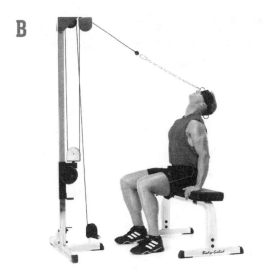

THE SECRETS TO PRESSING HUGE WEIGHTS

Years ago, the measure of a man among the Olympians was his ability to clean a weight and then press it overhead. More than a few of these behemoths pressed 500 pounds or more. Today, you'd be hard-pressed to find one guy in any gym who can press even 225 pounds.

Don't be fooled by appearances. Pressing huge weights is easy if you know a few key points.

Strengthen your legs. Pencil legs can't help you lift big weight. You need strong legs that can stabilize your body. When lifting, push your feet into the floor so that you "drive" through the legs.

Take a deep breath and hold it. You need maximum stability to move maximum weights. By holding a deep breath, you stabilize internal pressures, which allows you to exert more force. Warning: Don't use this technique if you've been diagnosed with high blood pressure.

Develop your lats. Well-developed back muscles help stabilize the scapula and provide support for you to press weights overhead.

Squeeze your shoulder blades together. Hold them in the squeezed position before unracking the weight. This draws your shoulders downward and reduces the distance the bar has to travel.

Keep your elbows under the bar. This allows you to transfer more force to lifting. If the elbows flare out to the sides, more force goes into working the chest, as opposed to lifting the bar.

Push the bar in a straight line. It shortens the distance it has to travel. Tilt your head back as the bar passes your face. Then bring the head back under the bar to complete the lockout.

Tilt the pelvis. Instead of arching your back, tilt your pelvis so that more stress is placed on your lower abdomen. This allows you to lean back without increasing torque in your lower back.

WEIGHTED NECK EXTENSION

This movement involves the use of a weight plate. It works all the muscles of the neck that bring the chin toward the chest (neck flexors).

A Place a folded towel on a weight plate, and lie facedown across a bench. Place the weight and towel on the back of your head. Support and balance the weight with both hands.

B Move your head up by hyperextending the neck. Return by bending the neck down until your chin touches the upper chest.

MAKE IT EASIER

- Use tubing or stretch bands. Loop tubing securely around head and hold other end of tubing in hands in front of chest. Adjust tension by pulling down more or less on tubing
- If you have any neck pain, shorten the range of motion.

DO IT HARDER

- Pause at three different positions on the way back. Hold each position for a count of 3.
- Use your hands to assist you, and lower the weight slowly.

A

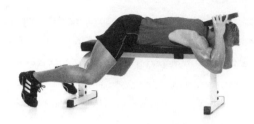

B

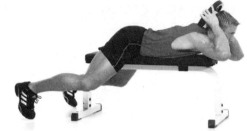

LEVEL 1 (FOCUS ON SIZE)

We've provided three different workouts for Level 1. One option is to do Workout #1 on Monday, Workout #2 on Wednesday, and Workout #3 on Friday. If you do this, do 2 warmup sets for the first exercise, followed by 3 sets of 6 repetitions using "real" weight. Do 3 sets of 10 reps for the second and third exercise, followed by 3 sets of 14 reps for the fourth exercise. Do only 1 set of the last exercise, for maximum reps.

Another option is to do just one of the workouts, three times a week. Vary the rep count daily. On Monday, for example, do 3 sets of 6 reps for the first four exercises; on Wednesday, do 3 sets of 10 reps for the first four; and on Friday, do 3 sets of 14 reps. Always start with 2 warmup sets for the first exercise (these don't go toward the final "count"). Do only 1 set of the last exercise, going for maximum reps. Pick a weight that will allow you to get 15 to 20 reps.

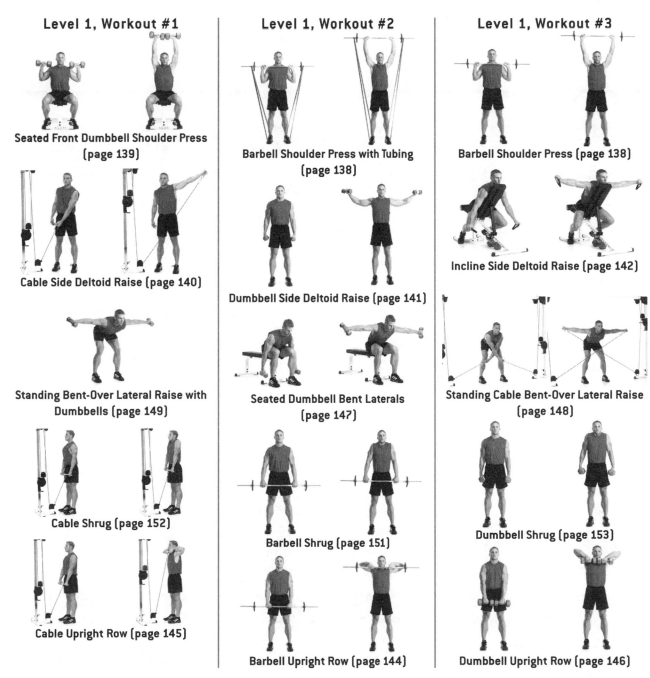

Level 1, Workout #1

Seated Front Dumbbell Shoulder Press (page 139)

Cable Side Deltoid Raise (page 140)

Standing Bent-Over Lateral Raise with Dumbbells (page 149)

Cable Shrug (page 152)

Cable Upright Row (page 145)

Level 1, Workout #2

Barbell Shoulder Press with Tubing (page 138)

Dumbbell Side Deltoid Raise (page 141)

Seated Dumbbell Bent Laterals (page 147)

Barbell Shrug (page 151)

Barbell Upright Row (page 144)

Level 1, Workout #3

Barbell Shoulder Press (page 138)

Incline Side Deltoid Raise (page 142)

Standing Cable Bent-Over Lateral Raise (page 148)

Dumbbell Shrug (page 153)

Dumbbell Upright Row (page 146)

LEVEL 2 (FOCUS ON STRENGTH)

Do one of the complete exercise programs as outlined below. Allow at least 1 day of rest between workouts.

Level 2, Workout #1

It's possible to increase your pressing strength by more than 20 percent in 9 weeks by following this routine. You only have to do it twice a week—a "light" day and a "heavy" day. First, determine your 1 repetition maximum (1RM) for the barbell shoulder press. (See page 14.) You can use the chart below to determine your barbell shoulder press weight, sets, and reps for a given workout. Round the weights to the nearest 5 pounds.

To stay limber (and safe), start each workout with two 5-rep warmup sets, using 50 percent and 70 percent of your 1RM. After you've done all sets and reps of your barbell shoulder press, complete the workouts with the additional exercises. Perform all sets for one exercise before moving to the next exercise. Take 1 to 2 minutes' rest between each set or exercise.

Level 2, Workout 1, Barbell Shoulder Press Cycle

WEEK	DAY	% 1RM	#SETS	#REPS
1	1	80	6	2
1	2	80	6	3
2	1	80	6	2
2	2	80	6	4
3	1	80	6	2
3	2	80	6	5
4	1	80	6	2
4	2	80	6	6
5	1	80	6	2
5	2	85	5	5
6	1	80	6	2
6	2	90	4	4
7	1	80	6	2
7	2	95	3	3
8	1	80	6	2
8	2	100	2	2
9	1	80	6	2
9	2	105	2	1 *

*AFTER THE 2 SETS AT TOP WEIGHT, KEEP DOING SINGLES, WITH 2 MINUTES' REST BETWEEN SETS. INCREASE THE WEIGHT 5 TO 10 POUNDS EACH TIME UNTIL YOU FIND YOUR NEW 1RM.

ADDITIONAL EXERCISES FOR WORKOUT #1

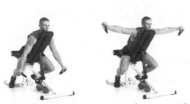

Barbell Shoulder Press (page 138)

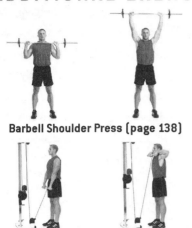

Cable Upright Row (page 145)

On both days, do 1 set to failure
for 10 to 15 reps.

Incline Side Deltoid Raise (page 142)

Same as exercise below.

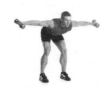

**Standing Bent-Over Lateral Raise with
Dumbbells (page 149)**

On Day 1, do 2 to 3 sets, 8 to 10 reps
each; on Day 2, do the same number
of sets, but only 4 to 6 reps.

Level 2, Workout #2

Do this workout three times a week. Perform 2 warmup sets for each exercise. Vary the rep count on successive days. For example, do 1 set of 3 reps on Monday, 1 set of 11 reps on Wednesday, and 1 set of 7 reps on Friday.

Each week, add 1 set to each exercise until you're up to 5 sets.

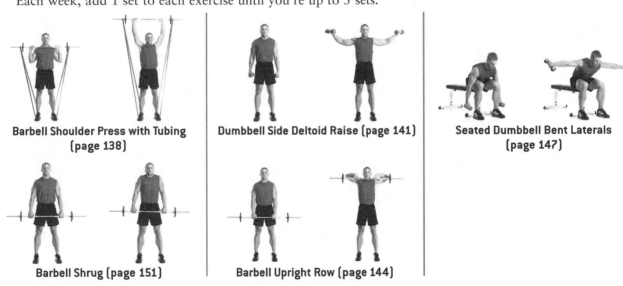

**Barbell Shoulder Press with Tubing
(page 138)**

Barbell Shrug (page 151)

Dumbbell Side Deltoid Raise (page 141)

Barbell Upright Row (page 144)

**Seated Dumbbell Bent Laterals
(page 147)**

Level 2, Workout #3

Do this workout three times a week. Perform 2 warmup sets for each exercise.

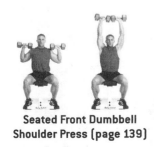

**Seated Front Dumbbell
Shoulder Press (page 139)**

Do 2 to 3 sets of 3 reps.

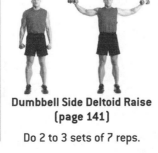

**Dumbbell Side Deltoid Raise
(page 141)**

Do 2 to 3 sets of 7 reps.

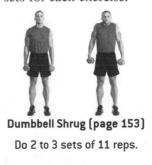

Dumbbell Shrug (page 153)

Do 2 to 3 sets of 11 reps.

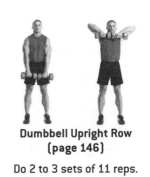

**Dumbbell Upright Row
(page 146)**

Do 2 to 3 sets of 11 reps.

LEVEL 3 (HYBRID TRAINING— SIZE AND STRENGTH)

We've provided three different workouts for Level 3. One option is to do all three workouts weekly. For example, do Workout #1 on Monday, Workout #2 on Wednesday, and Workout #3 on Friday. If you choose this option, do 2 warmup sets for the first exercise, lifting lighter-than-usual weights. Follow the warmup with 5 sets of 2 reps for the first exercise.

Next, do 2 sets of 6 reps for the second exercise, followed by 2 sets of 12 reps for the rest.

Another option is to do just one of the workouts, three times a week. Vary the rep count daily. On Monday, for example, do 3 sets of 2 reps for the first three exercises; on Wednesday, do 3 sets of 6 reps for the first three exercises; and on Friday, do 3 sets of 12 reps for the first three exercises.

Level 3, Workout #1

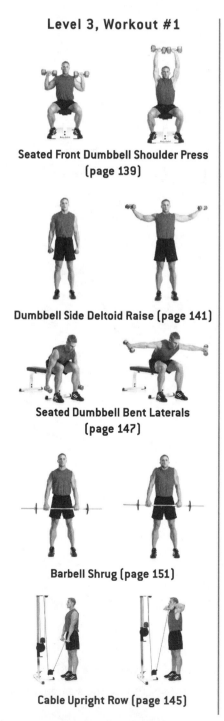

Seated Front Dumbbell Shoulder Press (page 139)

Dumbbell Side Deltoid Raise (page 141)

Seated Dumbbell Bent Laterals (page 147)

Barbell Shrug (page 151)

Cable Upright Row (page 145)

Level 3, Workout #2

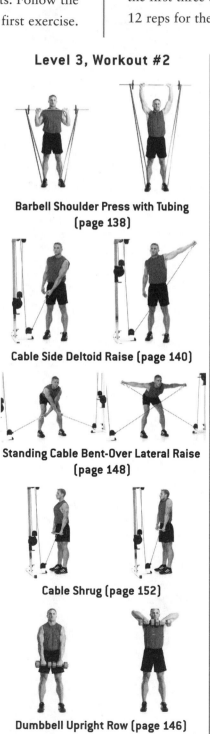

Barbell Shoulder Press with Tubing (page 138)

Cable Side Deltoid Raise (page 140)

Standing Cable Bent-Over Lateral Raise (page 148)

Cable Shrug (page 152)

Dumbbell Upright Row (page 146)

Level 3, Workout #3

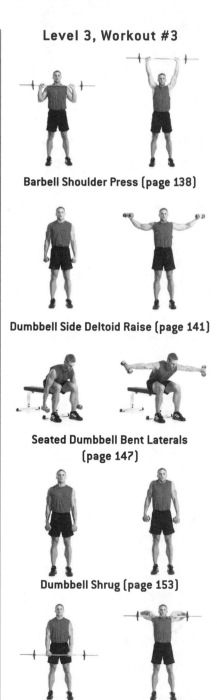

Barbell Shoulder Press (page 138)

Dumbbell Side Deltoid Raise (page 141)

Seated Dumbbell Bent Laterals (page 147)

Dumbbell Shrug (page 153)

Barbell Upright Row (page 144)

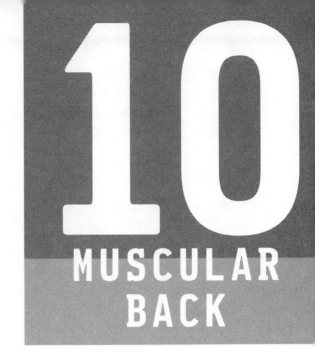

You'll never look really strong unless you commit to working the back. A "good" back has two qualities that can make a huge impact on your appearance: thickness and a V-taper shape. The thickness brings your shoulders back and gives more emphasis to a well-defined chest. The V-taper creates an optical illusion that makes the waist appear smaller and the shoulders larger.

If appearance alone isn't enough to get you motivated, here's another good reason to get more serious about your back workouts. About 80 percent of

men experience some degree of back pain at some point. Yet the majority of men can essentially eliminate chronic pain and vastly reduce the risk of injury just by keeping the back strong.

BACK EXPLAINED

Because the muscles of the back are involved in so many movements, you can work them to some degree just by keeping up with your usual routines. A lot of shoulder exercises, for example, give the upper back a solid workout. Deadlifts are often considered a hip exercise, but they exert a lot of tension on the lower back, as well.

You'll obviously want to design a dedicated back workout—though if you're really serious about getting stronger, you'll actually need a *series* of workouts. There are so many muscles in the back—including large muscles, such as the trapezius and

latissimus, and smaller muscles, such as the rhomboids—that it's impossible to hit them all in a meaningful way in a single workout.

When you're putting together a back program, keep in mind that you're hitting three distinct areas: the upper, middle, and lower back. You have to work all three areas to build strength, improve posture, and get the kind of shape you're looking for.

The Upper Back

This area includes the trapezius, teres major, and the rhomboids.

- The trapezius is a long, trapezoid-shaped muscle that runs down the upper section of the spinal cord. It starts at the base of the skull and attaches at the middle-to-lower back. The individual muscle fibers pull in three directions: up, down, and toward the centerline of the body.

The functions of the traps include scapular elevation (shrugging up), scapular adduction (drawing the shoulder blades together), and scapular depression (pulling the shoulder blades down).

- The teres major muscle originates on the outer (lateral) edge of the scapula and attaches to the upper arm. It works with the rotator cuff muscles to stabilize the shoulder joint, and with the latissimus dorsi to pull the arm back.

- The rhomboids (major and minor) originate on the spine and attach to the middle part of the scapula, or shoulder blades. The rhomboids bring the scapula in toward the spine, essentially squeezing the shoulder blades together.

The Middle Back

This area comprises one main muscle: the latissimus dorsi, or "lats." It originates on the spine and on top of the pelvic girdle, and connects to the upper arm bone. It's the largest back muscle, one that spreads out like a fan and provides force in an enormous range of body positions. The main job of the lats is to bring the upper arm bone (the humerus) down and behind the body. When your arm is fixed, such as during a pullup, the lats pull the entire weight of your body toward the arm.

The lats also stabilizes the torso during a variety of movements, including the barbell bench press. Since the lats has muscle fibers running at different angles, you'll want to do a variety of exercises that hit the muscles from different directions.

Men who want to develop back width, or "wings," utilize a variety of pullups and pulldowns, using different grip widths. The best exercises for working the lats involve bringing the arm toward the back of the body, such as barbell rows, one-arm dumbbell rows, T-bar rows, pulldowns, and cable rows.

The Lower Back

The erector spinae is a group of muscles that support the spinal column. They include the longissimus, the spinalis, and iliocostalis. The muscles of the erector spinae attach to the vertebrae, the ribs, and the pelvis. Basically, all these muscles do is support the spine and allow it to extend. Exercises that work this area include hyperextensions, deadlifts, and good mornings.

THE TOTAL BACK WORKOUT

You should do more exercises for your back than for any other muscle group. Remember, the back consists of three distinct areas. During a workout, choose exercises that hit the upper, middle, and lower back. Plan on doing at least the same number of exercises and sets for these combined areas that you'd do for the shoulders, chest, and abdominals.

Allow for downtime. The back muscles are one of the biggest muscle groups in your body. When trained really hard, they may require longer recovery periods between sets, exercises, and workouts. Some exercises, such as deadlifts, are often done only once a week by beginning and intermediate lifters, and only once every 10 to 14 days by more advanced lifters.

The harder you train, the more recovery time you will need between workouts. A general rule of thumb is to wait for at least 48 hours between each back workout.

Vary your pulldowns. This exercise is the keystone of any back workout. Don't get stuck in a rut: You want to be hitting muscles throughout the back, and especially the lats, from different angles with every training cycle. For example, vary handle attachments. Change your hand spacing. Use different pull angles. This approach will constantly challenge the different lat muscle fibers and lead to explosive gains in size and strength.

Here's how it might work. During one training cycle, use a wide-grip pulldown to the front, and maybe a close-grip cable row with a neutral handle. During the next training cycle, use a close-grip pulldown to the front, along with a wide-grip barbell row.

Do the same thing when gripping barbells. Change your grip regularly. If you perform barbell rows with a narrow, underhand grip during one training cycle, switch to a wide, overhand grip the next cycle.

Lift heavy early. If your goal is maximal strength, perform heavy lifting exercises, such as deadlifts, early in the workout. Your energy will be high and you can move heavier weights. Push yourself to the limit while you're still strong. On the other hand, if your goal is to boost size, start workouts with exercises that really push your weakest or smallest areas.

Dump the weight belt. Men love wearing these things, even though they don't make a whit of difference for most lifters, and can actually slow progress. The only time to wear a weight belt is when you're moving your absolute top weights in the strength phases of training. You don't need it the rest of the time. You're better off using your muscles to stabilize the spine. That's what you're at the gym for, remember?

Watch out for rounding. You'll see a lot of guys rounding their upper backs when they're finishing up a rep during pulldowns. Don't do it. Rounding the back brings the chest and shoulders into play and reduces tension on the back. A similar thing happens when you stick your head forward. It often causes the lower back to round. Keep your head in a neutral position. You'll get a better workout, and keep your spine healthier at the same time.

Keep a set of wrist straps in your gym bag. Your grip should be strong enough to let you handle the heaviest weights with ease. But getting a good grip on old equipment is another story. The handles used in back workouts invariably get smooth over time, making them hard to hold. Bust out a pair of wrist straps. They make it easier to lift top weights without the risk of slipping.

Stretch for safety. A lot of men have excessive lumbar arches (lordosis) and tight lats. Stretch the muscles well and often—with Pilates, yoga, and static stretching. Simply hanging from a bar can make a real difference.

You should definitely give yourself time to warm up before launching into heavy back exercises. Men have torn biceps doing exercises such as deadlifts and barbell rows. A few minutes of warmup will prime your muscles and get them ready for lifting. Perform a full-body warmup, followed by a dynamic warmup, followed by an exercise-specific warmup before lifting heavy weights.

Beware of bouncing. Don't bounce weights off the floor when deadlifting or doing barbell rows. Don't bounce the plates together in a weight stack when using a cable or pulley device. And finally, don't bounce the weights when doing machine rows.

Take advantage of specialty racks. They make it easier to set the bar at the right position.

Go it alone. When doing barbell deadlifts or barbell rows, don't depend on a spotter. Do as many reps as you can with good form. Then stop.

BARBELL ROW

This is a great overall exercise. It not only works muscles in the back, but also in the shoulders, butt, and the back of the thighs. Since the bent-over position requires you to keep your stomach tight and your back flat, it provides an ab and lower-back workout as well.

A Stand with your feet shoulder width apart, and your knees slightly bent. Bend at the waist until your upper body is parallel to the floor. Keeping your back flat, grip a barbell with your hands wider than shoulder width apart. Your palms should face your body.

B Pull the bar toward you until it touches your chest. Your elbows should be higher than your back. Hold for a second, then slowly lower the barbell to about the middle of your shins, and repeat.

MAKE IT EASIER

- Lift your torso up so that your back is above parallel with the floor. Pull the bar to your abdominal region.
- Use a wider grip to make it easier to pull.
- Use an underhand grip—or use a bar with parallel handles.

DO IT HARDER

- To challenge your balance, stand on one leg. You may want to start with an empty bar because the movement is difficult to do.
- Put sturdy collars on each end of the bar to hold the weights in place. Hold the bar at arm's length, with your hands more than shoulder width apart. Pull up on only one side of the bar until it touches your chest. Hold the bar at arm's length on the other side. Lower the "rowed" side, and switch. The movement will look like a seesaw, with each side taking turns going up.
- Pause at the bottom of the movement, squeeze your scapulas together, and pull the bar to your chest. Hold for 2 to 3 seconds, then slowly lower.

A

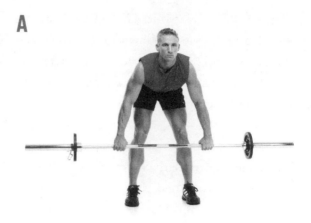

B

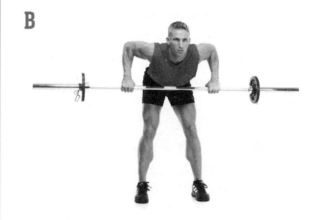

ONE-ARM CABLE ROW

This exercise isolates the latissimus dorsi (mid- and lower back) muscles, working each separately.

A Stand facing a D-handle low pulley cable. Grip the handle with one hand, your palm facing in and your arm fully extended. Lean forward, keeping your knees slightly bent and one foot forward of the other. Your back should remain straight. Brace your right hand against your right thigh.

B Pull the handle toward your side. You should feel your left lats contracting as your elbow travels past your side and moves inward toward your back. Pull until the handle lightly touches your chest. Pause, then slowly return to the starting position.

MAKE IT EASIER

- Use two hands.

DO IT HARDER

- Change the height of the pulley each set to stimulate different fibers.
- Rotate from an overhand to a neutral grip as you pull the handle toward your chest.
- Pause at the bottom of the movement, squeeze your scapulas together, and pull the handle to your chest. Hold for 2 to 3 seconds, then slowly lower.

A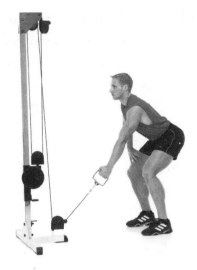

B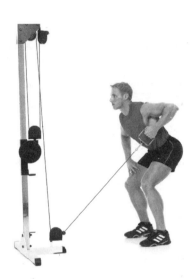

ALTERNATING GRIP CHINUP

This movement gives a superb upper back workout. The side using an underhand grip (biceps in a stronger position) has a mechanical advantage compared to the side with the overhand grip (biceps in a weaker position). It forces your upper back muscles to do more of the work.

A Grip a chinup bar with one hand, using an overhand grip. With the other hand, use an underhand grip. Your palms will face in opposite directions. Position your hands slightly wider than shoulder width apart. Hang from the bar with your legs slightly bent and your ankles crossed.

B Pull yourself up until your chin is over the bar. Hold for a second, then return to the starting position. Repeat without resting.

MAKE IT EASIER

- Switch both hands to an underhand grip.
- Use a closer grip.
- Hook your foot into a stretch band to help pull yourself up.

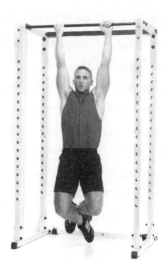

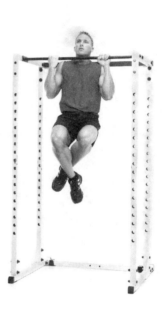

DO IT HARDER

- Use a wide grip and take turns pulling to one side, then the other.
- Throw a towel or thick rope over the bar and stagger your grip, so that one hand is higher than the other.
- Pause at three different positions on the way down.

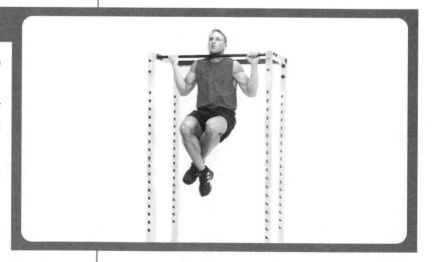

CHINUP

This movement works your arms as well as the lats. Space your hands shoulder width apart.

A Grip a chinup bar with your palms facing your body, and your hands wider than shoulder width apart. Hang from the bar with your legs slightly bent and your ankles crossed.

B Pull yourself up until your chin is over the bar. Hold for a second, then return to the starting position. Repeat without resting.

MAKE IT EASIER

- Use a closer grip.
- Have a bench under you. Use your feet to help push up.
- Hook your foot into a stretch band to help pull yourself up.

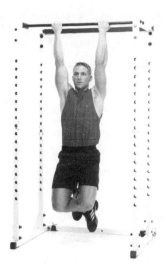

A

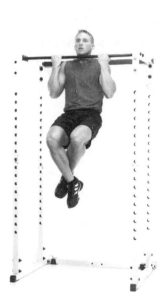

B

DO IT HARDER

- Use a wider grip.
- Throw a towel or thick rope over the bar and stagger your grip, so one hand is higher than the other.
- Pause at three different positions on the way down.

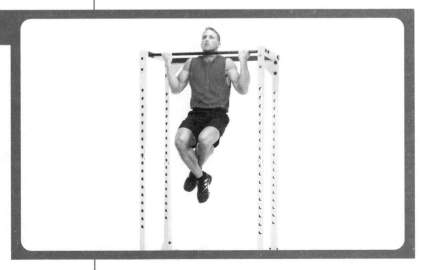

ONE-ARM DUMBBELL ROW

The advantage of this exercise is that it works one side of the back at a time, making it possible to isolate and strengthen the latissimus dorsi (mid- and lower back), rhomboid (upper back), and trapezius (upper back and neck) muscles individually.

A With a dumbbell in your right hand, rest your left knee and left hand on the centerline of a bench. Place your right foot firmly on the floor, your knee slightly bent. Keep your back straight and your eyes facing down. Let your right arm hang down. Your right elbow should remain unlocked, and your right palm should face in toward your right side.

B Pull the dumbbell up and in toward your torso, raising it as high toward your chest as possible. Your right elbow should point up toward the ceiling as you lift. Hold for a second, then return to the starting position. Complete the set, then switch sides.

MAKE IT EASIER

- Lift your torso up so your back is above parallel with the floor. Pull the dumbbell to your abdominal region.
- Do this standing with both feet on the floor, your back parallel to the floor, and one hand on a high bench or rack for support.
- Use a cable weight instead of a dumbbell.

DO IT HARDER

- To challenge your balance, stand on one leg. Extend the other leg directly back. Your back and free leg should be parallel to the floor. The dumbbell should be in the hand opposite the foot in contact with the floor.
- Pull the dumbbell up and out, away from the chest.
- Pause at the bottom of the movement, squeeze your scapulas together, and pull the handle to your chest. Hold for 2 to 3 seconds, then slowly lower.

A

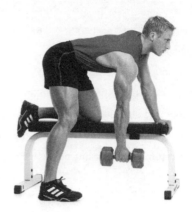

B

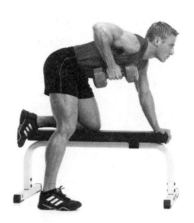

TWO-ARM DUMBBELL ROW

This exercise strengthens the latissimus dorsi (mid- and lower back), rhomboid (upper back), and trapezius (upper back and neck) muscles individually.

A With a dumbbell in each hand, stand with your knees bent and your back parallel to the floor. Let your arms hang down. Your elbows should remain unlocked, and your palms should face in toward your legs.

B Pull the dumbbells up and in toward your torso, raising them as high toward your chest as possible. Your elbows should point up toward the ceiling as you lift. Hold for a second, then return to the starting position.

MAKE IT EASIER

- Lift your torso up so that your back is above parallel with the floor. Pull the dumbbells to your abdominal region.
- Rest the dumbbells on a low bench between reps.
- Use an underhand grip (palms facing forward) to make it easier to pull.

DO IT HARDER

- To challenge your balance, stand on one leg. You may want to start with very light dumbbells because the movement is difficult to do.
- Hold the dumbbells at arm's length, and row them in an alternating fashion.
- Pause at the bottom of the movement, squeeze your scapulas together, and pull the handle to your chest. Hold for 2 to 3 seconds, then slowly lower.

A

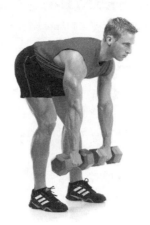

B

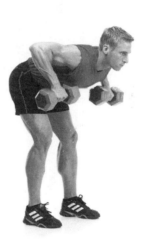

ONE-ARM TUBING ROW

This movement works the latissimus dorsi (upper back), rhomboids (upper back), and trapezius (upper back and neck) muscles.

A Wrap a length of exercise tubing around a stationary object. Keep wrapping until there is no slack. Stand with your knees slightly bent and one foot forward of the other. Keep your back straight. Hold the handle in one hand, with that arm extended. Your other elbow should remain unlocked, and your palm should face your side.

B Pull the handle up and in toward your torso, as far toward your chest as possible. Hold for a second, then return to the starting position. Complete the set, then switch sides.

MAKE IT EASIER

• Use an underhand grip. Or use a bar with parallel handles.

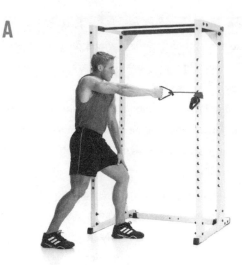

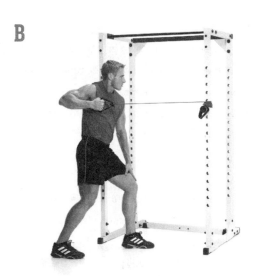

DO IT HARDER

• Set tubing above head height and pull while in a lunge.

• Stand up, pull with one arm, then quickly switch sides and pull with the other arm. This should be done very explosively. Alternate sides until you complete all your reps.

• Pause at the bottom of the movement, squeeze your scapulas together, and pull the handle to your chest. Hold for 2 to 3 seconds, then slowly lower.

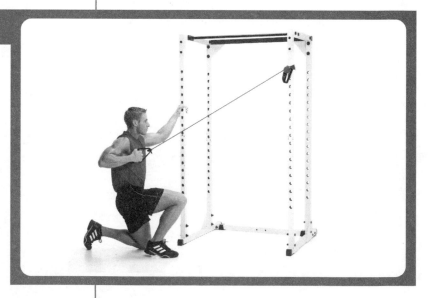

PULLUP

This exercise is a great workout for your rhomboid (upper back) and latissimus dorsi (mid- and lower back) muscles.

A Stand under a chinning bar. Grip the bar overhand, with your hands slightly wider than shoulder width apart.

B Pull yourself up until your chin is higher than the bar. Hold for a second, then slowly lower to the starting position. Don't let your feet touch the floor. Exhale on your way up, and inhale on your way down. Don't let your body swing.

MAKE IT EASIER

- Switch both hands to an underhand grip.
- Use a closer grip.
- Hook your foot in a stretch band to help pull yourself up.

DO IT HARDER

- Use a wide grip. Take turns pulling to one side and then the other.
- Throw a towel or a thick rope over the bar and stagger your grip, so that one hand is higher than the other.
- Pause at three different positions on the way down.

A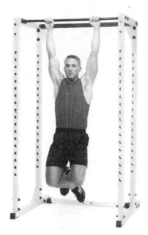

B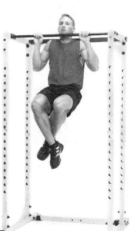

HOW TO DO MORE PULLUPS

The average guy can only do about 8 pullups before falling to the floor. It's worth doing better.

- Do them at your own pace. Men can do more pullups when they self-pace; forget the usual advice that calls for pulling up to a count of 2, and dropping to a count of 4.
- Find a hand spacing that feels comfortable. Usually this will maximize the amount of force that you can generate.
- Loop one end of a stretch band through the other end and wrap around the bar. When you get tired, stick one foot in the open end of the band and use the "spring" to complete more reps.
- As you get stronger, vary your grip: close , medium, wide, staggered, alternating, underhand, and neutral. The variety of angles will enable you to train more muscle fibers and pull more weight.
- Train progressively. In the first week, do as many pullups as you can in 5 seconds. Rest for 1 minute, then do another 5-second set. Rest for 1 minute, then do the final 5-second set. Do this two to three times a week. Each week, add 5 seconds to your pullup time. Reduce your rest time by 5 seconds. At the end of 12 weeks, you'll be doing pullups for 180 straight seconds—and your upper body will show the results.

PULLDOWN

This exercise primarily works the latissimus dorsi (mid- and lower back), teres major (below the shoulder blades), and the rhomboids (upper back). Because it is done with a machine, the movements are easy to control.

A Sit or kneel at a lat pulldown station. Grip the bar overhand, with your hands shoulder width or farther apart. Your palms should face away from your body. Keep your upper body straight and your eyes forward.

B Pull the bar down in front of your head until it reaches the top of your chest. Keep your upper body close to upright throughout the movement. Hold for a second, then slowly return your arms to the starting position.

MAKE IT EASIER

- Use an underhand grip.
- Use a neutral or parallel grip.
- Lean back slightly as you pull the bar down.

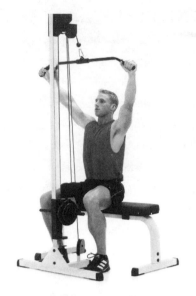

A

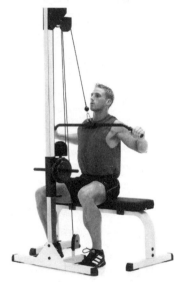

B

DO IT HARDER

- Using a cable, stand or kneel in front of the pulley and bring the bar from above your head down to your thighs, keeping your arms straight.
- Pause at three different positions on the way up with the bar.

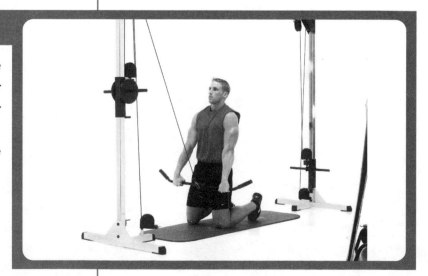

CABLE PULLOVER

This exercise works the muscles of the upper back. Because it is done with a machine, the movements are easier to control.

A Attach a bar handle to the low pulley on a weight machine. Set one end of the bench about 2 feet from the pulley. The cable, when extended, should bisect the bench. Lie on the bench, with your head toward the pulley. Reach behind you, grip the bar with an underhand grip, and hold the bar over your chest at almost arm's length. With your knees bent, place your feet on the floor, keeping your back from arching.

B Without bending your elbows beyond the starting angle, lower the handles behind your head until your arms are almost parallel to the floor. Pause, then return to the starting position.

MAKE IT EASIER

- Bend your elbows more.
- Don't lower the bar below the head.

DO IT HARDER

- Keep your elbows straighter.
- Lower the bar as far back as you can.
- Use a rope handle instead of a bar.
- Pause at the bottom of the movement.

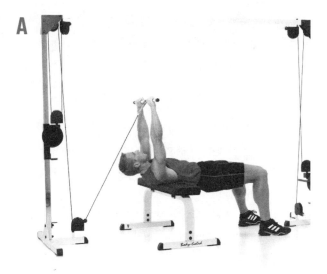

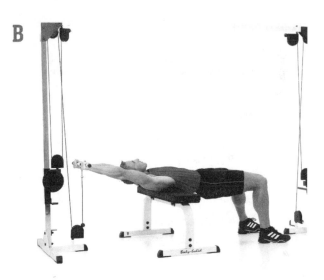

SEATED ROW

This is the perfect exercise for sculpting the entire back, especially the upper-middle back.

A Sit on a pulley row machine or facing a bar handle low pulley cable. With your knees slightly bent, anchor your feet. Keep your back straight as you lean forward. Grip the handle with a narrow overhand grip. Push backward with your feet until your arms are fully extended and you are leaning back slightly past 90 degrees.

B Pull the handle until it touches your abdominal region, bringing your body into an upright position. Your elbows should point behind you. Don't lock your knees. Hold for a second, then return to the starting position.

MAKE IT EASIER

- Use tubing instead.
- Use a wider grip attachment, or an underhand grip.

DO IT HARDER

- Pull back with two hands, but lower with one hand. These are called negatives.
- Lean forward slightly and pull the handle to your chest.
- Pause at the bottom of the movement, squeeze your scapulas together, and pull the handle to your chest. Hold for 2 to 3 seconds, then slowly lower.

BARBELL T-BAR ROW

This exercise strengthens the back and develops good posture and form. The movement works all the muscles of the back as well as the rear deltoid (shoulder) muscles.

A Using an Olympic-size (45-pound) bar, wedge one end in a corner and place a weight plate on the other end. Wrap two wrist straps or a V-handle around the bar just below the weight. Hold it with both hands so that it doesn't slide or wobble. Straddle the bar, keeping your knees slightly bent. Your chin should be up, your chest out, stomach in, shoulders down, and back flat.

A
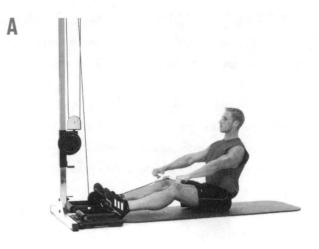

B
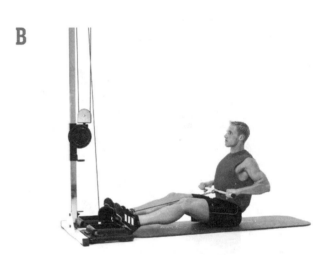

A
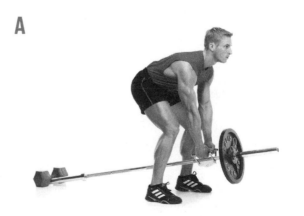

B Pull the bar to your chest, arching your back slightly and letting your elbows rise above your chest. Hold for a second, then slowly lower the bar to arm's length.

B

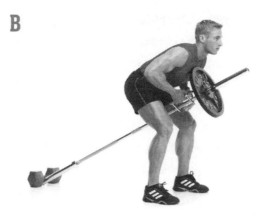

MAKE IT EASIER

- Pull the bar to your abdominal region.
- Use a wider grip to make it easier to pull.
- Place a parallel handle attachment under the bar.

DO IT HARDER

- Use a towel instead of a strap to pull.
- Use only one hand at a time.
- Pause at the bottom of the movement, squeeze your scapulas together, and pull the handle to your chest. Hold for 2 to 3 seconds, then slowly lower.

NO KIDDING?

WHAT'S BETTER: BACK-AND-CHEST OR BACK-AND-BICEPS WORKOUTS?

The conventional training advice is to combine chest and back workouts on the same days, an approach known as "push-pull." More recently, some trainers have begun recommending combined back and biceps workouts. Both approaches work—though the preponderance of evidence favors the back-chest strategy.

Studies show that you can significantly increase force, and the rate of muscle development, by training antagonistic muscles—the chest and back, in other words. That's the idea behind workouts that alternate antagonistic movements, such as rows followed by a bench press. Doing these exercises in opposition makes each more effective.

So what about training the back and biceps together? The research here isn't very convincing, even though it makes sense in theory. Most back exercises bring the biceps into play, often to a significant degree. Since the biceps get an "incidental" workout and are partly fatigued during the back portion of your workout, you're less likely to hammer them too hard during the biceps-only part. This can prevent overtraining.

Sports physiologists who have done the research lean more toward the back-chest strategy. The real-life difference between the two approaches, however, is probably less significant than it might appear in the lab. Both approaches add variety to your training, and that's one of the best ways to maximize results.

ROW WITH TUBING

In addition to the muscles in the back, this exercise works the deltoid (shoulder), gluteal (butt), and hamstring (back thigh) muscles.

A Stand with your feet shoulder width apart, your knees slightly bent. Bend at the waist until your upper body is parallel to the floor, keeping your back flat. Run a length of exercise tubing under your feet. Grip the handles with your hands wider than shoulder width apart. Your palms should face your body.

B Raise the handles until your elbows are higher than your back. Your forearms should be perpendicular to the floor. Hold for a second, then slowly lower the handles to about midshin, and repeat.

MAKE IT EASIER

- Lean forward so your torso is less than 90 degrees. Pull the handle to your abdominal region.
- Use a neutral-grip attachment.
- Use an underhand-grip position.

DO IT HARDER

- Lean back so your torso is past 90 degrees. Pull the handle to your chest region.
- Run a towel through the handle. Pull while holding one end of the towel in each hand.
- Pause at the bottom of the movement, squeeze your scapulas together, and pull the handle to your chest. Hold for 2 to 3 seconds, then slowly lower.

BACK HYPEREXTENSION (BACK ABOVE HIPS)

This all-purpose back exercise is especially good for your erector (lower back) muscles. It requires keeping your back slightly higher than your hips.

A Position yourself in a back extension machine, with your ankles locked behind the padded bars, and your groin area and upper thighs resting on the padded platform. Your hips should be over the edge of the platform. Bend over at the waist, with your upper torso lowered to a point a few inches above perpendicular to the floor. Put your hands behind your head.

A

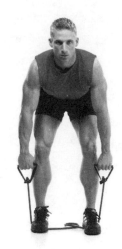

B

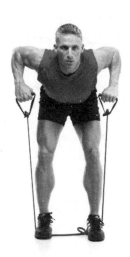

A

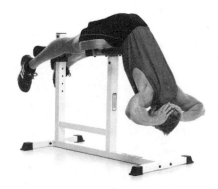

B Raise your upper body as high as you can by contracting your glutes. Do not arch the back excessively. Hold for a second, then return to the starting position.

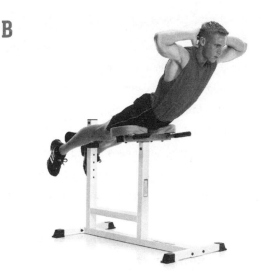

MAKE IT EASIER

- Move back so that more of your thigh is on the platform.
- Bend your knees more.
- Let your arms hang out in front of you.

DO IT HARDER

- Move forward so that less of your thigh is on the platform.
- Keep your knees straight, but not locked.
- Hold a dumbbell or weight plate across your chest.

HOW HELPFUL ARE FORCED REPETITIONS?

Forced repetitions means that you're getting assistance to lift a weight. For example, you might use one arm or leg to help the other limb do the work during the exertion phase. Or a spotter will help you lift the weight, then step back during the negative part of the movement.

There are good reasons to do forced repetitions. Recent research shows that well-trained men who perform 8 reps on their own, followed by 4 additional forced reps, have an improved hormonal response that generates increases in size and strength.

Forced reps are tough on the body, though. Trainers usually advise men to incorporate this technique rarely—say, during 1- or 2-week phases of their training.

Forced reps aren't so good if you're relatively new to lifting. You'll do better sticking to weights you can lift on your own. If you're working with a spotter and need assistance on the last few reps, lighten the load for the next round. Otherwise, you'll probably be dealing with some serious soreness, without a lot of gain.

If you're already at an advanced stage of strength training, forced reps can be a real boon. The usual approach is to lift a weight six to eight times "solo," followed by 2 to 4 forced reps.

DEADLIFT

This exercise strengthens nearly every muscle in your body, including the legs, back, shoulders, and arms.

A Stand upright, with a weighted barbell in front of you. Keeping your back straight, bend over the barbell and grip it with your hands shoulder width apart, using an alternating grip. When you are set up, your knees should be bent about 90 degrees or so. Keep your arms straight and your elbows unlocked. Your shoulders should be in front of or over the bar, but not behind the bar.

B Start the movement by driving your heels through the floor. Lift the bar past your knees with your legs. Then pull the bar to the top using your glutes and back. Your back and arms should be straight throughout the movement. Only your knees and hips should be moving. Hold for a second, then slowly lower the weight.

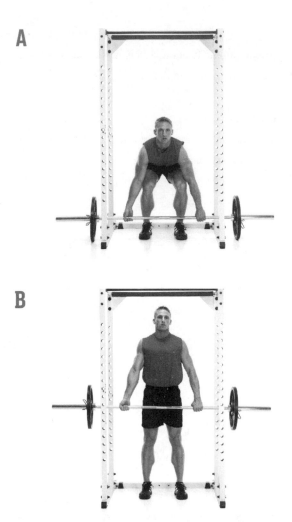

MAKE IT EASIER

- Use reverse band setup to make it easier to get the weight moving. Loop bands over top of the rack and around the bar.
- Use a trap bar.
- Start from the top instead of off the floor: Lift the bar off a rack, step backward, and then perform the deadlift.

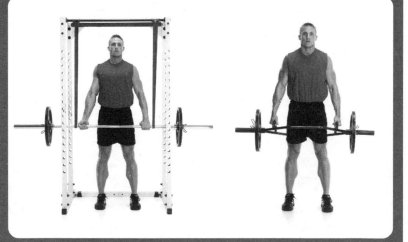

DO IT HARDER

- Stand on a platform so the bar is at ankle height. This will make you start from a lower position. Be careful not to round your back.
- Stand on one leg only. This is a very difficult movement.
- Use a very wide grip to involve more of the lats.
- Use a band to make it harder to lift as you come close to full extension. Loop each end of the band over the bar and stand on the middle of the band, as shown.

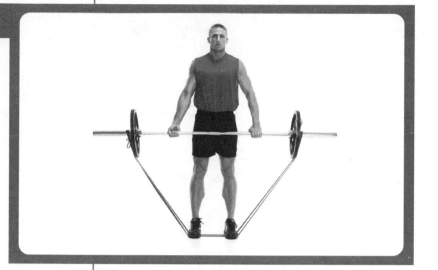

THE SECRETS TO A GOOD DEADLIFT

The deadlift really works your hips and back. It's actually a total-body exercise because just about every muscle group kicks in to support the weight and stabilize your body. To do it right:

- Take a deep breath and hold it. This stabilizes internal pressures and allows you to exert more force. Warning: Don't hold your breath if you have high blood pressure.

- Push your feet into the ground and drive the bar up with your legs. A good deadlift involves a leg press to get started, then a back extension to finish.

- Your knees should be bent at about 90 degrees or higher when you set up. Take the slack out of the bar before you pull it off the floor. When the bar starts to bend, pull it off the floor. This allows your body to really know what it has to lift. Rushing the start will throw your positioning off, and you'll have to work harder to lift the weight. You should feel a pull in your traps before the weight starts to move.

- Squeeze your shoulder blades together and hold them there before lifting the weight. This will help prevent your upper back from rounding—and will enable you to lift more weight.

- As you come off the ground, your shoulders and hips should rise at the same rate. If your hips rise faster, the weight is going forward—and you may miss the lift.

- Straighten the legs. That's what gets the deadlift started. Once the bar passes the knees, it's all about hip and back extension.

DUMBBELL DEADLIFT

This exercise is done with two dumbbells. It strengthens your back, arms, and thighs. Move slowly, lifting both dumbbells in a controlled manner.

A Place two dumbbells on the floor. Stand with your feet shoulder width apart. The dumbbells should be outside your feet. Keeping your back straight, bend at the knees and grip the dumbbells, with your palms facing in toward your legs. Keep the dumbbells in the same position (as if they were a barbell) throughout the movement.

B Lift the dumbbells to upper-thigh level. Keep your back, arms, and legs straight, and your knees unlocked. Hold for a second, then slowly return to the starting position.

MAKE IT EASIER

- Start with the dumbbells at a higher position. Rest them on a bench or platform.
- Position the dumbbells outside and lateral to your feet, so that your hands are in a neutral position for the entire lift.
- Start from the top instead of off the floor. Lift the dumbbells off a bench or rack, step backward, and then perform the deadlift.

DO IT HARDER

- Stand on a platform so that the dumbbells are at ankle height. This will make you start from a lower position. Be careful not to round your back.
- Stand on one leg only.
- Use a very wide hand spacing to involve more of the lats.

ONE-ARM DUMBBELL DEADLIFT BETWEEN THE LEGS

This movement works one side of the back at a time, making it easier to isolate and build the muscles.

A Standing with your feet shoulder width apart, place a dumbbell on the floor between your feet. Keeping your back straight, bend at the knees and grip the dumbbell with your left hand, using an overhand grip.

A
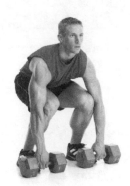

B
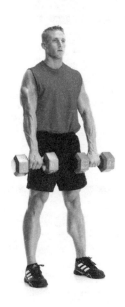

A
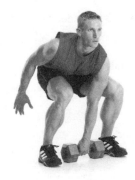

B Lift the dumbbell to upper-thigh level. Your back, arms, and legs should stay straight. Keep your knees unlocked. Hold for a second, then slowly lower the weight to the starting position. Repeat on the right side.

B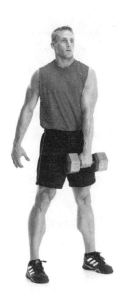

MAKE IT EASIER

- Start with the dumbbell at a higher position. Rest it on a bench or platform.
- Position the dumbbell so that your hand is in a neutral position for the entire lift.
- Start from the top instead of off the floor. Lift the dumbbell off a bench or rack, step backward, and then perform the deadlift.

DO IT HARDER

- Stand on a platform so that the dumbbell is at ankle height. This will make you start from a lower position. Be careful not to round your back.
- Stand on one leg only.
- Hook exercise tubing under your feet and attach the ends to the dumbbell so that the movement gets harder as you come to full hip extension.

DEADLIFTS AND BULGING DISCS

When deadlifting properly, you will get very strong and add serious muscle size. But deadlifting improperly can send you to a doctor, fast. This isn't an exaggeration. When the back is rounded under heavy loads, internal forces can push your spinal discs backward. If the forces are great enough, the discs can bulge or rupture and jam against nearby nerves. That's serious pain, and it can put you out of commission for months—or for good.

To deadlift safely:

- Don't round your lower back. Keep it flat.
- When lowering, your knees should be bent over the bar, not behind it.
- Keep the weight balanced over your shoulders; don't hold the weight in front of you.

ROMANIAN DEADLIFT

This all-purpose exercise strengthens not only your back, but also your arms, shoulders, and legs. Use less weight than for a regular deadlift.

A Hold a lightly weighted barbell at mid-thigh level, with your hands farther than shoulder width apart, palms facing your body. Keep the barbell against your legs, with your arms fully extended. Keep your back straight, your shoulders back, and your chest out.

B Bend from the hips, keeping the bar close to your thighs. Your back should stay straight, your knees slightly bent. Lower the bar slowly toward the floor, going as far as you comfortably can. With a slow, controlled movement, return to the starting position, keeping your back straight.

MAKE IT EASIER

- Start with the barbell at a higher position. Rest it on a bench or platform.
- Use a trap bar.
- Start from the top instead of off the floor. Lift the bar off a bench or rack, step backward, and then perform the deadlift.

DO IT HARDER

- Stand on a platform so the bar is at ankle height. This will make you start from a lower position. Be careful not to round your back.
- Stand on one leg only.
- Use a very wide grip to involve more of the lats.

A

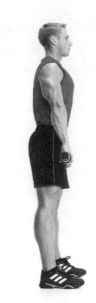

B

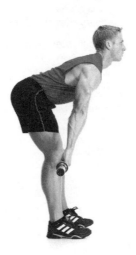

STIFF-LEG DEADLIFT

Want to hit your hams and glutes hard? This is the deadlift variation for you. This movement is similar to the conventional deadlift, except that the knees are straight but not locked out.

A Stand upright with a barbell in front of you. Bend at the hips and, with a flat back, grip the barbell with your hands shoulder width apart, your palms down. Balance your weight evenly on both feet. Take a deep breath.

B Exhale while extending the trunk to the top deadlift position. Keep the back flat and legs straight. Hold for a second, then slowly lower the weight.

MAKE IT EASIER

- Start with the barbell at a higher position. Rest it on a bench or platform.
- Use a trap bar.
- Start from the top instead of off the floor. Lift the bar off a bench or rack, step backward, and then perform the deadlift.

DO IT HARDER

- Stand on a platform so the bar is at ankle height. This will make you start from a lower position. Be careful not to round your back.
- Stand on one leg only.
- Use a very wide grip to involve more of the lats.

A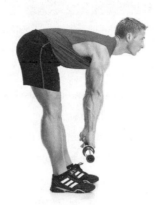

B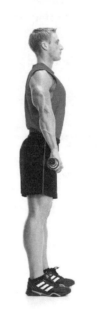

GOOD MORNING

This exercise is not recommended for beginners because it requires a strong lower back and good form. It provides an extensive mid-body workout. It works the hamstrings (back thigh), gluteal (butt), and all the back muscles, especially the erector spinae (lower back) muscle.

A Stand with your legs shoulder width apart, your knees unlocked. Hold a barbell across your shoulders, with your hands slightly farther than shoulder width apart, palms facing out. Keep your upper body straight, your shoulders back, and your chest out. Lean forward slightly at the waist.

B Bend slowly at the waist, keeping your back straight, until your upper body is parallel to the floor. You should be looking forward, not down. Hold for a second, then slowly return to the starting position.

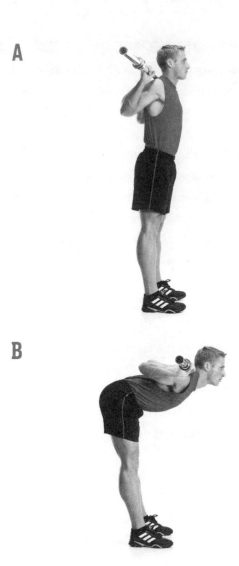

A

B

MAKE IT EASIER

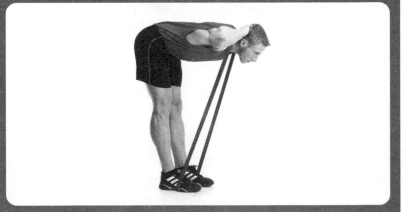

- Place the barbell lower on your traps.
- Don't go down as far.
- Instead of using a barbell, stand on exercise tubing and loop the other end behind your head as if you were holding a bar. Perform the exercise as described above.

DO IT HARDER

- Stand on one leg.
- Stand with a very wide stance.
- Stand with a very narrow stance.

REVERSE BACK HYPEREXTENSION

This exercise requires that you keep your feet above the hips. It will help strengthen the lower back.

A Lie facedown on a bench or table, with your hips at the edge, your legs together, your knees slightly bent, and your toes touching the floor. You can also lie on a stability ball on top of a bench. Grip the sides of the bench above your head to keep your upper body stable. Hold on firmly to avoid sliding off the bench.

B Raise your legs upward, keeping your feet together, toes pointed, as high as you can. Hold for a second, then slowly lower your legs to the starting position. Do not allow your feet to touch the floor until you have completed one set.

MAKE IT EASIER

- Use a low platform so you don't have to move as far.
- Bend your knees more.
- Do only one leg at a time.

DO IT HARDER

- Use a high platform so your feet don't touch the floor.
- Keep your knees straight, but not locked.
- Use ankle weights.

TOE TOUCH

This exercise will strengthen the lower back, the hamstrings (back thigh), and gluteal (butt) muscles. Work on increasing flexibility by doing more repetitions before you consider adding more weight.

A Hold a dumbbell in your right hand. Your feet should be shoulder width apart, with your knees unlocked.

A

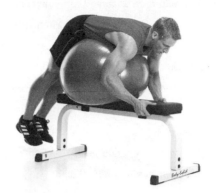

B

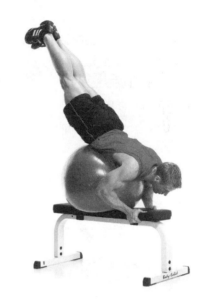

A

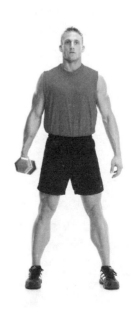

B Bend forward and to the left. Touch the dumbbell to your left foot. Hold for a second, then slowly return to the starting position. Finish the set, then switch sides.

B

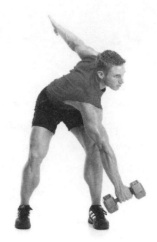

MAKE IT EASIER

- Instead of using a dumbbell, anchor exercise tubing by standing on it with your foot. Perform the exercise as described above.
- Instead of going to the floor, stop at a bench or step.
- Use a cable pulley set at a low height.

DO IT HARDER

- Stand on a platform so that the dumbbell goes below your ankle. This will make you start from a lower position. Be careful not to round your back.
- Stand on the opposite leg only. That is, if the dumbbell is in your left hand, stand on your right leg.
- Hold a dumbbell in each hand and alternate sides.

A NASTY ROW

Chances are, this painful scenario sounds familiar: You're determined to row some seriously heavy weight. You bend over, grab the barbell, and *wham!* There's a stabbing pain above your right elbow, and suddenly there's a new bulge where there didn't used to be one.

Congratulations. You've just torn your right biceps.

A couple of things caused this to happen. A sudden jerking motion in the elbow can cause it to hyperextend and overstretch the biceps. While this is happening, you're simultaneously contracting the muscle in order to pull the resistance toward your body. In other words, the muscle is trying to contract and expand at the same time. The internal forces basically go through the ceiling and exceed the ability of the tendon to hang on to its supporting bone. The biceps tendon tears free. That's about the time you almost pass out.

Lesson: Don't get too casual when you're moving heavy weights. An injury like that can cost you about 8 weeks in a cast, and another 5 to 8 weeks of rehab. All you had to do to prevent it was to warm up a little first, and definitely avoid jerking movements. *Always* move weights smoothly and with total control.

TWISTING REVERSE BACK HYPEREXTENSION

The abdominal and lower back muscles overlap and work together to move your trunk, whether for lifting or twisting. Sturdy lower back muscles are just as important as strong abs. These extensions are the best low back exercise you can do.

A Get in position on a back extension station. Your ankles should be locked behind the padded bars, with your upper thighs resting on the platform, and your hips over the edge. Put your hands behind your head. Bend at the waist, lowering your upper torso until it's almost perpendicular to the floor.

B Keeping your hands behind your head, raise your torso up and to one side, until it's slightly above parallel to the floor. Lower to the starting position, then raise your torso up and to the other side. Hold for a second, then return to the starting position, alternating sides with each rep.

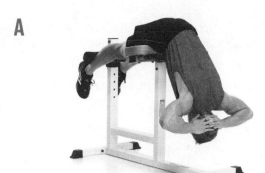

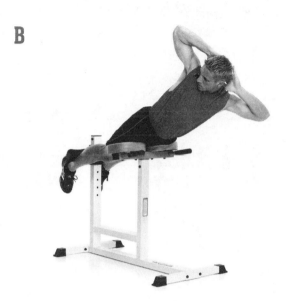

MAKE IT EASIER

- Move back so that more of your thigh is on the platform.
- Bend your knees more.
- Let your arms hang in front of you.

DO IT HARDER

- Move forward so that less of your thigh is on the platform.
- Keep your knees straight, but not locked.
- Hold a dumbbell or weight plate across your chest.

LEVEL 1 (FOCUS ON SIZE)

We've provided three different workouts for Level 1. Workout variations mean more size and strength—and less boredom.

One option is to do all three workouts weekly. For example, do Workout #1 on Monday, Workout #2 on Wednesday, and Workout #3 on Friday. If you choose this option, do 2 warmup sets for the first exercise, followed by 3 sets of 6 repetitions using "real" weight. Next, do 3 sets of 10 reps for the second exercise, followed by 3 sets of 14 reps for the third exercise. Do only 1 set of the last exercise, going for maximum reps.

Another option is to do just one of the workouts, three times a week. Vary the rep count daily. On Monday, for example, do 3 sets of 6 reps for the first three exercises; on Wednesday, do 3 sets of 10 reps for the first three exercises; and on Friday, do 3 sets of 14 reps for the first three exercises. Always start with 2 warmup sets for the first exercise (these don't go toward the final "count"). Do only 1 set of the last exercise, going for maximum reps. Pick a weight that will allow you to get 15 to 20 reps.

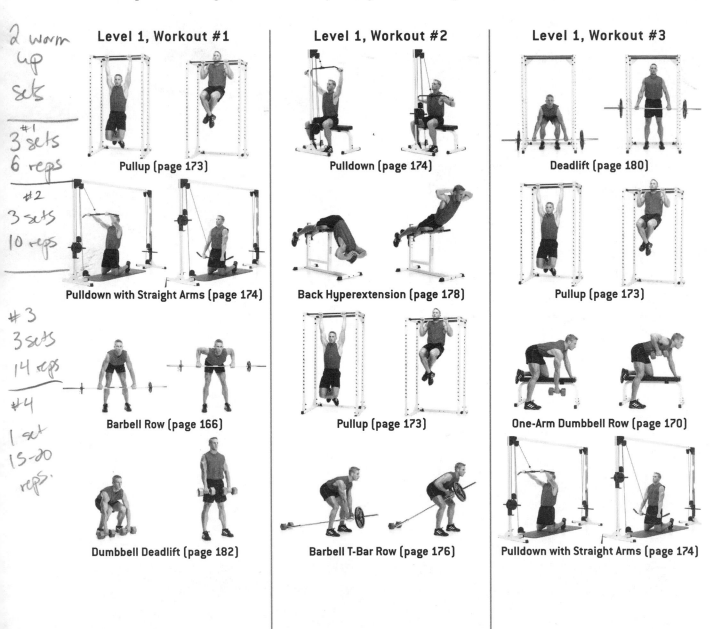

handwritten margin notes:
2 warm up sets
#1 3 sets 6 reps
#2 3 sets 10 reps
#3 3 sets 14 reps
#4 1 set 15-20 reps.

Level 1, Workout #1

Pullup (page 173)

Pulldown with Straight Arms (page 174)

Barbell Row (page 166)

Dumbbell Deadlift (page 182)

Level 1, Workout #2

Pulldown (page 174)

Back Hyperextension (page 178)

Pullup (page 173)

Barbell T-Bar Row (page 176)

Level 1, Workout #3

Deadlift (page 180)

Pullup (page 173)

One-Arm Dumbbell Row (page 170)

Pulldown with Straight Arms (page 174)

LEVEL 2 (FOCUS ON STRENGTH)

Level 2, Workout #1: Max Deadlift Routine

It's possible to increase your deadlift load by more than 60 pounds in less than 10 weeks by following this routine. You only have to do it twice a week—a "light" day and a "heavy" day. First, determine your 1 repetition maximum (1RM) for the deadlift. (See page 14.) Then use the chart below to determine your deadlift weight, sets, and reps for a given workout. Round the weights to the nearest 5 pounds.

To stay limber (and safe), start each workout with two 5-rep warmup sets, using 50 percent and 70 percent of your 1RM. After you've done all sets and reps of your deadlift, complete the workout with the additional exercises on the following page.

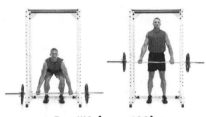

Deadlift (page 180)

Level 2, Workout 1, Deadlift Cycle

WEEK	DAY	% 1RM	#SETS	#REPS
1	1	80	6	2
1	2	80	6	3
2	1	80	6	2
2	2	80	6	4
3	1	80	6	2
3	2	80	6	5
4	1	80	6	2
4	2	80	6	6
5	1	80	6	2
5	2	85	5	5
6	1	80	6	2
6	2	90	4	4
7	1	80	6	2
7	2	95	3	3
8	1	80	6	2
8	2	100	2	2
9	1	80	6	2
9	2	105	2	1*

*AFTER THE 2 SETS AT TOP WEIGHT, KEEP DOING SINGLES WITH 2 MINUTES' REST BETWEEN SETS, INCREASING THE WEIGHT 5 TO 10 POUNDS EACH TIME, UNTIL YOU FIND YOUR NEW 1RM.

Level 2, Workout #1, Day 1

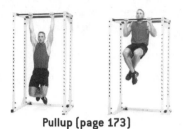

Pullup (page 173)

Do 2 to 3 sets, with 8 to 10 reps per set.

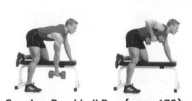

One-Arm Dumbbell Row (page 170)

Do 2 to 3 sets, with 8 to 10 reps per set.

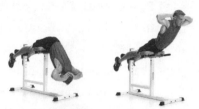

Back Hyperextension (page 178)

Do 1 set for maximum reps.

Level 2, Workout #1, Day 2

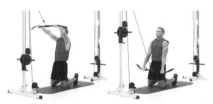

Pulldown with Straight Arms (page 174)

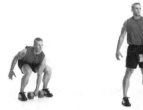

One-Arm Dumbbell Deadlift between the Legs (page 182)

Do 2 to 3 sets, with 4 to 6 reps per set.

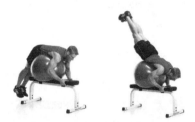

Reverse Back Hyperextension (page 187)

Do 1 set for maximum reps.

Level 2, Workout #2

Do this workout three times a week. Perform 2 warmup sets for each exercise. Vary the rep count on successive days. For example, do 1 set of 3 reps on Monday, 1 set of 11 reps on Wednesday, and 1 set of 7 reps on Friday.

Each week, add 1 set to each exercise until you're up to 5 sets. If you're feeling excessive soreness, reduce the number of sets for each exercise.

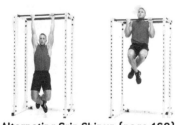

Alternating Grip Chinup (page 168)

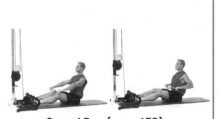

Seated Row (page 176)

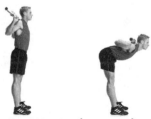

Good Morning (page 186)

Level 2, Workout #3

Do this workout three times a week. Perform 2 warmup sets for each exercise. If you're feeling excessive soreness, reduce the number of sets for each exercise.

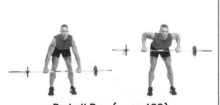

Barbell Row (page 166)

Do 2 to 3 sets, with 3 reps per set.

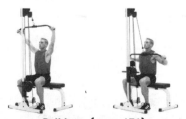

Pulldown (page 174)

Do 2 to 3 sets, with 7 reps per set.

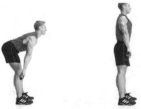

Romanian Deadlift (page 184)

Do 2 to 3 sets, with 11 reps per set.

LEVEL 3 (HYBRID TRAINING—FOCUS ON SIZE AND STRENGTH)

We've provided three different programs for the Level 3 back workouts. You can stick to one program throughout the week. Or shake things up and do different programs on different days. The number of sets and repetitions you'll do in each workout depends on the approach you take. Here are the two main options.

Option A

- Perform all three workouts in a single week. For example, do Workout #1 on Monday, Workout #2 on Wednesday, and Workout #3 on Friday.

- After a general warmup, do 2 warmup sets for the first exercise, lifting lighter-than-usual weights.

- Do 5 sets of 2 reps for the first exercise.

- Next, do 2 sets of 6 reps for the second exercise.

- Do 2 sets of 12 reps for the third exercise.

Option B

- Pick one of the workouts and stick with it all week.

- After a general warmup, do 2 warmup sets for the first exercise, lifting lighter-than-usual weights.

- Vary the rep count on each day. For example, do 3 sets of 2 reps for the first three exercises on Monday. On Wednesday, do 3 sets of 6 reps for the first three exercises. On Friday, do 3 sets of 12 reps for the first three exercises.

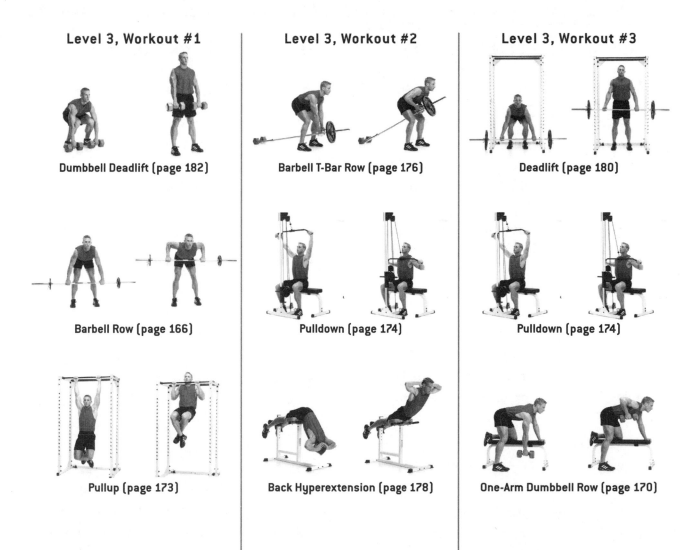

Level 3, Workout #1

Dumbbell Deadlift (page 182)

Barbell Row (page 166)

Pullup (page 173)

Level 3, Workout #2

Barbell T-Bar Row (page 176)

Pulldown (page 174)

Back Hyperextension (page 178)

Level 3, Workout #3

Deadlift (page 180)

Pulldown (page 174)

One-Arm Dumbbell Row (page 170)

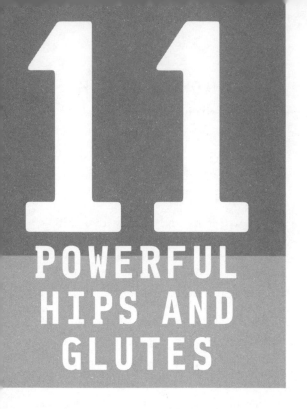

11
POWERFUL HIPS AND GLUTES

Ask the average woman which body part she finds most attractive in a guy, and she'll probably say the butt. You'd think the average guy, in turn, would dedicate a heck of a lot of his workouts to this potentially eye-catching part. But the butt—or the gluteal muscles, to be more precise—often gets left out.

That's a mistake, and not only because you might be missing out on the occasional female eye. Your butt is only one part of the muscles that make up the hips. Without strong hips—well, you can't do much of anything. They're the muscles that provide speed and endurance when you're running, walking, cycling, or just moving around. They help you stand up straight. They also provide the foundation for your lower body. Strong hips and glutes mean you move better and stand stronger.

HIPS AND GLUTES EXPLAINED

The hip joint is formed by the femurs (upper leg bones) where they mesh with the pelvic girdle. The three bones of the pelvic girdle—the ilium, ischium, and pubis—come together in such a way that six basic movements are possible.

- Flexion. When the feet are fixed, this movement allows you to bend at the waist. When the torso is fixed, it allows you to do leg raises.

- Extension. When the feet are fixed, extension allows you to stand straight from a bent-over position. When the torso is fixed, it lets you bring the thighs away from the chest, such as when doing the negative phase in leg raises.

- Abduction. This means moving your legs away from your side.

- Adduction. This is bringing your legs together.

- Internal rotation. This movement is when you rotate one foot toward the other. When you pivot inward on one foot, you're doing an internal rotation.

- External rotation. This is when you rotate one foot away from the other, so your toes are pointing out.

Since the hip joint can move in so many different directions—and because of this it's inherently unstable—it is protected by a variety of muscles. Some of these muscles are very large; others are on the small side. These muscles consist of six basic groups.

For starters, there are three different hip flexors. They function to bring the torso toward the thighs, or the thighs toward the torso.

Then there are the hip extensors, which bring the torso away from the thighs, or the thighs away from the torso. These include the gluteus maximus, the large muscle that makes up a substantial part of the butt. On the outside of the hips are the abductors, the muscles that bring the legs apart. The glutes play a role here, as well.

There are lot of other hip muscles that come into play. We won't discuss them all in detail. Suffice it to say that while most hip and glute exercises hit the major muscles, no single exercise will hit all of them. Once again, variety is the key word. The more variety you incorporate in your workouts, the more muscles you'll build and strengthen. If you want to maximize glute development for a firm butt, shift more of your energy to heavy movements, such as squats, deadlifts, and lunges. If you're more interested in building general size and strength, or if your butt development is already in line with the rest of your body, minimize the heavy lifting and stick with lighter weights and higher reps.

THE TOTAL HIP AND GLUTE WORKOUT

Since most men experience back pain on occasion, and because most men tend to neglect the hips and glutes during workouts, this is about the time to make the connection. Tight hip flexors frequently contribute to lower back pain by causing the pelvis to tilt forward. To counteract this, you need to stretch the hip flexors and strengthen the lower back and abdominal muscles. This will reduce pelvic tilt and decrease lower back pain by improving the balance between the muscles of the hip region.

While we're on the topic of pain, it's worth mentioning a small muscle called the piriformis that's buried deep inside the hip. When this muscle is tight

and understrengthened, it has a tendency to press against the sciatic nerve. This condition, known as piriformis syndrome, is notorious for causing howling pain that frequently travels through the buttocks and down the back of the thigh. When the muscle is *really* tight, it can pull on the sacrum and interfere with movement where it meets the pelvis. If your forward bends are limited, there's a good chance you're having piriformis trouble. Definitely work on your hamstrings, and include a few hip rotator stretches, which are basic moves in any yoga class. It should clear things up.

Here are a few additional tips for working this vital area.

Emphasize body-weight or free weights. Cable, tubing, and machine training generally don't recruit as many muscle fibers as body-weight exercises or free weights. If you're really trying to get big faster, use dumbbells, barbells, and plates. For an extra blast, squeeze your butt at the top of each movement. This recruits still more fibers and is an easy shortcut to bigger size.

Press through your heels. That probably doesn't make a lot of sense when you see it on the page, but you can feel it when you're doing squats, leg presses, lunges, hack squats, and deadlifts. Driving power through your heels maximizes hip involvement and promotes more muscle stimulation.

Add variety. Incorporate both isolation exercises and compound exercises to work the hips more effectively. In addition, perform squats with a variety of stances. For example, change the space between your feet, the angle of the toes pointing out, and the angle of the ankle joint. While you're at it, frequently change your lineup of reps, sets, rest between sets, speed of movement, and so on.

Don't forget about hip balance. Most guys favor workouts for hip extension and hip external rotation, but basically forget about the other four hip movements. This kind of lopsided training leads to joint problems. Don't make that mistake. Balance your training and pick exercises that work all hip movements. You can probably do this with any four or six of the basic exercises we've included.

Change lunge angles. Lunges are among the best hip and glute workouts you can do. You can make them better by shifting angles rather than always doing them straight-ahead. Include rear, side, and transverse lunges in your workouts. Lunges can be tricky at first, so do them with body weight only for starters. When you're confident with balance, you can begin adding weights.

When performing lunges, make sure that the ankles and knees are in alignment. The knee should be moving in the same direction as the ankle. Sometimes guys get sloppy, and the knee moves in or out instead of staying directly over the ankle.

Add some weight. It's simple to add additional weight to lunges, stepups, and other body-weight exercises. You can balance a barbell across your shoulders, for example, or hold a dumbbell in each hand. Or you can switch from two-legged exercises to one-leg-only to make the workouts harder.

Get hot and heavy. Before lifting heavy weights, perform a full-body warmup, followed by a dynamic warmup, followed by an exercise-specific warmup.

Don't take shortcuts. For most guys, squats and deadlifts are all they need to build strong, well-shaped hips and glutes. However, if you want hips that are also functional, don't depend only on these basics. Plan on incorporating lunges, one-legged movements, and other exercises.

You'll still want to perform squats and deadlifts, of course. For more impact, do them at the beginning of your workout, when you're rested and can move the most weight. Then move on to isolation movements, such as hip adductions or hip flexions.

Tighten your gut. Keeping the abs tight during hip exercises will counter some of the spinal forces that can wrench that stack of vertebrae where it's not supposed to go.

Straighten up—and don't overwork. You want to stand up straight when doing most hip and glute exercises. It's the only way to move the muscles through their full range of motion.

When you're planning your program, be sure not to overemphasize hip adduction movements. Men who do this tend to get excessive muscle size in the inner thighs. Apart from making you look out of whack, it can lead to skin rubbing or chafing if the muscles on the right and left legs come together.

Play it safe. Take advantage of safety racks—and use a spotter when possible.

Don't bounce weights off the ground. Lower the weight under control and lift up with a little more speed.

Go it alone. Don't depend on a spotter when doing barbell deadlifts or barbell rows. Do as many reps as you can with good form. Then stop.

Back up to the previous chapter and get a leg up in the next. Many of the back and leg exercises also work the hips in a variety of ways. For complete hip training, they should be incorporated into your workouts, as well.

HIP EXTENSION WITH BENT KNEE

This exercise isolates the glutes and gives them a solid workout. If you want more intensity, add a pair of light ankle weights.

A Get down on your hands and knees. Your wrists should be under your shoulders, and your knees under your hips. Raise your right knee a few inches off the floor.

B Slowly push your right leg up and back, keeping it bent at a 90-degree angle, and pressing your heel toward the ceiling. Feel your gluteal muscles contract as you push up. Don't let your thigh go beyond parallel to the floor. Hold for a second, then slowly lower your leg to the starting position. Finish the set and switch legs.

MAKE IT EASIER

- Don't come up as high with your heel.
- Put a mat under your knees and hands.
- Keep your head, neck, and back parallel to the floor.

DO IT HARDER

- Extend the arm that's opposite the lifting leg in front of you. Hold the arm, then lift the leg.
- Add ankle weights.
- Attach tubing to ankle by hooking on foot as shown and holding other end down with hand (as shown at top right).
- Attach to ankle attachment on cable machine (middle right).
- Perform the exercise with a straight leg (bottom right).
- Perform the exercise with a straight leg and attach tubing to ankle by hooking on foot and holding other end down with hand.
- Perform the exercise with a straight leg and attach to ankle attachment on cable machine.

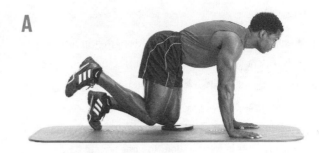

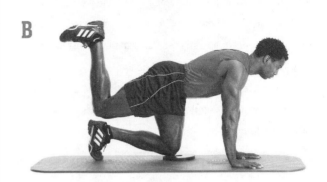

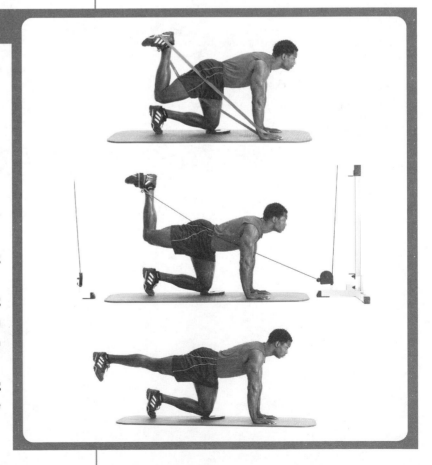

CLEAN PULL

This exercise improves your grip strength and makes your legs, hips, and lower back more powerful. The initial position is similar to a deadlift, except that you use a hook grip and keep your hips lower.

A   Stand with your feet shoulder width apart, with a barbell on the floor in front of you. The bar should be over your feet and close to your shins. Keeping your back straight, your head up, and your shoulders directly over or a little ahead of the bar, squat down and grip the bar with your arms extended and positioned just outside your knees.

B   Do not let your hips kick up past your shoulders at the start from the floor. Pull the bar past your knees to the lower third of the thigh.

C   Move your knees and hips forward.

D   Extend explosively into a top shrug position. You should be able to hold the top position, with your ankles, knees, and hips fully extended. If you fall forward or backward, you're not pulling in a straight line.

MAKE IT EASIER

- Use wrist straps, looping them over the hands and barbell.
- Pull the barbell off blocks set above knee height.
- Initially, move the bar slowly, so that you hit the optimal mechanical positions. As your technique improves, increase the speed.

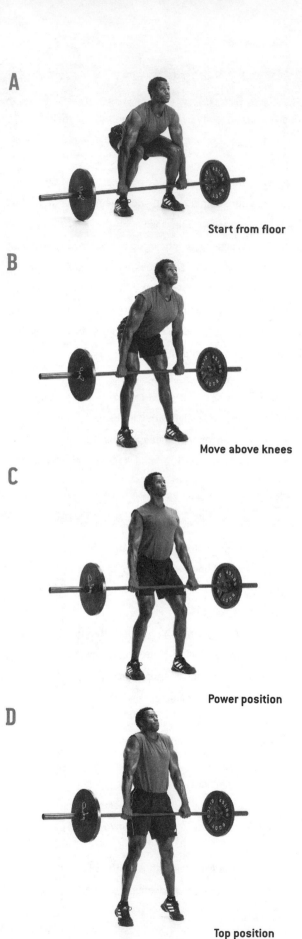

A

Start from floor

B

Move above knees

C

Power position

D

Top position

DO IT HARDER

- Power clean the weight to the rack position.
- Hold the top position for a 3-count, without falling forward or backward.
- To increase resistance, attach tubing to the barbell (either in the center or on each end) and a low stationary object.

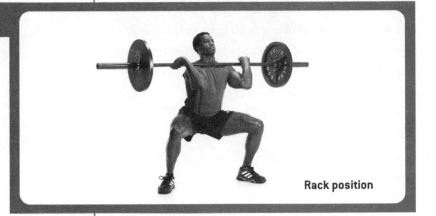

Rack position

BARBELL DUCK SQUAT

This unique exercise works the gluteal (butt), adductor (inner thigh), and quadriceps (front thigh) muscles at angles that are different from any other exercise.

A Stand with your feet more than shoulder width apart, your toes pointing out. Unrack a barbell behind your neck resting on your traps. Your chest should be out, your shoulders back, and abs tight, and back straight. Keep your head in line with your spine and look straight ahead. There will be a forward lean to your body.

B Squat as low as you can without rounding your lower or upper back. Don't bounce and don't let your knees turn in. Hold for a second. Then, keeping your feet flat on the floor and driving through your heels, rise with your hips slightly forward and your abs tight.

MAKE IT EASIER

- Don't squat as low.
- Perform bench squats. Squat until your butt hits a bench.
- Wear lifting shoes with a heel. It makes squatting easier.

DO IT HARDER

- Hook exercise tubing under your feet and hold it in your hand while squatting, along with the dumbbell. It increases tension as you ascend.

A

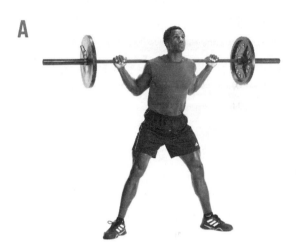

B

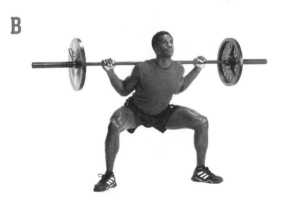

TWO-HAND DUMBBELL CLEAN

This exercise improves your grip strength and makes your legs, hips, and lower back more powerful. The initial position is similar to a deadlift, except that you use a hook grip and position heavy dumbbells in front of your feet.

A Stand with your feet shoulder width apart, with two dumbbells on the floor in front of you. Keeping your back straight, your head up, and your shoulders directly over or a little ahead of the dumbbells, squat down and grab the dumbbells with your arms extended and positioned just outside your knees.

B Do not let your hips kick up past your shoulders at the start from the floor. Pull the dumbbells past your knees to the lower third of the thigh.

C Move your knees and hips forward.

D, E Extend explosively into a top shrug position just before you shuffle your feet laterally and go into a half-squat position to catch the dumbbells.

If you fall forward or backward, you're not pulling in a straight line. Alternate arms every rep.

MAKE IT EASIER

- Use wrist straps, looping them over the hands and dumbbells.
- Pull dumbbells off blocks set above knee height.
- Initially, move the dumbbells slowly, so that you hit the optimal mechanical positions. As your technique improves, increase the speed.

A

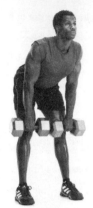

Start from floor

B

Move above knees

C

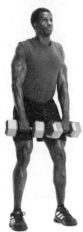

Power position

D

Top position

E

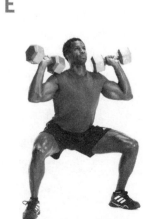

Rack position

DO IT HARDER

- Use two heavier dumbbells and perform a two-hand dumbbell power shrug from the floor. Set up the dumbbells outside of each leg and extend upward as fast as you can (using good technique).
- Clean only one dumbbell at a time.
- If dumbbells get too easy, use a 7-foot barbell. See power clean (page 199).

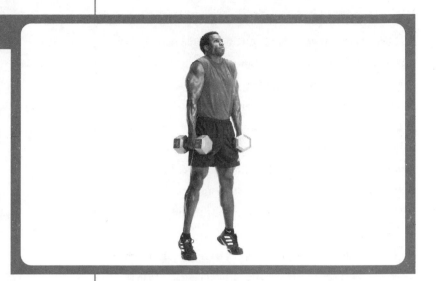

HOW TO ENHANCE HIP MOBILITY

Have you ever watched a guy pick something up? Chances are, he bends at the waist with his legs straight, hardly even bending the knees. If you do this long enough, your hips will get progressively tighter. Then, when you really need them to move, they don't.

Movement in the hips is called mobility. This refers to the normal range of motion you have in the hip joint. For some men, though, "normal" becomes a pretty sorry sight. Whatever your current range of motion, it's not a prison sentence. There are a number of ways to increase hip mobility, prevent injury, and, while you're at it, improve your lifting techniques.

- Beware of "gluteal amnesia." A colleague of mine, Alwyn Cosgrove, came up with this term to describe men who don't really know how to contract, or "fire," their glutes. When working on hip extension exercises, start out doing the movement a little slower than usual. Focus on squeezing the glutes. Your butt should be so tight you could hold a piece of paper between the cheeks. This move helps open up the front part of the hips, where men are usually tight.

- Most men have stronger external rotators compared to their internal rotators. Watch the average man walk. Do his feet point in or out? Most of the time they point out. This subtle little imbalance in the hip musculature creates forces that pull on the body and can eventually cause problems in the hip, ankle, or knee joints. To get back in balance, use a stretch band or tubing that pulls against the weak muscle. For example, if your internal rotators are weak, set up a stretch band that pulls the knee out while you're doing a stationary lunge. It will force you to activate more of the muscles on the medial side and strengthen the weak muscles around your hip.

- Tight or weak adductors? Try this little strategy on for size. Set up in front of a power rack or other fixed object. Move both feet sideways as far as you can comfortably go. Hold the position for a 5-count, while you rotate your weight from the outside to the inside of the foot, trying to lift your body up. Relax, then do it again. Repeat a few times. Doing this movement will help increase strength and mobility in hip adduction. It works quickly, too. Use the rack for support in case you have balance problems, or need help to come out of the position.

ONE-ARM DUMBBELL SNATCH

This exercise improves your grip strength and makes your legs, hips, and lower back more powerful. The initial position is similar to a deadlift, except that you use a hook grip and position a heavy dumbbell between your feet.

A Stand with your feet shoulder width apart, with a dumbbell on the floor in front of you. Keeping your back straight, your head up, and your shoulders directly over or a little ahead of the dumbbell, squat down and grab the dumbbell with your right arm extended and positioned just inside your right knee.

B Do not let your hips kick up past your shoulders at the start from the floor. Pull the dumbbell past your knees to the lower third of the thigh.

C Move your knees and hips forward.

D Extend explosively into a top shrug position just before you shuffle your feet laterally.

E Receive the dumbbell in a half-squat position. If you fall forward or backward, you're not pulling in a straight line. Alternate arms every rep.

MAKE IT EASIER

- Use a wrist strap, looping it over the hand and dumbbell.
- Pull the dumbbell off blocks set above knee height.
- Initially, move the dumbbell slowly, so that you hit the optimal mechanical positions. As your technique improves, increase the speed.

DO IT HARDER

- Stand on a platform so that you have to pull the dumbbell up farther.
- Set up two dumbbells 10 feet apart. Clean one dumbbell, put it back down, shuffle laterally to the other dumbbell, and clean it. Repeat for the desired reps.
- Use a 7-foot barbell. See power snatch (page 211).

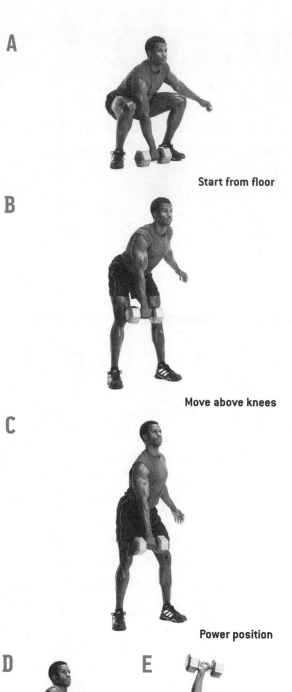

A Start from floor

B Move above knees

C Power position

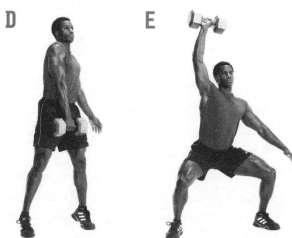

D Top position

E Rack position

ALTERNATING LUNGE

This dynamic exercise builds strength and coordination while working the quadriceps (front thigh), hamstring (back thigh), gluteal (butt), and hip flexor (front hip) muscles.

A Stand with your feet shoulder width apart and your hands at your sides. Keep your upper body upright and your head in line with your spine.

B Take a long step forward with your left foot. Plant your left foot firmly on the floor and bend your knee until your left thigh is parallel to the floor. Don't let your left knee extend past your left foot. Your right leg should be extended behind you, the knee slightly bent, and the heel raised. Immediately step back with your left foot, pressing your right heel to the floor. Your feet should be shoulder width apart. Repeat the exercise with your right foot. You have now completed 1 repetition.

MAKE IT EASIER

- Don't bend your front knee as far.
- Take a smaller step forward.
- Perform body-weight squats with both legs. (Follow directions for the Barbell Squat on page 220, without the barbell.)

DO IT HARDER

- Hold a dumbbell in each hand at your sides.
- Place the front foot on a platform.
- Hold a barbell for extra resistance (set up as if you're doing a squat).

A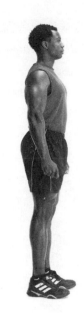

B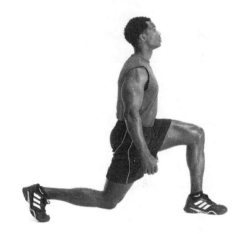

LATERAL LUNGE

This lunge strengthens the adductor (inner thigh), abductor (outer thigh), hamstring (back thigh), and gluteal (butt) muscles. It improves lateral movement for activities such as tennis, volleyball, and even dancing.

A Stand with your feet slightly more than shoulder width apart and your hands at your sides. Keep your knees unlocked, your toes pointing out slightly, chest out, shoulders back, stomach tight, and back straight. Your head should be in line with your spine.

B Step to your left. Landing heel to toe, press your hips down until your left thigh is parallel to the floor. Your left foot should point to the side; don't let your left knee extend past your toes. Keep your right leg extended, and your right foot planted firmly on the floor, pointing forward. Your torso should face the front. Hold for a second, then push with your left leg and return to the starting position. Lunge to the left until you complete 1 set, then switch sides.

MAKE IT EASIER

- Don't lunge as deeply.
- Take a smaller step.
- Perform body-weight squats with both legs. (Follow directions for the Barbell Squat on page 220, without the barbell.)

DO IT HARDER

- Hold a dumbbell in each hand at your sides.
- Place the lunging foot on a platform.
- Hold a barbell for extra resistance (set up as if you're doing a squat).

A

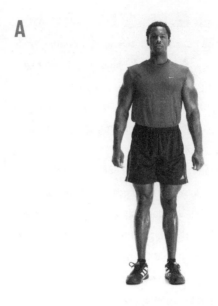

B

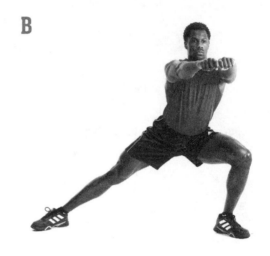

STATIONARY LUNGE/ SPLIT SQUAT

This is an excellent exercise that works the gluteal (butt), quadriceps (front thigh), and hamstring (back thigh) muscles.

A Stand with your head in line with your spine, your back straight, and your feet shoulder width apart. Place your hands on your hips.

B Take a long step forward with your left foot. Bend your leg until your left thigh is parallel to the floor. Your right leg should extend back, with your right knee slightly bent and almost touching the floor. Hold this position for a second. Keep your left foot stationary as you slowly straighten your left leg. Continue bending and straightening your leg until you finish the set, then switch legs.

MAKE IT EASIER

- Don't bend your front knee as far.
- Take a smaller step.
- Perform body-weight squats with both legs instead. (Follow directions for the Barbell Squat on page 220, without the barbell.)

DO IT HARDER

- Hold a dumbbell in each hand at your sides.
- Place the front foot on a platform.
- Hold a barbell for extra resistance (set up as if you're doing a squat).

A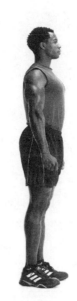

B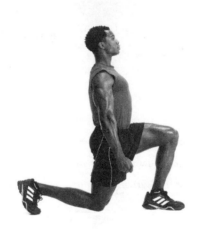

WALKING LUNGE

This is an excellent exercise that works the gluteal (butt), quadriceps (front thigh), hamstring (back thigh), and calf muscles.

A Stand with your head in line with your spine, your back straight, your feet shoulder width apart, and your hands at your sides.

B Take a long step forward with your right foot. Bend your leg until your right thigh is parallel to the floor. Your left leg should extend back, with your left knee slightly bent and almost touching the floor. Your step should be long enough so that your back leg becomes almost straight.

C From this position, push off of your front foot (right), raise your back leg (left), and step forward with it, so that it becomes the lead leg (left now in front). Continue lunging in this fashion until you reach the predetermined point that you planned on "walking" to.

MAKE IT EASIER
- Don't bend your front knee as far.
- Take a smaller step.
- Perform body-weight squats with both legs. (Follow directions for the Barbell Squat on page 220, without the barbell.)

DO IT HARDER
- Hold a dumbbell in each hand at your sides.
- Place your front foot on a platform.
- Use a barbell for extra resistance (set up as if you're doing a squat).

DOUBLE LEG SUPINE HIP LIFT ON FLOOR

This exercise strengthens the hamstrings (back of thigh), gluteal (butt), lower back, and abdominal muscles.

A Lie on your back on the floor. Bend your knees, placing your feet close to your buttocks, hip width apart. Your arms should be alongside your torso, palms down.

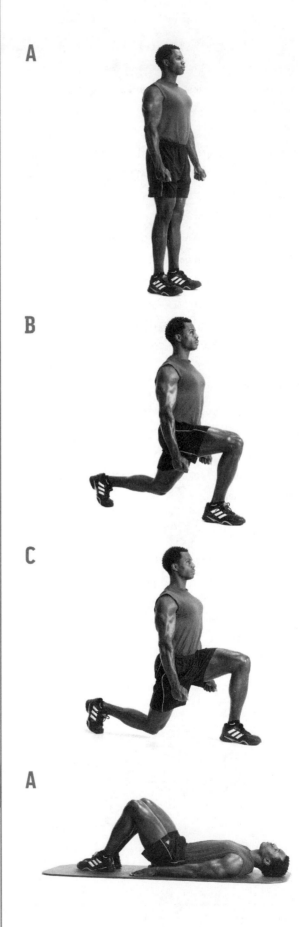

A

B

C

A

B Lift your hips up toward the ceiling. Keep your knees over your ankles and your shoulders on the floor. Hold for a second, lower, and repeat.

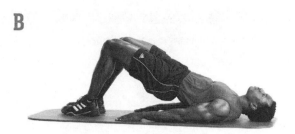

B

MAKE IT EASIER

- Don't bring your heels as far back toward your butt.
- Spread your arms out for more support.
- Don't lift your hips as high.

DO IT HARDER

- Place your feet on a platform or stability ball.
- Hold a weight plate on your torso.
- Use one leg, either on the floor, on a platform, or on a stability ball.

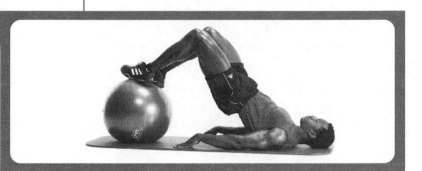

NO KIDDING?

HOW IMPORTANT ARE PELVIC TILTS?

Trainers often advise men to tilt the pelvis one way or the other to maximize the effects of an exercise. They talk so much about it that you'd think they'd know how to give you the level of practical detail that would actually, you know, let you *do* it.

Don't hold your breath waiting for clear answers. It's true that the pelvis can move either forward (anterior pelvic tilt) or backward (posterior tilt). It does make sense to tilt the pelvis backward or forward, depending on the exercise, because it can marginally reduce spinal pressures. For example, a posterior tilt, in which you press your lower back to the floor, is good for ab workouts. An anterior tilt helps maintain an arch in the spine when doing deadlifts.

This all seems to make sense—until you realize that the pelvis never stays in one spot. The tilt changes throughout a lifting movement. In other words, even though some pelvis positions are correct in theory, it's impossible to maintain them when you're actually moving.

Don't worry about pelvic tilts. To keep things simple, focus on maintaining a flat back when doing hip exercises, such as squats or deadlifts. It's not a bad approach when doing ab workouts as well. That's all you have to do to help avoid excessive strain on the hip or spinal ligaments or muscles.

ROMANIAN DEADLIFT

This all-purpose exercise strengthens the back, arms, shoulders, and legs. Use less weight than you would for a regular deadlift.

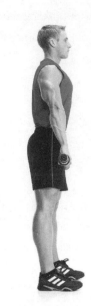

A Hold a lightly weighted barbell at mid-thigh level, with your hands farther than shoulder width apart, your palms facing your body. Keep the barbell against your legs with your arms fully extended, your back straight, shoulders back, and chest out. Pause for a second.

B Slowly bend over from the hips, keeping the bar close to your thighs. Your back should stay straight, with your knees slightly bent. Lower the bar slowly toward the floor, going as far as you comfortably can. With a slow, controlled movement, keeping your back straight, return to the starting position.

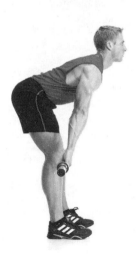

MAKE IT EASIER

- Use wrist straps.
- Pull the bar off blocks set above knee height.
- Initially, move the bar slowly, so that you hit the optimal mechanical positions. As your technique improves, increase the speed.

DO IT HARDER

- Stand on a platform so that you have to pull the bar farther.
- Perform the movement using only one leg. This is very difficult, so reduce the weight by 60 percent to 70 percent.
- Attach tubing to the barbell, either in the center or on each end, and to a stationary object that's low to the ground.

HIP PAIN ISN'T ALWAYS WHAT YOU THINK

If you're doing serious hip and glute work, sooner or later you'll probably wake up one day with a killer ache in the hip. Your doctor will tell you you've strained some muscle you've never heard of and advise you to take it easy. Maybe you do, maybe you don't. The pain gets a little better, but it never goes away. So you do the usual guy thing and ignore it.

Bad choice. Your joints shouldn't make noises and they shouldn't ache. Nor does the problem always originate where the pain is.

A lot of men who complain about hip pain, for example, actually have flat fleet. The excessive ankle motion caused by flat feet generates extra torque on the knee, which transfers more torque to the hip. Over time, the body adapts to the extra forces by strengthening one side of the hip relative to the other. In other words, you get increasingly im-balanced, due to an uneven distribution of forces along the "kinetic chain."

Unless you recognize what's happening, sooner or later something will give—and that something might be your hip. See your doctor. If he or she can't give you a clear answer, make an appointment to see a sports physician. Don't ignore any joint pain. If you do, it will almost always get worse.

SNATCH PULL

This exercise improves your grip strength and makes your legs, hips, and lower back more powerful. The initial position is similar to a deadlift, except that you use a hook grip and keep your hips lower.

A Stand with your feet shoulder width apart, with a barbell on the floor in front of you. The bar should be over your feet and close to your shins. Keeping your back straight, your head up, and your shoulders directly over or a little ahead of the bar, squat down and grip the bar with your arms extended and positioned just outside your knees.

B Do not let your hips kick up past your shoulders at the start from the floor. Pull the bar past your knees to the lower third of your thighs.

C Move your knees and hips forward.

D Extend explosively into a top shrug position. You should be able to hold the top position, with your ankles, knees, and hips fully extended. If you fall forward or backward, you're not pulling in a straight line.

MAKE IT EASIER

- Use wrist straps.
- Pull the bar off blocks set above knee height.
- Initially, move the bar slowly, so that you hit the optimal mechanical positions. As your technique improves, increase the speed.

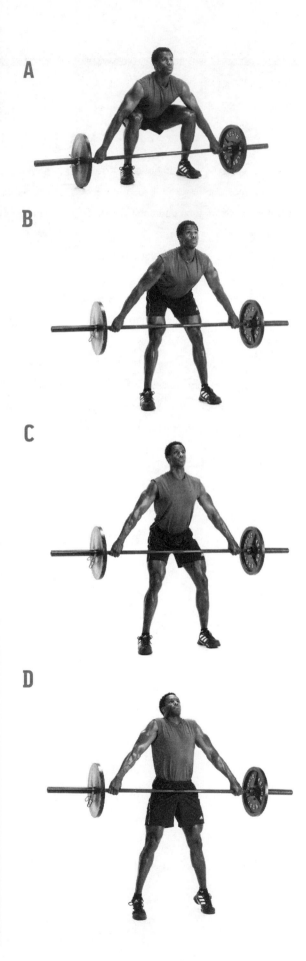

A

B

C

D

- Perform a power snatch.
- Hold the top position for a 3-count, without falling forward or backward.
- Attach tubing to the barbell, either in the center or on each end, and to a stationary object that's low to the ground.

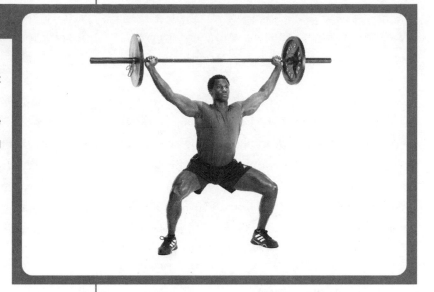

LEVEL 1 (FOCUS ON SIZE)

We've provided three different workouts for Level 1. Workout variations mean more strength and size—and less boredom.

One option is to do all three workouts weekly. For example, do Workout #1 on Monday, Workout #2 on Wednesday, and Workout #3 on Friday. If you choose this option, do 2 warmup sets for the first exercise, followed by 3 sets of 6 repetitions using "real" weight. Next, do 3 sets of 10 reps for the second exercise, followed by 3 sets of 14 reps for the third exercise. Do only 1 set of the last exercise, going for maximum reps.

Another option is to do just one of the workouts, three times a week. Vary the rep count daily. On Monday, for example, do 3 sets of 6 reps for the first three exercises; on Wednesday, do 3 sets of 10 reps for the first three exercises; and on Friday, do 3 sets of 14 reps for the first three exercises. Always start with 2 warmup sets for the first exercise (these don't go toward the final "count"). Do only 1 set of the last exercise, going for maximum reps.

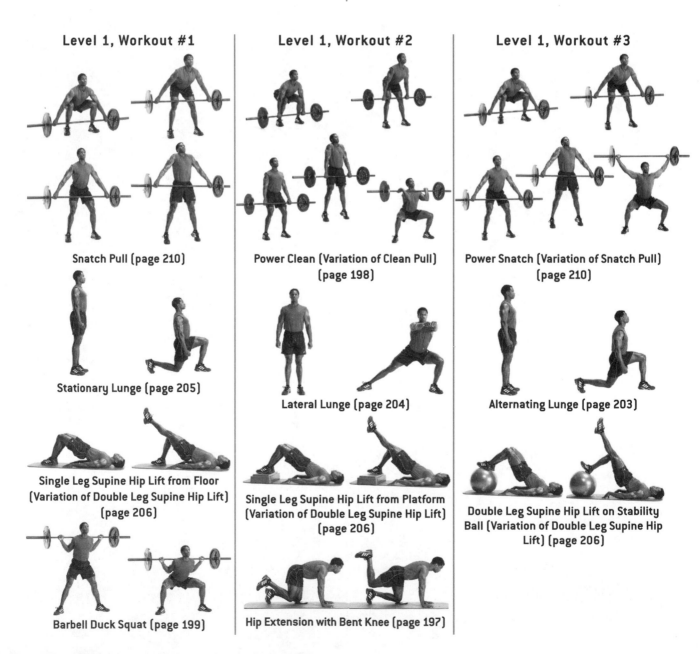

Level 1, Workout #1

Snatch Pull (page 210)

Stationary Lunge (page 205)

Single Leg Supine Hip Lift from Floor (Variation of Double Leg Supine Hip Lift) (page 206)

Barbell Duck Squat (page 199)

Level 1, Workout #2

Power Clean (Variation of Clean Pull) (page 198)

Lateral Lunge (page 204)

Single Leg Supine Hip Lift from Platform (Variation of Double Leg Supine Hip Lift) (page 206)

Hip Extension with Bent Knee (page 197)

Level 1, Workout #3

Power Snatch (Variation of Snatch Pull) (page 210)

Alternating Lunge (page 203)

Double Leg Supine Hip Lift on Stability Ball (Variation of Double Leg Supine Hip Lift) (page 206)

LEVEL 2 (FOCUS ON STRENGTH)

Level 2, Workout #1
Max Romanian Deadlift (RDL) Routine

It's possible to increase your Romanian Deadlift (rDL) load by more than 60 pounds in less than 10 weeks by following this routine. You only have to do it twice a week—a "light" day and a "heavy" day. First, determine your 1 repetition maximum (1RM) for the Romanian Deadlift. (See page 14.) Then use the chart below to determine your Romanian Deadlift weight for a given workout. Round the weights to the nearest 5 pounds.

To stay limber (and safe), start each workout with two 5-rep warmup sets, using 50 percent and 70 percent of your 1RM. After you've done all your sets and reps of your Romanian Deadlift, complete the workout with the addtional exercises on the following page.

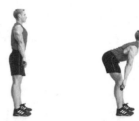

Romanian Deadlift (page 208)

Level 2, Workout #1, Romanian Deadlift Cycle

WEEK	DAY	% 1RM	#SETS	#REPS
1	1	80	6	2
1	2	80	6	3
2	1	80	6	2
2	2	80	6	4
3	1	80	6	2
3	2	80	6	5
4	1	80	6	2
4	2	80	6	6
5	1	80	6	2
5	2	85	5	5
6	1	80	6	2
6	2	90	4	4
7	1	80	6	2
7	2	95	3	3
8	1	80	6	2
8	2	100	2	2
9	1	80	6	2
9	2	105	2	1 *

*AFTER THE 2 SETS AT TOP WEIGHT, KEEP DOING SINGLES WITH 2 MINUTES' REST BETWEEN SETS, INCREASING THE WEIGHT 5 TO 10 POUNDS EACH TIME, UNTIL YOU FIND YOUR NEW 1RM.

ADDITIONAL EXERCISES FOR WORKOUT #1, DAY 1

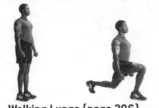

Walking Lunge (page 206)

Do 2 to 3 sets with 8 to 10 reps per set.

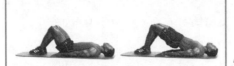

Double Leg Supine Hip Lift on Floor (page 206)

Do 2 to 3 sets with 8 to 10 reps per set.

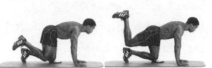

Hip Extension with Bent Knee (page 197)

Do 1 set with maximum reps.

ADDITIONAL EXERCISES FOR WORKOUT #1, DAY 2

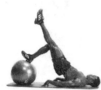

Single Leg Supine Hip Lift on Stability Ball (Variation of Double Leg Supine Hip Lift) (page 207)

Do 2 to 3 sets with 4 to 6 reps per set.

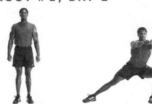

Lateral Lunge (page 204)

Do 2 to 3 sets with 4 to 6 reps per set.

Alternating Lunge (page 203)

Do 1 set with maximum reps.

Level 2, Workout #2

Do this three times a week. Do two warmup sets per exercise. Vary the reps on successive days. For example, do 1 set of 3 reps on Monday, 1 set of 11 reps on Wednesday, and 1 set of 7 reps on Friday. Each week, add 1 set to each exercise until you're up to 5 sets. For excessive soreness, reduce the sets per exercise.

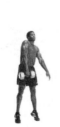

One-Arm Dumbbell Clean (page 202)

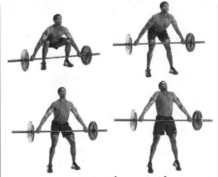

Snatch Pull (page 210)

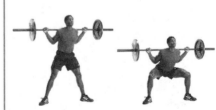

Barbell Duck Squat (page 199)

Level 2, Workout #3

Do this three times a week. Do 2 warmup sets per exercise. For excessive soreness, reduce the sets per exercise.

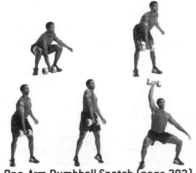

One-Arm Dumbbell Snatch (page 202)

Do 2 to 3 sets of 3 reps.

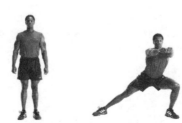

Lateral Lunge (page 204)

Do 2 to 3 sets with 7 reps per set.

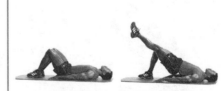

Single Leg Supine Hip Lift from Floor (Variation of Double Leg Supine Hip Lift) (page 207)

LEVEL 3 (HYBRID TRAINING—FOCUS ON SIZE AND STRENGTH)

Option A

- Perform all three workouts in a single week. For example, do Workout #1 on Monday, Workout #2 on Wednesday, and Workout #3 on Friday.

- After a general warmup, do 2 warmup sets for the first exercise, lifting lighter-than-usual weights.

- Do 5 sets of 2 reps for the first exercise.

- Next, do 2 sets of 6 reps for the second exercise.

- Do 2 sets of 12 reps for the third exercise.

Option B

- Stick with one workout all week.

- After a general warmup, do 2 warmup sets for the first exercise, lifting lighter-than-usual weights.

- Vary the rep count on each day. For example, do 3 sets of 2 reps for the first three exercises on Monday. On Wednesday, do 3 sets of 6 reps for the first three exercises. On Friday, do 3 sets of 12 reps for the first three exercises.

Level 3, Workout #1

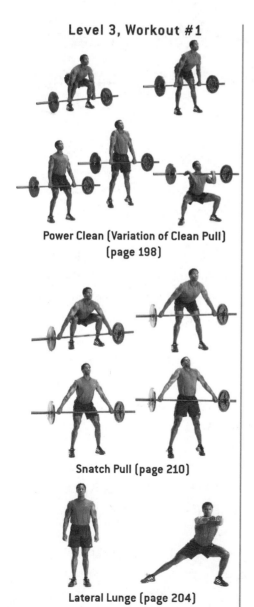

Power Clean (Variation of Clean Pull) (page 198)

Snatch Pull (page 210)

Lateral Lunge (page 204)

Level 3, Workout #2

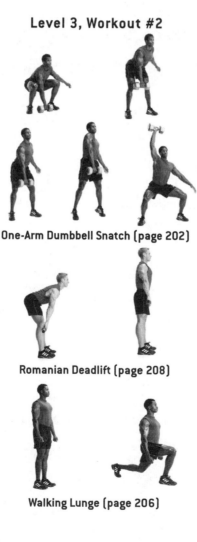

One-Arm Dumbbell Snatch (page 202)

Romanian Deadlift (page 208)

Walking Lunge (page 206)

Level 3, Workout #3

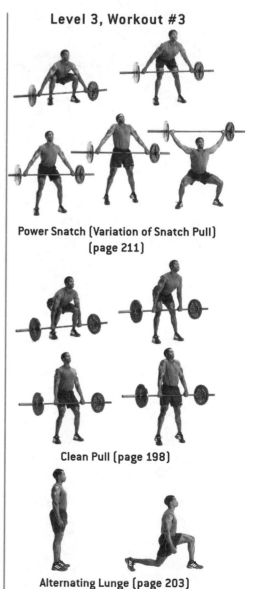

Power Snatch (Variation of Snatch Pull) (page 211)

Clean Pull (page 198)

Alternating Lunge (page 203)

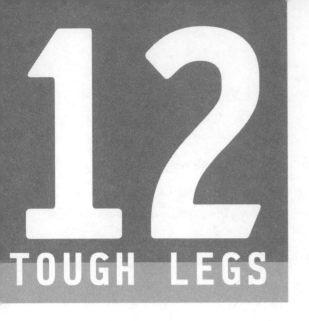

12

TOUGH LEGS

he legs of a well-built man make up about 60 percent of his total muscle mass. Those legs can generate tremendous force—force for better sports performance and more endurance. Not to mention just getting around better.

If you're trying to lose weight, or keep from gaining it, leg workouts are a good investment because all of that muscle mass acts like a calorie furnace. Strong legs also make your physique look more complete. Nothing looks sillier than a guy with a massive upper body standing on pencil legs.

Yet you see that look a lot in the gym. Leg exercises are hard work, so it's easy to understand why a lot of men put them off until the end of the workout—and then "forget" them.

Don't make the same mistake. If you want to get in optimal shape, you can't neglect the legs.

We'll talk about all sorts of leg exercises in the coming pages. Keep in mind, though, that the legs consist of very different (and almost independent) muscle groups. Exercises that work the thighs or hamstrings won't have much effect on the calves. To make things easy, we've divided the workouts and workout tips into the main muscle groups: the quadriceps (thighs), hamstrings (back of the thigh), and the calves. Also keep in mind that many of the back and hip exercises also work the legs in a variety of ways. For complete leg training, those exercises should be incorporated as well.

QUADRICEPS EXPLAINED

The quadriceps is a group of four muscles on the anterior (front) of the thigh. The four muscles are the vastus medialis, vastus intermedius, vastus lateralis, and rectus femoris. The first three attach to the front of the tibia and originate at the top of the femur. The rectus femoris crosses the hip joint and originates on the pelvis.

The primary function of the quadriceps is to extend (straighten) the knee joint. The rectus femoris also extends the knee, and because it crosses the hip joint, it flexes the hips.

THE TOTAL QUAD WORKOUT

Exercises that work the quadriceps are all movements that require you to straighten the legs against resistance. This includes all varieties of leg presses, squats, and lunges. In general, you can recruit more muscle fibers and build size faster with free weights. However, leg extensions are more effective when you use machines.

Watch your toe position. Leg extensions are a good exercise for building muscle on the outer part of the thigh. But you have to watch your form. Turning the toes in or pointing them straight ahead maximizes the use of the vastus lateralis muscle. Turning the toes out makes leg extensions less effective for working this particular muscle. However, a good training program will include each of these options. Changing your toe position hits muscle fibers from a lot of different angles.

Work the inner thigh. The best exercise for building the vastus medialis is the front squat. Follow this exercise with leg extensions with the toes out or pointed straight ahead.

Don't forget the middle. The best exercises for building the rectus femoris in the middle of the thigh are leg extensions with toes straight or turned out, hack squats, and front squats.

Save the belt for tough lifting. The job of the muscles around the spine is to hold it stable. Wearing a weight belt can rob these muscles of the stress they need to grow. Yet wearing a belt can help you lift more weight, which you need for greater size and strength. What's the compromise? Warm up and perform light sets without a belt. Only put it on when you're lifting your top weights of the day. As you get stronger, you'll find you're able to lift progressively heavier weights without the belt.

Lose the knee wraps. A lot of serious lifters wrap their knees when doing squats or presses. The rationale is that wrapping helps protect the joints. Not true. Wearing a knee wrap will enable you to lift heavier weights, which creates *more* compressive force on the joint. That's not a bad thing. Force is what pushes muscles to grow. The problem with wearing a wrap is that it prevents knee tendons and ligaments from getting their share out of the work. That can impede your progress, not move it forward. Unless you're competing on the weight circuit, don't bother with knee wraps.

Don't pre-exhaust the quads. Search through your dad's old lifting magazines and you'll probably come across a lot of articles on pre-exhaustion training. This is when you follow one exercise with another exercise for the same muscles. For example,

LEGS WORKOUT CHECKLIST

No matter which of the three main leg muscle groups you're working, remember the following:

- When doing body-weight exercises, always start with two-leg movement patterns. Then progress to one leg when you can do all your reps with good form.

- Don't bounce weights. Lower weight slowly with full control. Lift weight with a little more speed.

- Take advantage of safety racks—and use a spotter when possible. The exception is when doing barbell deadlifts or barbell rows: Don't depend on a spotter; instead, do as many reps as you can with good form, then stop.

- Before lifting heavy weights, perform a full-body warmup, followed by a dynamic warmup, followed by an exercise-specific warmup.

trainers used to recommend doing an isolation movement, such as leg extensions, followed by a compound movement, such as a leg press. Research has shown that this actually reduces the amount of weight you can lift, as well as the level of muscle activation. That's the opposite of what any serious lifter wants. You'll be better off alternating exercises that work *opposing* muscle groups—for example, the quads first, followed by the hamstrings.

Be careful with the Smith machine. It's an effective device for leg training when you're doing squats, but it also robs you of the benefits of balance training. There's something to be said for keeping a wobbly bar steady using nothing but your own muscles.

Besides, it's common for men using the Smith machine to set up with their feet too far forward. This causes them to round their lower backs in the bottom position, which places a lot of stress on the spine. This might explain why squats done using a Smith machine have one of the highest injury rates of any exercise.

Plant your butt. It's tempting to lift your butt off the seat when doing leg presses—especially if you're pushing more weight than your legs are prepared to handle. Don't do it. For one thing,

raising the butt robs the legs of some of the benefits. Worse, it puts a lot of stress on the lower back.

Go for motion over weight. Don't be the weight-room fool who loads up the leg press with a ton of iron and then only moves it a few inches. This does very little to work the quads. Instead, drop the weight to the point that you can still complete a full range of motion.

Watch those angles. When doing any leg exercise, be careful that the hip, knee, and ankle line up in the same plane. Some guys get sloppy and let their knees move in or out relative to their ankle joints. This creates excessive stress on the knee and can lead to all sorts of problems. Can you say "surgery"?

While you're thinking about form, get in the habit of keeping the lower back flattened and arched while you lift. It should never be rounded when you're doing leg exercises.

Check your strength ratio. Your quads should *always* be stronger than your hamstrings. If they're not, there's something wrong with your workout. Make sure that you balance knee extension and knee flexion movements. In general, plan on doing at least the same volume, or maybe a little more, for the quads as you do for the hamstrings.

BARBELL HACK SQUAT

This squat puts relatively little pressure on the knees and lower back. It strengthens the knees, hamstrings (back of thigh), quadriceps (front of thigh), and gluteal (butt) muscles.

A With your feet hip width apart, stand with a barbell placed directly behind your heels. Squat down and grip the bar with your palms facing away from your body. Your hands should be slightly more than shoulder width apart. Stand up, holding the bar at arm's length behind your thighs. Keep your head in line with your body.

A

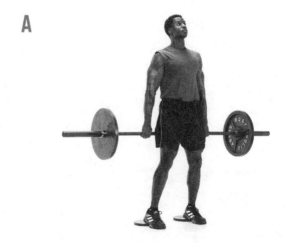

B Squat down until your thighs are close to parallel with the floor. Do not allow your knees to extend over your toes. Hold for a second, then rise, keeping your arms fully extended.

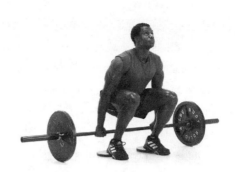

B

MAKE IT EASIER

- Use dumbbells instead of a bar.
- Use a Smith machine.
- Don't squat down as far.

DO IT HARDER

- Stand on the balls of your feet.
- Stand on a platform so that the plates go below your feet as you squat down.
- Add bands or heavy chains to the bar so that it gets heavier as you squat up.

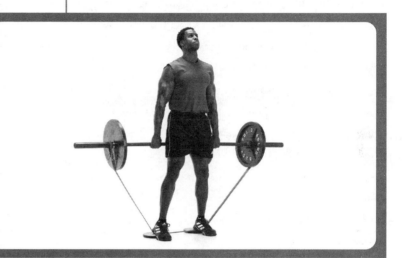

NO KIDDING?

DOES STANCE AFFECT SQUATS?

Altering foot position is often recommended for isolating various muscles. This is true for a lot of workouts, but it doesn't seem to make much of a difference with squats.

More than a few trainers are convinced that a wide-stance squat works the hips more, while a close-stance squat works more of the quads. If this were true, you'd expect to find greater muscle activity in the rectus femoris, vastus medialis, and vastus lateralis when standing with the feet closer, and greater adductor activity with the feet wider.

A wide stance does increase adductor, glute, and hamstring activation. A narrow stance, however, has little or no extra effects on the quads.

If you want your quads to grow, you have to lift heavy. Changing your squat stance won't make much of a difference. If you want to build the medial thigh and buttocks, a slightly wider stance might make a difference.

BARBELL SQUAT

This exercise essentially provides a whole-body workout. It strengthens the quadriceps (front thigh), gluteal (butt), and hamstring (back thigh) muscles, along with the shoulders, back, and arms.

A Place a barbell at shoulder level on a squat rack. Grip the bar with your hands slightly farther than shoulder width apart, palms facing forward. Step under the bar so that it is positioned evenly across your upper back and shoulders. Stand upright, with your feet hip width apart, toes pointing slightly out. Don't drop your head; it should be in line with your torso, with your eyes looking ahead.

B Keeping your feet flat and your torso straight, bend your knees slightly and squat down under control. Don't round your back or let your knees extend past your toes. Squat until your thighs are almost parallel with the floor. Pause, then rise to the starting position.

MAKE IT EASIER

- Use dumbbells instead of a bar.
- Use a Smith machine.
- Only squat down until your hips touch a padded bench.

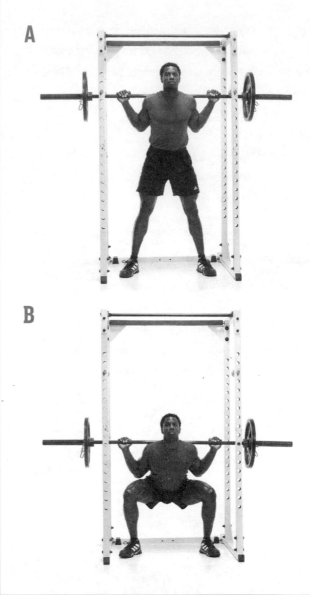

A

B

DO IT HARDER

- Stand on the balls of your feet.
- Squat down below parallel.
- Add bands or heavy chains to the bar so that it gets heavier as you squat up.
- Attach bands to top of rack by looping one end through the other end around the frame and pulling tight. Attach the open end onto the bar by pulling down on the band and forcing the open end onto the barbell. Squat as described above and shown at right. This makes the weight lighter as you squat deeper.

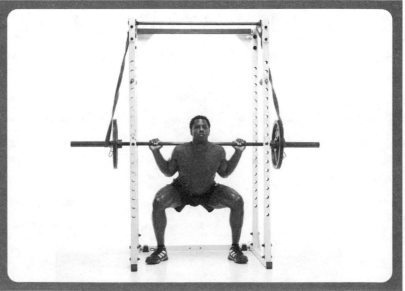

STEPUP

This is a good dual-purpose exercise. It provides an aerobic workout while increasing strength and flexibility. It works the quadriceps (front thigh), gluteal (butt), hamstring (back thigh), hip flexor (front hip), and adductor (inner thigh) muscles.

A Stand upright about a foot away from a sturdy box, platform, or bench that is 12 to 18 inches high. Keeping your upper body straight, step forward with your left foot, placing it on the center of the bench.

B Complete the step by bringing your right foot next to your left. Step backward with your right foot and use your left leg to lower your body. Step down with your left foot to bring it back to the starting position. Repeat the steps, this time leading with the right foot.

MAKE IT EASIER

- Use a lower step.
- Hold on to a stationary object like a power rack for support.

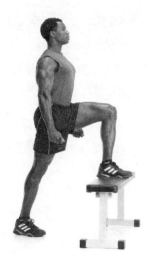

A

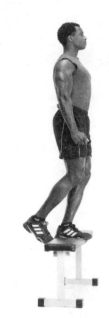

B

DO IT HARDER

- Set the step at knee height.
- Step up and down on one leg for all your reps, only allowing your free foot to lightly touch the floor.
- Step up on an air pad or other balance device.
- Hold a barbell behind your neck, with your hands slightly wider than shoulder width apart.
- Hold dumbbells at your sides.

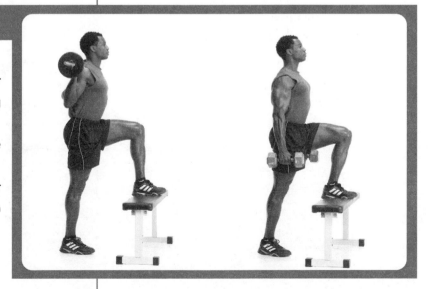

BULGARIAN SPLIT SQUAT

This exercise works the quadriceps (front thigh), gluteal (butt), and adductor (inner thigh) muscles. An alternate method is to perform the movement holding a dumbbell in each hand.

A Stand about 3 feet in front of a bench. Place your left foot behind you on the bench so that only your instep is resting on it.

B Lower your body until your right knee is bent 90 degrees and your left knee nearly touches the floor. Your right lower leg should be perpendicular to the floor and your torso should remain upright. Push yourself back to the starting position as quickly as you can. Finish all of your repetitions, then repeat the lift, this time with your right foot resting on the bench while your left leg does the work.

MAKE IT EASIER

- Use resistance tubing instead. Attach it to a low stationary object under or behind you and hold the ends of the tubing with your hands. Perform the exercise as described above.
- Use a lower bench.

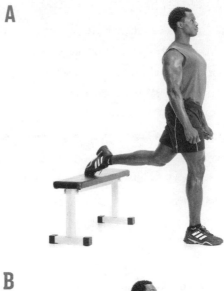

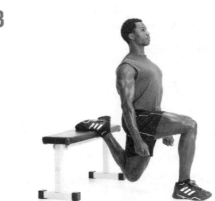

DO IT HARDER

- Stand on the ball of the front foot.
- Pause at the bottom position.
- Using an overhand grip, hold a barbell so that it rests comfortably on your upper back (not on your neck).
- Stand on an air pad or other balance device.

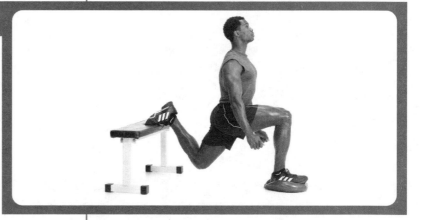

DUMBBELL SQUAT

This movement improves balance while strengthening the quadriceps (front thigh) and gluteal (butt) muscles.

A Grip the end of a dumbbell with both hands, with your thumbs around the bar and the weight resting on your palms. Your arms should be fully extended at your sides, palms in. Keep your feet hip width apart and your torso upright. Maintain a natural curve in your lower back.

B Keeping your torso straight, bend your knees and squat down until your thighs are parallel to the floor. Your heels may lift off the floor slightly as you roll onto the balls of the feet. Don't bounce. As you come up, squeeze your quadriceps and your butt muscles as much as you can.

MAKE IT EASIER

- Use resistance tubing instead. Attach it to a low stationary object behind you or stand on the tubing and hold the ends of the tubing with your hands. Perform the exercise as described above, or use a Smith machine.
- Don't squat down as far. Or squat down only until your hips touch a padded bench.

DO IT HARDER

- Stand on the balls of your feet.
- Squat down below parallel.
- Stand on a balance board or air pad.

A

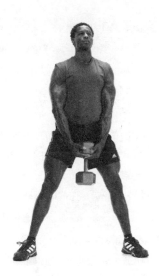

B

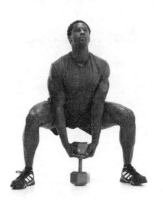

FRONT SQUAT

This move strengthens the quads, knees, hips, and lower back. It's a superb choice for preventing sports injuries. It's difficult to do, so use less weight than you would with a regular squat.

A   Place a barbell at midchest level on a squat rack. Walk in toward the bar until it rests on top of the front of your shoulders. Grip the bar with your hands slightly farther than shoulder width apart, palms facing in. Stand up straight, fully supporting the bar with your arms and shoulders; keep your elbows high. Take one step back from the rack. Your feet should be flat on the floor, about shoulder width apart. Keep your upper body straight, and your head in line with your spine.

B   Squat down until your thighs are parallel with the floor. Don't let your knees extend past your toes. Keep your torso straight, your eyes looking forward. Hold for a second, then rise to the starting position.

MAKE IT EASIER

- Use dumbbells or a Smith machine instead.
- Don't squat down as far. Or squat down only until your hips touch a padded bench.

A
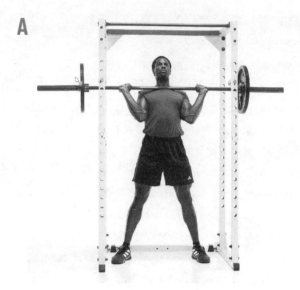

B
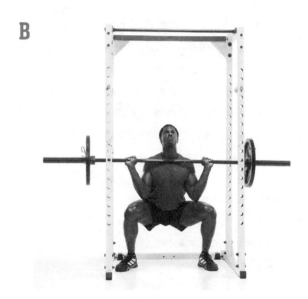

DO IT HARDER

- Stand on the balls of your feet.
- Squat down below parallel.
- Add bands or heavy chains to the bar so that it gets heavier as you squat up.
- Attach bands to a stationary object or heavy dumbbell and attach the other end to the bar.
- Attach bands to the top of a rack or heavy dumbbell and attach the other end to the bar.

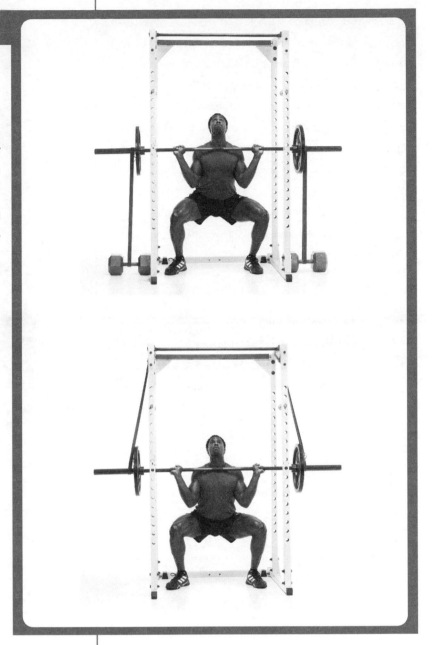

INCLINE LEG PRESS

This is a good choice for those with back problems or limited flexibility. It works the hamstring (back thigh), quadriceps (front thigh), and hip flexor (front hip) muscles.

A Sit in an incline leg press machine, making sure that the seat is adjusted so your hips are bent at a 90-degree angle or less. Place your feet shoulder width apart, toes turned out slightly. Grip the handlebars and press your lower back to the pad.

B Push forward on the foot plate to straighten your legs. Once you are set at the top position, lower the weight under control and return to the starting position.

MAKE IT EASIER

- Space your feet wider apart.
- Move your feet higher on the platform.
- Position your feet so that your knees are at a 90-degree angle and touch your chest when you come down all the way.

DO IT HARDER

- Use a staggered stance, with one foot higher than the other. Be sure to do the same number of sets with each foot forward.
- Position your feet so that your knees go past your chest in the bottom position.
- Use only one leg at a time.

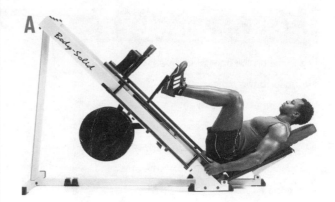

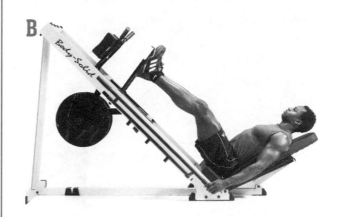

LATERAL BARBELL SQUAT

These squats will help keep your joints, tendons, and ligaments strong and agile. They work the quadriceps (front thigh), hip flexors (front hip), and two of the three gluteal (butt) muscles. They also work the tensor fascia latae, the band of muscles that runs down the side of the thigh.

A Stand up straight and hold a barbell evenly across your upper back and shoulders. Your hands should be slightly farther than shoulder width apart, palms facing forward. Place your feet in a wide stance, with your toes pointing forward. Your head should stay in line with your body.

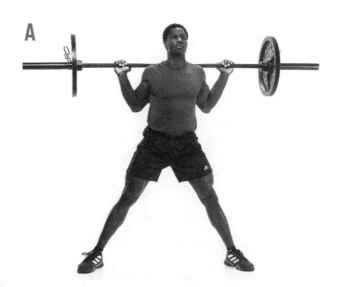

B Turn your left foot to the right as you bend your left knee in the direction of your toes. Keep going until your thigh is parallel to the floor. Your knee should be directly over your ankle. Don't let the knee turn in. Put most of your weight on your left leg, keeping your right leg extended and the knee slightly bent. Hold for a second, then return to the starting position by extending your left leg and bringing your torso up to center. Then, turn the right foot out and repeat on the right side. That makes 1 repetition.

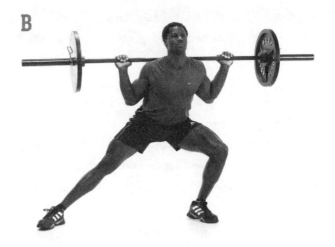

MAKE IT EASIER

- Use a medium-wide stance.
- Don't squat laterally as far.
- Squat down until your hips touch a padded bench.

DO IT HARDER

- Stand on the balls of your feet.
- Squat down below parallel.
- Add bands or heavy chains to the bar so that it gets heavier as you squat up.

POOR SQUAT FORM AND MENISCAL TEARS

The meniscus is a C-shaped piece of fibrocartilage in the outer part of the knee joint. Most of the meniscus has no blood supply, which means it doesn't readily heal from routine damage. As men get older, the meniscus naturally begins to degenerate, which makes it susceptible to tears.

Approximately 36 percent of all meniscal tears occur when people rise up from a squatting position—not just in the gym, but from *any* squat, such as when you're working in the yard or toasting wieners at a campfire.

As you'd expect, gym squats are especially risky because of the massive weights involved. You don't want to tear your meniscus. The usual treatment is surgery, 6 weeks of restricted activity, and possibly months before your knee really feels strong again.

Twisting movements of the knee are the main cause of meniscal tears. When you're coming out of a squat, don't twist or turn or let your knee move outward.

LATERAL STEPUP

This is an excellent exercise for building the hamstrings (back thigh), quadriceps (front thigh), and the gluteal (butt) muscles.

A Stand sideways to a bench. Step up laterally with the right foot onto the bench.

B Extend your right knee and pull up your left foot.

C Step down by extending your left leg toward the floor. Before all reps, change direction, and repeat on the other side.

MAKE IT EASIER

- Use a lower bench.
- Hold on to a stationary object like a power rack for support.

DO IT HARDER

- Perform as above using a barbell.
- Perform as above, using dumbbells.
- Set the bench at knee height.
- Use two benches. Stand between them and step up and down on one and then the other for each rep..

A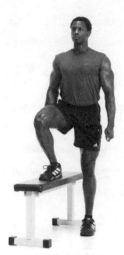

B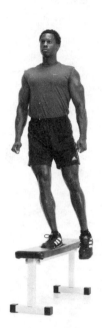

C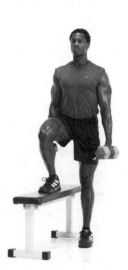

LEG EXTENSION

This exercise will really work your quadriceps. Altering the position of your foot—pointing the toes in or out, for example—will change the way the muscles are worked.

A Sit in a leg extension machine, with your legs behind the padded lifting bars, and your hands gripping the handles at the sides of the bench. Your knees should be bent 90 degrees or more, with your toes pointing in front of you.

B Using the machine handles for support, straighten your legs by lifting with your ankles and contracting your quadriceps. At full extension, straighten your legs as far as you can. Your toes should point straight ahead. Hold for a second, then return to the starting position.

MAKE IT EASIER

- Use a smaller range of motion.
- Turn the toes out to work more of the vastus medialis (muscle on the inside of the knee).
- Turn the toes in to work more of the vastus lateralis (muscle on the lateral side of the knee).

DO IT HARDER

- Train only one leg at a time.
- Lift with two legs and lower with one leg. Do the same number of lowering reps for each leg.
- Pause at three positions on the way down and contract the quadriceps at each position.

A
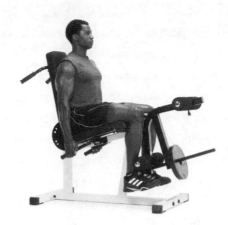

B
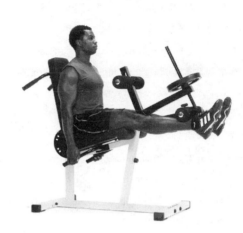

PARTIAL SPLIT SQUAT

While not as difficult as Bulgarian split squats, these lunges are a challenge for even experienced lifters.

A Step forward with your left leg, taking a bigger-than-normal step. Keep your upper body upright and your arms at your sides. Bend your left leg to 90 degrees, keeping your left knee in line with your ankle. Lower your back leg (right leg) until your knee touches the floor. Place your right hand on the inside of the front (left) knee, and put your left hand on the butt muscle of the left leg. Raise your back knee 1 inch off the floor. This is the starting position.

B Raise yourself up by extending both legs; you'll feel tension in your knee and butt. The movement is completed when you no longer feel these muscles contracting. Pause, then return to the starting position, with your knee 1 inch off the floor. Complete a set, then repeat on the other side.

MAKE IT EASIER

- Use a smaller range of motion.
- Place padding or a towel under your knee.
- Hold on to something stable for balance, such as the side of a squat rack.

DO IT HARDER

- Use a larger range of motion.
- Lower yourself more slowly.
- Wear a weighted vest.

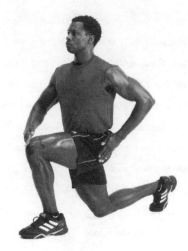

A

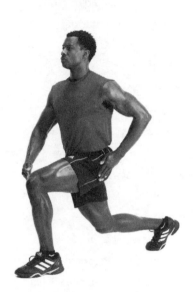

B

BACKWARD (REVERSE) LUNGE

Reverse lunges work the same muscles as forward lunges, but without putting additional stress on the knees.

A Stand up straight, with your feet hip width apart. Your hands should be slightly farther than shoulder width apart, palms facing forward.

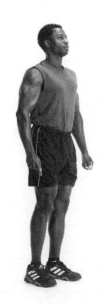

A

B Take a lunging stride backward, so that only the ball of the foot rests on the floor. Simultaneously, sit back into the lunge until your back knee is an inch or two from the floor. Your front leg should be bent no more than 90 degrees, with the thigh parallel to the floor, and your knee directly over your ankle. Push off from your front leg to return to the starting position, then repeat on the other side. That completes 1 repetition.

MAKE IT EASIER

- Use a smaller range of motion.
- Hold on to a stationary object like a power rack for support.

DO IT HARDER

- Use a larger range of motion.
- Use dumbbells or a barbell.
- Step down off a 2- to 4-inch platform.

B

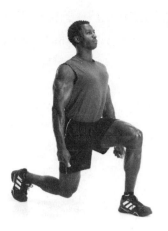

SQUATS AND LOWER-BACK INJURIES

If you squat with the bar on your clavicle, it's a front squat. If you squat with the bar on your traps, it's a back squat. Front squats put more emphasis on your knees, making them great for quadriceps development. Back squats place more emphasis on your hips, making them great for glute and lower-back development.

The general gym view is that back squats are more likely to cause lower-back injury. But studies have shown that the risks are about the same for both forms of squats. What does increase the risk is how much you lean. The more you lean forward—what's known as "leaning forward trunk inclination"—the more likely you are to get hurt.

If you're doing squats and feel your hips moving up faster than your shoulders, you probably have too much forward lean. Ideally, stay as upright as possible when squatting. This is another reason that maintaining good form is priceless.

Even when your back is acting up a little, there's a safe way to do squats. All you need is a little-known device called a safety squat bar, which lowers the center of mass of the load you're lifting. The bar is designed to balance itself on your upper body even when you aren't holding on. All you have to do is grip the handles that are set at chest height and run parallel to the floor. You'll find that you're able to squat while staying almost perfectly upright. This mechanical position minimizes shear forces on the lower back, and at the same time it really targets the quads.

Many lifters with back problems can perform safety squats without any pain whatsoever. You still need some common sense, of course. Don't pile on so much weight that you have to call on your upper body to rise back up. Use the handles as guides only; let your lower body do the work.

SINGLE LEG SQUAT

In addition to improving balance and coordination, this movement also works the legs, hips, and butt.

A Stand upright, with your feet shoulder width apart and your knees slightly bent. Position a sturdy chair or other support on your right side. Rest your hand on it for balance.

B Begin to squat on your right leg, while extending your left leg in front of you. Keep your back straight. As soon as your right thigh is parallel to the floor, press yourself back up to the starting position. Don't pause between repetitions; you should look like a piston, pumping up and down. Finish the set, then switch sides.

DO IT HARDER

- Use a larger range of motion.
- Use dumbbells or a barbell.

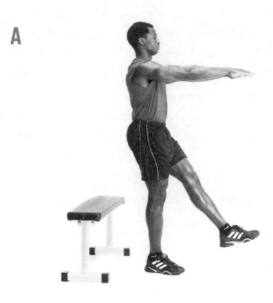

A

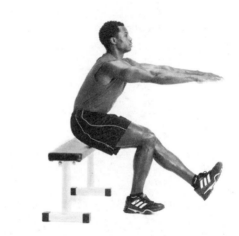

B

MAKE IT EASIER

- Use two legs.
- Squat down on one leg to a large stability ball wedged against a bench or wall so it won't roll. As this becomes easy, switch to a smaller stability ball. Over time you will be able to squat down without a stability ball.
- Use reverse bands or hold on to a railing for assistance. Attach bands to the top of a rack and hook one arm through each band so that the bands come under the armpits. This will make you "lighter" as you squat down, making the exercise easier.

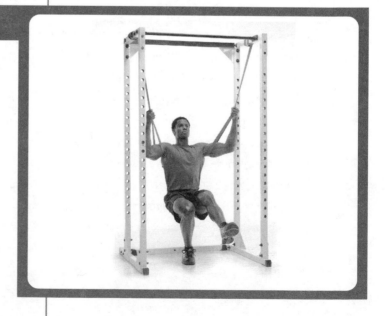

HAMSTRINGS EXPLAINED

The hamstrings in the back of the thigh consist of three separate muscles: the biceps femoris, the semi-tendinosus, and the semimembranosus. Each of these muscles originates just underneath the gluteus maximus (the main butt muscle) on the pelvic bone and attaches to the tibia.

The primary functions of the hamstrings are knee flexion (bringing the heel toward the butt) and hip extension (moving the leg to the rear).

THE TOTAL HAMSTRING WORKOUT

The hamstrings are primarily fast-twitch muscles. They respond well to exercises that involve low reps and powerful movements. Any exercise that flexes the knee or extends the hips against resistance will work the hamstrings. Some of the best workouts include all varieties of leg curls, stiff-legged deadlifts, lunges, and squats.

Hit the outer muscles. The best exercises for working the outer part of the back of the legs are standing and lying leg curls. Seated leg curls and deadlifts also work these muscles, but not as well as the standing and lying variations.

Hit the inner muscles. The best exercises for this part of the hamstrings are seated leg curls, followed by standing and lying leg curls. Deadlifts will build them to some extent, but not as much as the curls.

Point your toes for strength, not for size. When you point your toes while doing leg curls, you activate the gastrocnemius, a muscle that also crosses the knee. Activating this muscle during curls will give the greatest gains in hamstring strength. If you're going for size more than strength, pull the toes in toward your shins rather than pointing them.

Don't forget to breathe. It sounds obvious, but a lot of men hold their breath when doing leg curls. Bad idea. Holding your breath increases internal pressure. When combined with extra blood flow to the head from lying down, you're looking at a recipe for stroke. Follow the usual guidelines: Breathe in while lowering weights, and breathe out during the exertion phase.

Allow plenty of warmup time. The hamstrings are naturally a little stiff in most men. Don't push them too hard or too fast. If you can't move all the way through a full range of motion on your first set—for example, you can't touch the bar to the floor when doing stiff-leg deadlifts—don't push yourself. Only go as far as your form (and hamstrings) will allow. As you warm up, go lower with the bar.

Stretch after, not before, your workout. You never want to perform static stretches of the hamstrings before you lift. This makes them weaker and will prevent you from progressing to the kinds of weight you need to build maximal size. As a pre-workout warmup, do leg swings or other dynamic movements. Save the static stretches for the end of your workout.

BODY-WEIGHT LEG CURL

You'll need a partner or a sturdy support to hold your lower body in order to perform this hamstring strengthener.

A Lie on your stomach on a bench or on a mat on the floor. Start with both legs straight out. Your knees should be just over the edge of the bench, or resting on the mat. Have your partner push down around the back of your ankles so that they can't move. Or hook your feet under something solid.

B Perform a body-weight leg curl by flexing the knee joint. Since your ankles are fixed, you have to bring your butt to your ankles. Use your hands to help start the movement by performing a pushup. Then use your hamstrings to finish the movement. Hold at the top, then slowly lower your body.

MAKE IT EASIER

- Push off the bench with more force to make it easier to start.
- Start with the bench at 45 degrees instead of flat.

DO IT HARDER

- Lift with two legs and lower using the muscles of just one leg.
- Use just one leg at a time.
- Wear a weighted vest.

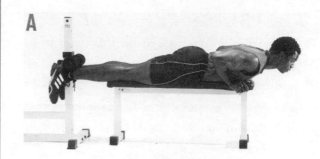

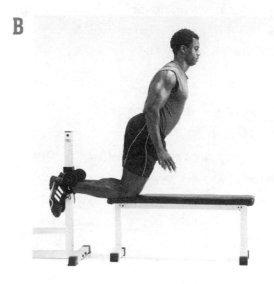

LEG CURL WITH ANKLE WEIGHT

In addition to strengthening the hamstrings, this exercise will also work the lower back.

A Lie on your stomach on a bench, with both legs straight out and an ankle weight on each ankle. Your knees should be just over the edge of the bench. If necessary, hold the legs of the bench for support.

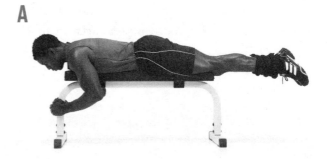

B Keeping your feet together and pointed out, raise your heels toward your butt until your legs are about at a 90-degree angle. Point your toes up, but don't arch your back; your pelvis should remain against the bench. Hold for a second, then return to the starting position.

MAKE IT EASIER

- Take off the ankle weights.
- Do machine leg curls on a machine (page 236).
- Start with the bench at 45 degrees instead of flat.

DO IT HARDER

- Do body-weight leg curls.
- Hold a dumbbell between your feet.
- Hook exercise tubing to an ankle attachment, with the other end attached to a fixed object behind you. Perform the exercise as described above.

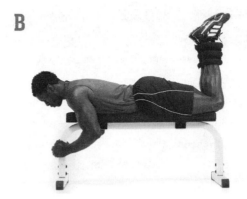

QUICK-BLAST TO LEG STRENGTH

Want to *instantly* increase your squat weight anywhere from 15 to 30 pounds? You can do it—with plyometrics. Plyometrics are movements that involve a quick stretch of a muscle, followed by a quick contraction. An example is a depth jump. You step off a platform about 20 inches high. When you land on the ground, you instantly, and explosively, try to jump as high as you can. Regular jumping won't cut it; it has to be explosive, or plyometric: quick lengthening followed by a quick contraction.

Here's an easy program to really blast your squat strength.

- Warm up with 5 minutes of light cycling.
- Do 3 to 5 sets of squats, with progressively increasing weights and decreasing reps.
- When you're approaching your top squat weight, do 2 depth jumps 30 seconds before each set.

You should see your top squat weight increase at least 15 pounds, and possibly a lot more.

MACHINE LEG CURL (LYING LEG CURL)

This is among the most common, and popular, ways of training the hamstrings.

A Lie on your stomach on a leg curl machine and hook your ankles behind the pads. Your knees should be just over the edge of the bench. Grip the handles or the side of the bench for support. Your legs should be fully extended, with your knees slightly bent.

B Keeping your pelvis against the bench and using the handles for support, raise your heels toward your butt until your legs are just short of a 90-degree angle. Return to the starting position, keeping your hamstrings tense through the entire range of motion.

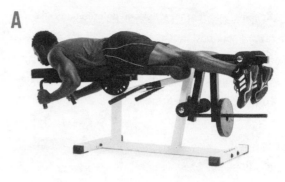

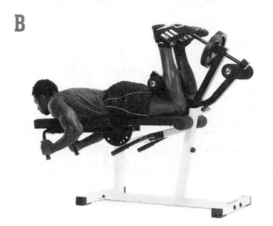

MAKE IT EASIER

- Try using ankle weights instead.
- Shorten the range of motion.
- Don't use any resistance.

DO IT HARDER

- Lift with two legs and lower using the muscles of just one leg.
- Use only one leg at a time.
- Use a larger range of motion.

STIFF-LEG DEADLIFT

Want to hit your hams and glutes hard? This is the deadlift variation for you. This movement is similar to the conventional deadlift, except that the knees are straight but not locked out.

A Stand upright with a barbell in front of you. Bend at the hips and, with a flat back, grip the barbell with your hands shoulder width apart, your palms down. Balance your weight evenly on both feet. Take a deep breath.

B Exhale while extending the trunk to the top deadlift position. Keep the back flat and legs straight. Hold for a second, then slowly lower the weight.

MAKE IT EASIER

- Use tubing for resistance, instead of a barbell. Run the tubing under your feet and grip the handles overhand. Perform the exercise as described above.
- Shorten the range of motion.
- Don't use any resistance.

DO IT HARDER

- Lift with two legs and lower using the muscles of just one leg.
- Use only one leg at a time.
- Gain a larger range of motion by standing on a platform.

A

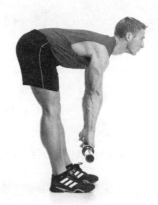

B

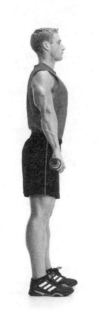

SUPINE LEG CURL ON STABILITY BALL

Changing the position of your toes in this exercise will alter the effects. Putting your toes in the up position will enhance the activation of the calf muscles. Pointing the toes will emphasize the hamstrings.

A Lie on your back, with your heels on a stability ball. Rise up on your shoulders, using your arms for limited support. Extend the hips.

B Using your heels, roll the ball toward your buttocks as far as you can without letting the hips drop. Return to the starting position under full control. Start with two legs, then progress to using one leg at a time while keeping the other leg extended (**C**).

MAKE IT EASIER

- Try using ankle weights or a leg curl machine instead.
- Shorten the range of motion.

DO IT HARDER

- Lift with two legs and lower using the muscles of just one leg.
- Use only one leg at a time.
- Use a larger range of motion.

A

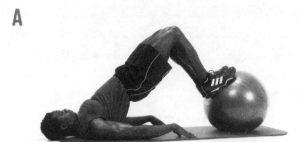

B

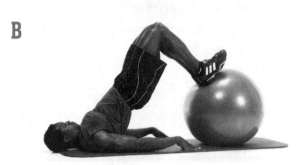

C

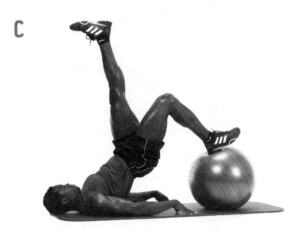

TUBING LEG CURL

This simple exercise is very effective for building your hamstring (back thigh) muscles. Use less resistance for this move than you would for a leg extension.

A Wrap a length of exercise tubing around the bottom of a weight bench. Place the tubing handles around the balls of your feet. Lie facedown on a weight bench, with your knees just over the edge. Hold the legs of the bench for support.

B Keeping your pelvis against the bench and your feet together, raise your heels toward your butt until your legs are at about a 90-degree angle. Hold for a second, then return to the starting position. Keep your hamstrings tense throughout the entire range of motion.

MAKE IT EASIER

• Try using ankle weights or a leg curl machine instead.
• Shorten the range of motion.

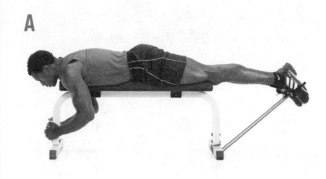

A

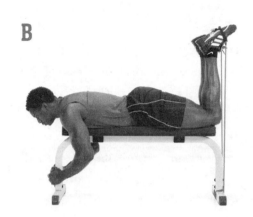

B

DO IT HARDER

• Do body-weight leg curls instead (page 234).
• Hold a dumbbell between your feet.
• Hook an ankle attachment to a cable machine instead of using tubing.

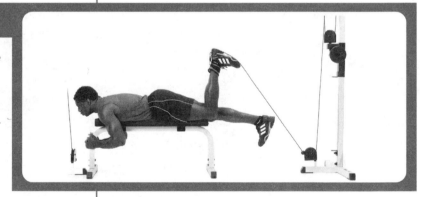

CALVES EXPLAINED

The primary muscles of the calves are the gastrocnemius, the soleus, and the anterior tibialis.

The gastrocnemius is the muscle that you see. It attaches to the heel with the Achilles tendon and originates behind the knee on the femur. Its job is to elevate the heel, a movement called plantar flexion.

The soleus lies underneath the gastrocnemius on the rear of the lower leg. It does the same job as the gastrocnemius: raising the heel. The only difference is that it works in a different position, when your knee is bent. The best exercise for working the soleus is the seated heel raise. For the gastrocnemius, good exercises include standing heel raises and donkey calf raises.

Finally, there's the anterior tibialis, a small muscle group on the front side of your lower leg. Its main function is flexing the foot upward. Walking works this muscle; many hard-core walkers experience shin pain when they increase their speed or distance. Forefoot raises will help keep the anterior tibialis in top shape.

TOTAL CALF WORKOUT

The calves are easier to work than most other leg muscles because they aren't that big to begin with, and only a few exercises have a significant impact on calf size.

Vary your foot position. The calves need a variety of exercise angles to really grow. When doing calf workouts, you can build the inside of the calf by squeezing up on your big toe. To hit the outside of the calf, squeeze on your little toe.

Pile on the weight. The gastrocnemius requires a lot of weight as well as a lot of reps to achieve any kind of serious size. Don't shortchange your calf workouts; go to the limit. The best exercises are donkey calf raises and standing single-leg heel raises. After that, standing two-leg heel raises and seated calf raises are good picks.

Pause to grow. Nearly every exercise gets extra octane when you pause for a moment at the top of the movement. This is particularly true of calf workouts. Always hold the top position for at least 1 second. Three seconds is better.

Put your feet in gear. Walking and climbing stairs are two of the best everyday movements for strengthening the calves. You'll need weights if you're really going to pack on the size, but walking and climbing keep the muscles primed and make it easier to put on extra bulk.

Check your shoe strategy. Even if you have weak ankles, avoid three-quarter or high-top athletic shoes on days you're working your calves. They'll limit your range of motion.

BODY-WEIGHT DONKEY CALF RAISE

This is a great move for strengthening the gastrocnemius muscle in the calf.

A Stand on the edge of a 2- to 4-inch platform, with your heels hanging off the edge. Your legs should be shoulder width apart, your toes pointed forward. Bend forward at the waist until your upper body is roughly parallel to the floor. Extend your arms straight and lean on something in front of you, such as a rack. Keep your knees slightly bent.

B Lift yourself up as high as possible on the balls of the feet. Hold for a second, then lower your heels as far as they will go.

MAKE IT EASIER

- Try a standing heel raise (page 242) with body weight only.
- Shorten the range of motion.
- Try an incline toe press (page 244) without weight.

DO IT HARDER

- Use only one leg.

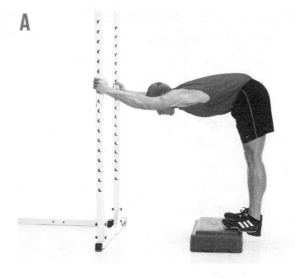

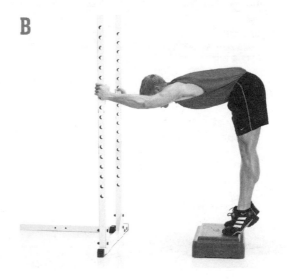

STANDING HEEL RAISE

This is one of the best exercises for building the calf muscles.

A Stand with your feet hip width apart and place your hands on your hips. Place your toes on a platform that's a couple of inches off the floor. Your heels should hang off the platform and your weight should be on the balls of your feet. You'll lean slightly forward.

B Rise all the way up on your toes. Feel the contraction in your calves, then pause briefly at the top. Lower yourself to the starting position.

MAKE IT EASIER

- Shorten the range of motion.
- Try an incline toe press (page 244) without weight.

DO IT HARDER

- Use only one leg.
- Try dumbbell standing heel raises (page 243) or donkey calf raises (page 241) with weight.

A

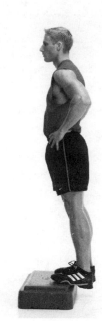

B

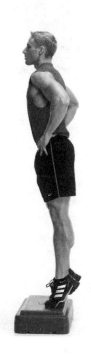

DUMBBELL STANDING HEEL RAISE

This is another good move for really blasting the calves.

A Stand with a dumbbell in each hand, with your feet hip width apart. Place your toes on a platform that's a couple of inches off the floor. Your heels should hang off the platform, with your weight on the balls of your feet. You'll lean slightly forward. Hold the dumbbells at your sides, with your arms extended down.

B Rise all the way up onto your toes. Feel the contraction in your calves, then pause briefly at the top. Your arms should remain extended at your sides, with your body upright. Lower yourself to the starting position.

MAKE IT EASIER

- Try a standing heel raise with body weight only.
- Shorten the range of motion.
- Try an incline toe press (page 244) without weight.

DO IT HARDER

- Use only one leg.
- Try standing heel raises (page 242) or donkey calf raises (page 241) with weight.

A

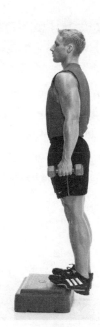

B

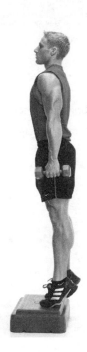

INCLINE TOE PRESS

This exercise works the muscles in the calves that allow the feet and ankles to flex.

A Sit straight in a leg press machine, making sure that the small of your back is pressed firmly against the pad. Adjust the seat so that the balls of your feet rest comfortably on the foot plate, 4 to 6 inches apart. Your toes should be pointing up, and your legs should be slightly bent.

B Push down with the balls of your feet, pointing your toes as much as you can. Hold for a second, then return to the starting position.

MAKE IT EASIER
- Try a standing heel raise (page 242) with body weight only.
- Shorten the range of motion.
- Try an incline toe press without weight.

DO IT HARDER
- Use only one leg.
- Try dumbbell standing heel raises (page 243) or donkey calf raises (page 241) with weight.

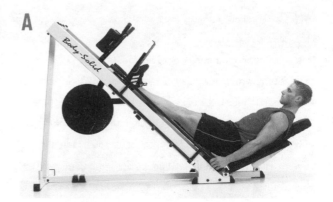

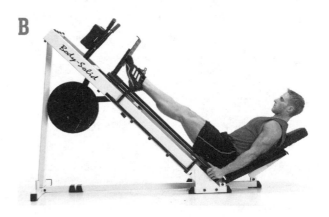

MACHINE STANDING HEEL RAISE

This is one of the most common exercises for building the calf muscles.

A Stand with your feet hip width apart. Stand under the shoulder pads of a standing calf machine and lift your body into position so that your heels are off the edge of the toe block. Your hands should be slightly farther than shoulder width apart, your palms facing inward. Your heels should be on the floor, and your weight on the balls of your feet.

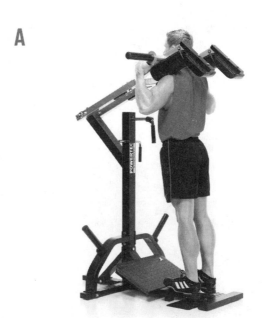

B Rise all the way up on your toes. Feel the contraction in your calves, then pause briefly at the top. Lower yourself to the starting position.

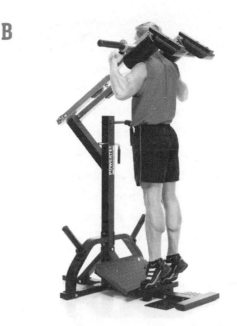

MAKE IT EASIER

- Try a standing heel raise (page 242) with body weight only.
- Shorten the range of motion.
- Try an incline toe press (page 244) without weight.

DO IT HARDER

- Use only one leg.
- Try dumbbell standing heel raises (page 243) or donkey calf raises (page 241) with weight.

SINGLE LEG HEEL RAISE

This exercise isolates each leg separately, allowing you to build your calf muscles to the size and strength you want.

A Hold a dumbbell in each hand and stand with your legs hip width apart. Put the toes of your left foot on a platform that's a couple of inches high. Keep the left heel hanging off the platform and your weight on the ball of the foot, so that you lean slightly forward. Tuck your right foot behind your left calf. If you need to, put your arms in front of you for balance.

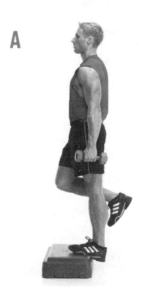

B Rise all the way up on the toes of your left foot. Feel the contraction in your calf, then pause briefly at the top. Try to keep your arms at your sides, with your body upright. Lower yourself to the starting position. Finish the set, then switch sides.

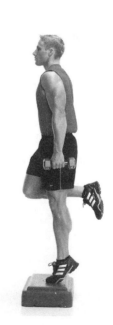

MAKE IT EASIER

- Try a standing heel raise (page 242) with body weight only.
- Shorten the range of motion.
- Try an incline toe press (page 244) without weight.

DO IT HARDER

- Try standing heel raises (page 242) or dumbbell standing heel raises (page 243).
- Try donkey calf raises (page 241) with weight.

SMITH MACHINE STANDING HEEL RAISE

This exercise is very effective at building the calf muscles.

A Facing a Smith machine, position the bar at upper-chest height. Place a platform that's a few inches high under the bar. Step under the bar so that it rests across the upper back and shoulders. Grip the bar with your hands slightly farther than shoulder width apart, your palms facing forward. Position your toes and the balls of your feet on the step, with your heels extending toward the floor. Disengage the bar. Stand straight by extending your knees and hips.

B Rise all the way up on your toes. Feel the contraction in your calves, then pause briefly at the top. Keep your knees straight throughout the movement; bend them only slightly during the stretch. Lower yourself to the starting position and repeat.

MAKE IT EASIER
- Try a standing heel raise (page 242) with body weight only.
- Shorten the range of motion.
- Try an incline toe press (page 244) without weight.

DO IT HARDER
- Try standing heel raises (page 242) or dumbbell standing heel raises (page 243).
- Try donkey calf raises (page 241) with weight.

A

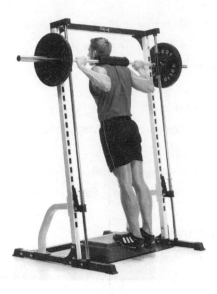

B

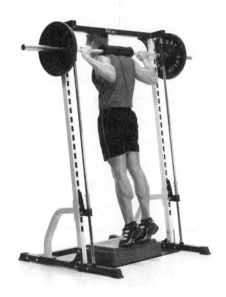

BARBELL SEATED HEEL RAISE

The calves are considered the most difficult muscle group in the body to develop. This movement works the entire calf, especially the soleus muscle in the lower part of the calf.

A Sit straight on the side of a bench. Rest the balls of your feet on a 6- to 8-inch platform, allowing your heels to stretch down as far as they will go. Hold a barbell across your thighs, a few inches from your knees.

B Raise your heels as high as possible by pressing your toes into the step. Your hands should only steady the bar; don't use them to support or lift the weight. Hold for a moment, then return to the starting position.

MAKE IT EASIER

- Try a seated heel raise without weight.
- Shorten the range of motion.
- Try an incline toe press (page 244) without weight.

DO IT HARDER

- Use only one leg.
- Try machine seated heel raises (page 248).
- Use dumbbells instead of a barbell.

A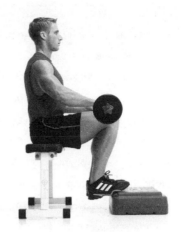

B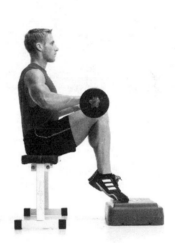

MACHINE SEATED HEEL RAISE

The calves are considered the most difficult muscle group in the body to develop. This movement works the entire calf, especially the soleus muscle in the lower part of the calf.

A Sit straight on a seated calf machine bench. Rest the balls of your feet on the toe platform, allowing your heels to stretch down as far as they will go. Position your knees under the thigh pads and unrack the weight.

B Raise your heels as high as possible by pressing your toes into the toe platform. Your hands should only steady the load; don't use them to support or lift the weight. Hold for a moment, then return to the starting position.

MAKE IT EASIER

- Try a seated heel raise without weight.
- Shorten the range of motion.
- Try standing heel raises (page 242) with a little knee bend.

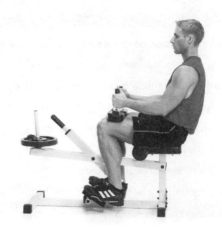

A

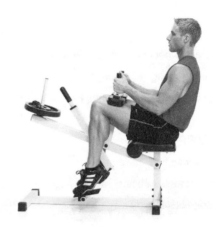

B

DO IT HARDER

- Try standing heel raises (page 242).
- Use dumbbells instead, holding them at your sides.

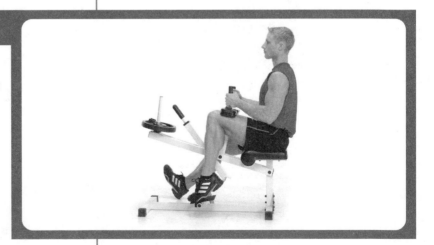

ANKLE FLEXION WITH CABLE

This exercise works your dorsiflexors, the foot muscles that help you lift your foot and toes.

A Position one end of a bench a few inches from a low pulley with an ankle strap. Stand to the left of the bench with your left knee slightly bent. Put your right heel on the edge of the bench closest to the pulley. The bottom of your foot should be level with or slightly below the bench. Fasten the ankle strap snugly around the toes of your right foot.

B Curl your toes as high as possible while keeping your heel planted firmly on the bench. Rest your arms on your right thigh for balance, but keep your back straight. Pause, then return to the starting position. Finish the set, then switch sides.

MAKE IT EASIER

- Try ankle flexion with tubing (page 250).
- Shorten the range of motion.
- Try using only a towel for resistance.

DO IT HARDER

- Try ankle flexion with weight plate (page 250).
- Do heel walks (page 251).
- Use dumbbells, holding them at your sides.

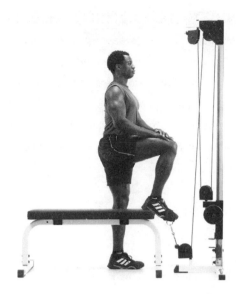

A

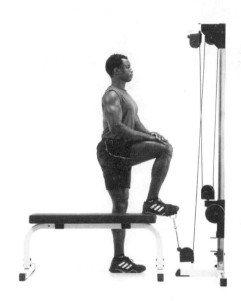

B

ANKLE FLEXION WITH TUBING

This is another exercise for working the foot muscles.

A Sit on the floor, with your right leg straight in front of you. Secure a length of exercise tubing around a stable piece of equipment, such as a weight machine. Place the tubing handle around your foot, so that the top of the handle rests on your instep. Move backward until there is tension on the tubing.

B Curl your toes and pull your foot toward your face, stretching the tubing. Return to the starting position.

MAKE IT EASIER

- Shorten the range of motion.
- Use only a towel for resistance.

DO IT HARDER

- Do ankle flexion with weight plate (below).
- Rest a dumbbell on the top of your fore-foot and curl toward your shin.
- Do heel walks (page 251).

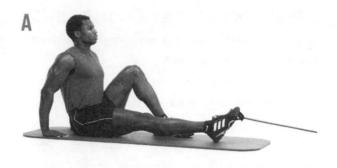

A

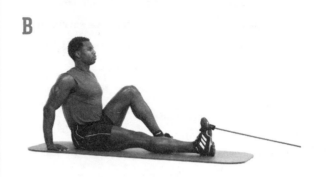

B

ANKLE FLEXION
WITH WEIGHT PLATE

This is probably the best exercise for isolating and working the dorsiflexors, the four muscles that enable you to lift your foot and toes.

A Sit on the end of a bench, with your legs together and your feet flat on the floor. Your knees should be bent at a 90-degree angle. Keeping your back straight, lean forward slightly from the waist, holding a weight plate that is resting across the base of your toes.

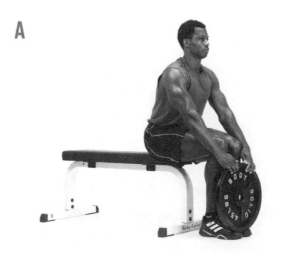

A

B Lift your toes as high as you can, keeping the weight balanced. Hold for a second, then lower your feet and the weight to the starting position.

MAKE IT EASIER

- Try ankle flexion with tubing (page 250).
- Shorten the range of motion.
- Use only a towel for resistance.

DO IT HARDER

- Try ankle flexion with cable (page 249).
- Do heel walks (below).
- Rest a dumbbell on the top of your forefoot and curl toward your shin.

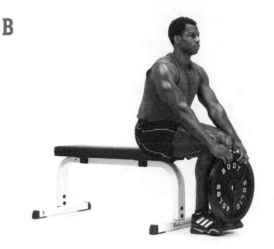

HEEL WALK

This simple movement strengthens the front part of the lower leg.

Standing upright, lift your toes so that your weight rests on your heels. Walk 20 to 30 steps, using the muscles at the front of your lower leg to maintain your position and balance. Rest for 30 seconds, then repeat.

MAKE IT EASIER

- Try ankle flexion with tubing (page 250).
- Shorten the range of motion.

DO IT HARDER

- Do ankle flexion with weight plate (page 250) or ankle flexion with cable (page 249).
- Try using dumbbells, holding them at your sides.

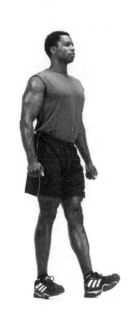

LEVEL 1 WORKOUTS

We've provided three different workouts for Level 1. One option is to do all three workouts weekly. For example, do Workout #1 on Monday, Workout #2 on Wednesday, and Workout #3 on Friday. If you choose this option, do two warmup sets for the first exercise, followed by 3 sets of 6 repetitions using "real" weight. Next, do 3 sets of 10 reps for the second exercise, followed by 3 sets of 14 reps for the next three exercises.

Another option is to do just one of the workouts, three times a week. Vary the rep count daily. On Monday, for example, do 3 sets of 5 reps for all the exercises; on Wednesday, do 3 sets of 10 reps for all the exercises; and on Friday, do 3 sets of 14 reps for all the exercises. Always start with 2 warmup sets for the first exercise (these don't go toward the final "count").

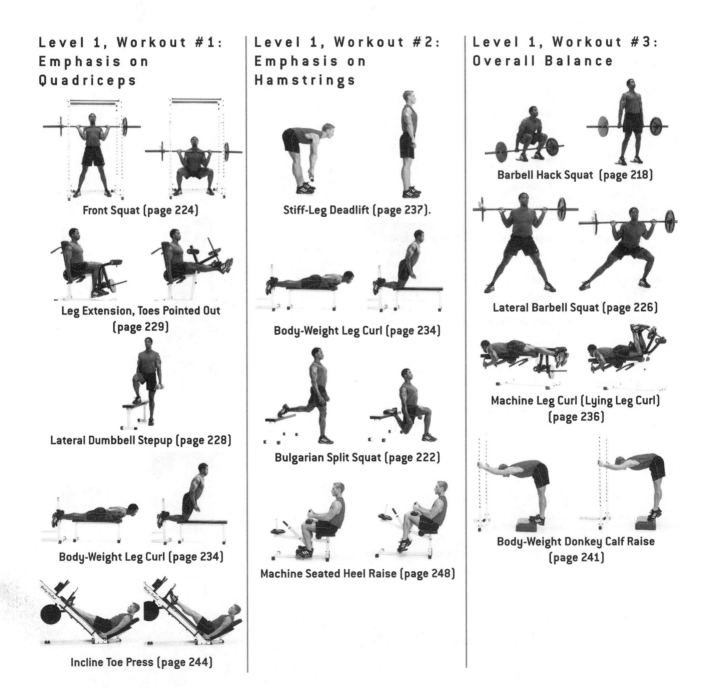

Level 1, Workout #1: Emphasis on Quadriceps

Front Squat (page 224)

Leg Extension, Toes Pointed Out (page 229)

Lateral Dumbbell Stepup (page 228)

Body-Weight Leg Curl (page 234)

Incline Toe Press (page 244)

Level 1, Workout #2: Emphasis on Hamstrings

Stiff-Leg Deadlift (page 237).

Body-Weight Leg Curl (page 234)

Bulgarian Split Squat (page 222)

Machine Seated Heel Raise (page 248)

Level 1, Workout #3: Overall Balance

Barbell Hack Squat (page 218)

Lateral Barbell Squat (page 226)

Machine Leg Curl (Lying Leg Curl) (page 236)

Body-Weight Donkey Calf Raise (page 241)

LEVEL 2 (FOCUS ON STRENGTH)

Level 2, Workout #1

MAX BARBELL SQUAT (BS) ROUTINE

It's possible to increase your squat load by more than 60 pounds in less than 10 weeks by following this routine. You only have to do it twice a week—a "light" day and a "heavy" day. First, determine your 1 repetition maximum (1RM) for the squat. (See page 14.) Then use the chart below to determine your Barbell Squat weight, sets, and reps for a given workout. Round the weights to the nearest 5 pounds.

To stay limber (and safe), start each workout with two 5-rep warmup sets, using 50 percent and 70 percent of your 1RM. After you've done all sets and reps of your Barbell Squat, complete the workout with the additional exercises on the following page.

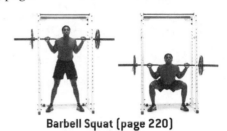

Barbell Squat (page 220)

Level 2, Workout #1, Barbell Squat Routine

WEEK	DAY	% 1RM	#SETS	#REPS
1	1	80	6	2
1	2	80	6	3
2	1	80	6	2
2	2	80	6	4
3	1	80	6	2
3	2	80	6	5
4	1	80	6	2
4	2	80	6	6
5	1	80	6	2
5	2	85	5	5
6	1	80	6	2
6	2	90	4	4
7	1	80	6	2
7	2	95	3	3
8	1	80	6	2
8	2	100	2	2
9	1	80	6	2
9	2	105	2	1 *

*AFTER THE 2 SETS AT TOP WEIGHT, KEEP DOING SINGLES WITH 2 MINUTES' REST BETWEEN SETS, INCREASING THE WEIGHT 5 TO 10 POUNDS EACH TIME, UNTIL YOU FIND YOUR NEW 1RM.

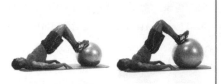

Supine Leg Curl on Stability Ball (page 238)

Do 2 to 3 sets, with 8 to 10 reps per set.

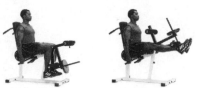

Leg Extension (page 229)

Keep your toes pointed straight. Do 2 to 3 sets, with 8 to 10 reps per set.

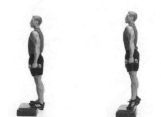

Dumbbell Standing Heel Raise (page 243)

Do 1 set with maximum reps.

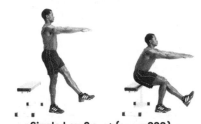

Single Leg Squat (page 232)

Do 2 to 3 sets, with 4 to 6 reps per set.

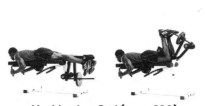

Machine Leg Curl (page 236)

Do 2 to 3 sets, with 4 to 6 reps per set.

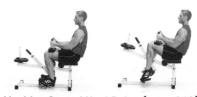

Machine Seated Heel Raise (page 248)

Do 1 set with maximum reps.

Level 2, Workout #2

Do this workout three times a week. Perform 2 warmup sets for each exercise. Vary the rep count on successive days. For example, do 1 set of 3 reps on Monday, 1 set of 11 reps on Wednesday, and 1 set of 7 reps on Friday.

Each week, add 1 set to each exercise until you're up to 5 sets. If you're feeling excessive soreness, reduce the number of sets for each exercise.

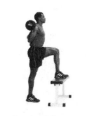

Barbell Stepup (Variation of Stepup) (page 221)

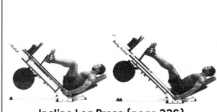

Incline Leg Press (page 226)

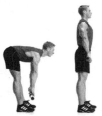

Stiff-Leg Deadlift (page 237)

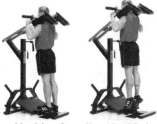

Machine Standing Heel Raise (page 244)

Level 2, Workout #3

Do this workout three times a week. Perform 2 warmup sets for each exercise. If you're feeling excessive soreness, reduce the number of sets for each exercise.

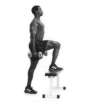

Dumbbell Stepup (Variation of Stepup) (page 221)

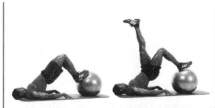

Supine Leg Curl on Stability Ball— Use Only One Leg (page 238)

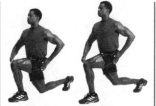

Partial Split Squat (page 230)

Do 2 to 3 sets of 11 reps each.

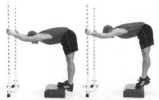

Body-Weight Donkey Calf Raise (page 241)

Do 2 to 3 sets of 11 reps each.

LEVEL 3 (FOCUS ON SIZE AND STRENGTH)

We've provided three different programs for the Level 3 leg workouts. You can stick to one program throughout the week. Or shake things up and do different programs on different days. The number of sets and repetitions you'll do in each workout depends on the approach you take. Here are the two main options.

Option A

- Perform all three workouts in a single week. For example, do Workout #1 on Monday, Workout #2 on Wednesday, and Workout #3 on Friday.

- After a general warmup, do 2 warmup sets for the first exercise, lifting lighter-than-usual weights.

- Do 5 sets of 2 reps for the first exercise.

- Next, do 2 sets of 6 reps for the second exercise.

- Do 2 sets of 12 reps for the third exercise.

- Do 2 sets of 12 reps for the fourth exercise.

Option B

- Pick one of the workouts and stick with it all week.

- After a general warmup, do 2 warmup sets for the first exercise, lifting lighter-than-usual weights.

- Vary the rep count on each day. For example, do 3 sets of 2 reps for all the exercises on Monday. On Wednesday, do 3 sets of 6 reps for all the exercises. On Friday, do 2 sets of 12 reps for all the exercises.

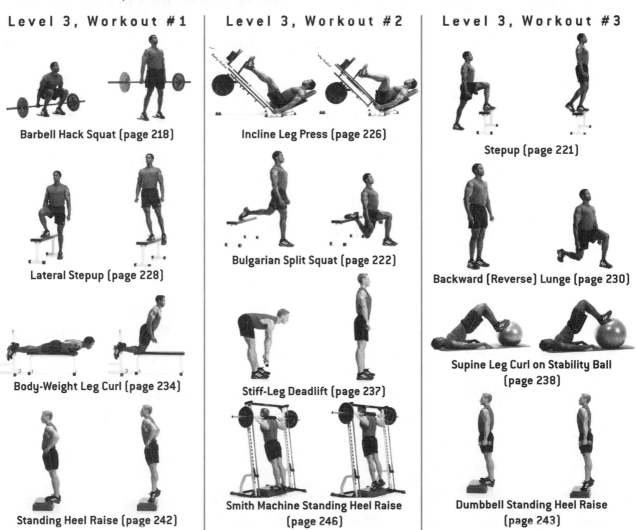

Level 3, Workout #1

Barbell Hack Squat (page 218)

Lateral Stepup (page 228)

Body-Weight Leg Curl (page 234)

Standing Heel Raise (page 242)

Level 3, Workout #2

Incline Leg Press (page 226)

Bulgarian Split Squat (page 222)

Stiff-Leg Deadlift (page 237)

Smith Machine Standing Heel Raise (page 246)

Level 3, Workout #3

Stepup (page 221)

Backward (Reverse) Lunge (page 230)

Supine Leg Curl on Stability Ball (page 238)

Dumbbell Standing Heel Raise (page 243)

13

TOTAL HARD BODY

The *science* of lifting is cutting-edge stuff. Most men don't have the inclination, or the time, to really master the advanced material that can take you to a whole different level of training—and dramatic improvements in size and strength—in as little as 12 weeks.

In the following pages, we'll walk you through the most important strategies for *advanced training.* You already know how to lift. You know how to put together a reasonably effective workout routine. You know how to quickly tear down muscles so they'll come back with impressive new size. That's just the beginning.

If you want to go beyond the basics, you have to get a handle on the newest training concepts—concepts that are being used every day by top-rated coaches and athletes.

FOCUS ON PATTERNS

Years ago, trainers used to advise men to structure their workouts around individual muscle groups. Now, the best advice is to work on muscle *patterns.* Athletes have been doing this for quite a few years. A tennis player, for example, will structure his workouts around sport-specific movements: building the legs to allow for stronger lateral movements, say, or working the arms to swing a racket with explosive force. This is light-years beyond old-style bodybuilding, in which the goal was simply to gain muscle. Muscle-pattern workouts, also known as movement-based approaches, involve analyzing

your movements to identify weak spots, and then designing workouts to improve those specific movements. This can work for everything from swinging a tennis racket with more force to shoving more iron on the bench press.

Reproducing the movements people perform daily, and then turning them into high-efficiency exercises, is the basis of movement-based training. Traditional bodybuilding consists of one-dimensional movements. Think of the barbell squat. You squat down and stand up, always staying in the same plane of motion. But this isn't the way we squat in real life. You bend down diagonally to pick up a sock. Simultaneously, you might be twisting to reach for a protein drink and keep a grip on the phone that's balanced next to your ear.

The best workouts simulate the kinds of multidimensional movements that we do every day. Men who design their plans with this principle in mind essentially get multiple payoffs for the price of one. They get bigger in less time because these workouts are optimal for really tearing down and building up muscle tissue. At the same time, they gain in "real" life. When you do the same motion thousands of times a day—and supplement these motions with targeted workouts—you get through life with more power and less fatigue. You move more efficiently, which means you won't be spilling your drinks or hanging up the phone by mistake.

A big part of muscle-pattern workouts centers on strengthening the muscles around the joints from a variety of angles, including working individual muscles and joints so that they're inherently more stable. Consider single-leg exercises, such as single-leg squats. They force you to optimize balance in a variety of directions at one time. This strengthens the smaller, stabilization muscles around the ankle, knee, and hip joints.

At the same time, though, you need to maintain the ability to lift heavy loads, so you can keep your muscle mass. The solution? Training programs that provide the loading of one movement with the balance-enhancing effects of another movement.

Each of the workouts in this book is based on this premise. Muscle-pattern workouts are absolutely what you want to do. In addition, if you want to really blast your way to bigger size, you have to have at least a passing familiarity with the latest approaches and techniques—what we might call the "science of size." Some of the concepts might sound familiar; others have only moved out of the laboratory and into the gym in the last few years. To make things easy, we've pulled together the latest thinking, along with specific techniques that will make it possible to put the concepts to work *today*.

LIFT FOR LEANNESS

While you're erasing the concept of one-dimensional training, it's worth opening your mind to a relatively new concept in weight loss—or, if you're already lean, weight maintenance. To maintain an optimal weight, you focus on training your muscles, not the cardiovascular system.

The purpose of bodybuilding is to improve muscle size and definition. Of course, this also means cutting fat as much as possible. Traditionally, this has been done by performing 30 to 45 minutes of "cardio" three to four times a week. You can lose weight with cardio. But build muscle at the same time? Nope. Have you ever seen any large, bulky runners or aerobics instructors? There's a good reason for that. The two approaches are contradictory.

You stimulate totally different muscle fibers and body systems for bodybuilding and aerobic exercise. The two are so completely different from each other that doing both at the same time basically makes them both ineffective.

Here's a better approach: functional circuit training. It's a way to get and stay lean, improve your cardiovascular health, *and* maintain (and improve) hard-earned muscle. Think of it as metabolic-type training. Circuit training totally fires up fuel consumption by muscle cells. That's the process that gets fat burning. Along the way, it's also the process that takes you directly to greater size.

Circuit training involves doing relatively high numbers of reps at relatively low weights. For example, one workout might consist of just a few exercises—say, single-leg squats, alternating dumbbell bench presses, alternating single-leg dumbbell rows, and abdominal crunches. You might do up to 10 "circuits"—a complete series of exercises—in a single workout, never lifting more than about 50 to 60 percent of your max weight. It takes a half hour or less. Do it three or four times a week, and you'll find that your weight drops faster than you ever thought possible. You'll have a lot more muscle, too.

Here's how it might work.

- Design a circuit that includes exercises for your lower body, chest and shoulders, upper back, and abdomen. All told, you might line up 10 different exercises.

- For each exercise, choose a weight that you can normally lift 10 times. For your circuit, however, you're only going to perform 5 reps.

- Go from one exercise to the next without stopping. For example, after you finish a set of 5 lunges, immediately start a set of bench presses. Do 5 reps, then immediately move on to the next exercise. Keep going until you finish every exercise in the circuit.

- After completing the first circuit, start from the beginning. Work all the way through the exercises again.

You'll probably want to stop at 4 or 5 circuits when you're starting out. You'll be blowing hard, believe it. As you get in better shape, keep increasing the number of circuits. Ten is a good goal. For variety, throw in some sprints, jumps, pushups, and pullups. These short, simple circuits will promote incredible cardiovascular improvements, without gnawing away at your hard-won size.

Circuits aren't a substitute for your other workouts. You might want to alternate circuit-based cardio days with your regular, all-out workouts. Whatever you do, don't jack up the weights for circuit training. That's not the goal. The idea of circuits isn't to train to lift weights, but to get a solid aerobic workout by lifting.

THE OLYMPIC EDGE

Consider three types of elite lifters, all in the same weight class: a bodybuilder, power lifter, and Olympic lifter. The bodybuilder is clearly the most muscular. The power lifter is probably the strongest, and the Olympic lifter is the most powerful. Athletes in each of these sports perform many of the same ex-

ercises. So why is the Olympic lifter so much more powerful?

Apart from the sheer dedication required to reach Olympic rank, the Olympic lifter performs exercises in a very explosive fashion. The core of his workouts consists of snatches, cleans, jerks, pulls, and squats, or variations and combinations of all of them. What are explosive movements? The athlete attempts to move the weights as quickly as possible. The result of this type of training is more power, what scientists define as force times velocity. The benefits go beyond weight competitions. Explosive workouts improve your ability to jump and sprint, or simply to move quickly in real-life situations.

Bodybuilders are usually in great shape. But because they tend to perform the same type of training all the time, they often lose (or never achieve) their athletic potential even while they're gaining size. So it makes sense to incorporate variations of Olympic and power lifts into your routine. You'll still gain tremendously in size, while honing other physical attributes at the same time.

New research, incidentally, shows that fast-twitch muscle fibers are more capable of hypertrophy (enlargement) than slow-twitch fibers. Adding power movements to your training activates more of these fast-twitch fibers. Bottom line: You can have a buff build *and* more of the athletic skill to use it!

Explosive movements, such as power snatches and power cleans, can be added to most bodybuilding programs. Here are a few things to keep in mind.

- Power exercises require a higher degree of skill than simpler exercises like barbell curls or shoulder presses. Work with an experienced trainer to get started—and spend time learning how to do the movement with light weights.

- It's best to do power exercises first in your workout. If you are just learning how to do a new exercise, perform it first so that fatigue from previous movements does not interfere. Even if you're experienced with these movements, doing them first makes it easier to work on improving your maximal power while you are still fresh. Once you're fatigued, there's no way you'll perform explosive movements to the best of your ability.

- Focus on form, not weight. Most men add weight too quickly. Moving more weight than you can handle almost guarantees bad form. Lifting large weights is certainly gratifying, but improper technique doesn't allow you to develop power or maximize what you can lift.

- Watch yourself in a mirror initially. This makes it easier to spot mistakes in form.

- Quit looking in the mirror as you get more experienced. It will slow you down.

- Initially, focus on learning the *pulling* motion for these exercises. Once you understand the transitional movements that the knees, hips, and other joints undergo throughout the pull, then focus on performing the lift *faster*. When you can perform the pulling motion quickly, progress to more advanced movements.

BAND TRAINING

Band training is a strategy that can vastly expand your training horizons. It's not easy, but the results can be dramatic. Doing a bench press or squat with band resistance requires that you move very fast— but with less risk than when you're working with free weights. Normally, when you try to accelerate the bar in an exercise like the squat or bench press, you have to slow down at some point before you reach full extension of the knee or elbow. If you don't, you run the risk of hyperextending the joint. When you use bands—attaching one end of the band to a fixed object and the other end to a bar—

the force required to complete the movement increases. Since you're working against more tension, you can move the bar in a squat or bench press as fast as possible without being likely to hyperextend a joint. As your mechanical advantage increases in the movement, the tension in the band also increases. That keeps you in a safety zone.

There are all kinds of elastic products available for weight training. These include bungee cords, elastic tubes, and elastic bands. Bungee cords are inexpensive, but don't stretch very far. Elastic tubes aren't always convenient to attach. The elastic bands generally work best. They can be stretched to many times their original length; you don't have to worry about running out the "stretch" as your training progresses. They are basically just giant rubber bands. The ends are easy to attach to the end of a barbell. They come in different widths, with the larger widths providing more tension.

You can do dozens of exercises with bands. Two good choices are the squat and bench press. In both cases, you set up one or more bands on each side of the bar running perpendicular to the ground, and directly under the bar at the start position. If the bands aren't set properly, one side will have more tension than the other, causing the bar to shift toward one side during the movement.

A good approach is to take a block of wood— say, a block of 4-by-4 that's about a foot long. Place a short block of 2-by-4 on each end of one side, so the big blocks rest on the ground, with the 2-by-4 sections touching the floor and the 4-by-4 section on top. You can make grooves on the top side of the 4-by-4 so that two heavy dumbbells can rest in them. Now you have a stable base you can attach a band to.

You simply loop the band around the block, and then through the other end of the band. Then, take the open end and hook it up to the barbell. Make sure to have someone hold the center of the bar to prevent it from falling off an upright. If you are squatting or benching in a power rack, and there are crossbeams at the bottom, you may be able to hook the bands to them, as well.

Sample Band Workout Routines

A popular strategy is to do 8 sets of 3 reps of a particular exercise with the bands. Research indicates that the optimal load for generating mechanical power can vary from 30 percent to 60 percent of the top weight you can lift for that movement. Most men arbitrarily choose 45 to 50 percent of their maximum bench press or squat. If you want to be really precise about determining what your optimal load is, stop by the human performance lab at your local university.

That's more precision than you're likely to need, of course. Just remember that it all boils down to using the best combination of force (weight plus band tension) and velocity to yield maximal power. In the workout plan below, you can do some guesstimating to figure out the 1RM (1 repetition maximum) percentages.

Below is a bench cycle that you can use for 7 weeks. Start by figuring out your maximum bench press (1RM) weight. To calculate your 1RM, see page 14. You can perform one other chest movement in the same workout, and one other triceps movement. You can perform other chest exercises during the second chest workout of the week. On your band bench workouts, always try to move the weights as fast as possible. At the end of the last workout, try a new max bench. You should see a major increase.

REVERSE BAND TRAINING: LIFT BONE-CRUSHING POUNDS WITH EASE!

I compete in Strongman competitions. One of the more common events is the log press. It hadn't been one of my best events. I was stuck at 220 pounds for 1 rep. Most guys I know can do 8 to 10 reps of the same weight. One day, someone suggested I try Reverse Band Log Presses. I gave it a try. Now, I'm log pressing 310 pounds.

SAMPLE BENCH CYCLE

Week	Workout	Band Tension (Wt at top of movement)	on Bar	Total Load (Wt at top of movement)	Reps	Sets
1	1	10% of 1RM	20% of 1RM	30% of 1RM	3	8
2	1	10% of 1RM	25% of 1RM	35% of 1RM	3	8
3	1	15% of 1RM	25% of 1RM	40% of 1RM	3	8
4	1	15% of 1RM	30% of 1RM	45% of 1RM	3	8
5	1	15% of 1RM	35% of 1 RM	50% of 1RM	3	8
6	1	20% of 1RM	35% of 1RM	55% of 1RM	3	8
7	1	20% of 1RM	40% of 1RM	60% of 1RM	3	8

Even if you don't see log pressing in your future, you can still use reverse band training for military presses, squats, and other movements that move the bar fairly straight up and down.

- The bands are looped around the crossbeam at the top of the frame on each side of a power rack. The open ends that hang down are then hooked over the ends of a barbell.

- Test it. Make sure that the tension on both sides is about equal. When everything is set up properly, you should notice that the weight seems lighter at the start of a pressing movement and gets harder as you press upward. During a squat, the weight will feel heavier at the top of the movement, and lighter as you squat down.

- Roughly speaking, the loads are lighter during mechanically weak positions, and heavier during mechanically stronger positions. To keep the weight from stalling out, you have to move the weight very fast.

Sample Reverse Band Workout Routines

The training protocol I use is simple. I perform 8 sets of 3 reps of a particular exercise with the bands. There are no clear-cut guidelines, so you will have to use a little trial and error. If you are military pressing 200 pounds, you may want to start out with a load that is equal to 30 percent of your usual top weight, or 60 pounds at the top.

The rule of thumb is to handle a weight that allows you to perform 3 repetitions in 3 seconds. Have a training partner time you. Have him give the "Start" command and start the timer. The movement will begin with the bar resting on your clavicle. You should lock it out 3 times in 3 seconds. Be careful not to hyperextend your elbow if the weight is too light.

If you finish in under 3 seconds, try adding more weight. Usually 5 to 10 pounds more will be plenty. It should feel easy at the beginning so you can accelerate the weight upward. Of course, as you move up, it gets heavier and becomes harder to press.

SAMPLE MILITARY PRESS CYCLE

Week	Workout	Wt at Bottom of Press	Wt at Top of Press	Reps	Sets
1	1	20% of 1RM	30% of 1RM	3	8
2	1	25% of 1RM	35% of 1RM	3	8
3	1	30% of 1RM	40% of 1RM	3	8
Test your max press					
4	1	45% of 1RM	45% of 1RM	3	8
5	1	40% of 1RM	50% of 1RM	3	8
6	1	45% of 1RM	55% of 1RM	3	8
7	1	50% of 1RM	60% of 1RM	3	8
Test your max press					

On the previous page is a sample cycle that you will use for 7 weeks. You should know your maximum military press weight in order to calculate the loads to use. The idea here is to allow the weight to increase by about 10 percent as you press the weight upward. If you can only set up the bands to get 8 percent or 11 percent, don't worry about it.

You can perform one other shoulder movement in the same workout, and one other triceps movement (if you train shoulders and triceps together). Make sure that your shoulders are fresh; don't train your chest or triceps the day before you use this program. You can perform other shoulder exercises during the second shoulder workout of the week. On your band workouts, always try to move the weights as fast as possible. At the end of the last workout, try a new max. You should see a major increase.

THE POWER RACK: THE TOOL OF CHOICE FOR STRENGTH TRAINING

Whether you're a beginner or an advanced lifter, the power rack has a lot to offer. It makes lifting safer, for one thing. If you're creative, it's a good platform to set up equipment for dozens of different movements. Every gym has at least one power rack. If you're thinking of setting up workout space at home, it's well worth the money.

When popping for a power rack, here are a few points to consider.

- Is the frame tall enough? If you plan to do standing overhead presses inside the rack, the bar should be able to move freely without hitting the top of the rack. For most guys, 84 inches is high enough. If the bar does hit the top of the rack, you may have to perform some of your exercises in a seated position, or set them up outside of the rack.
- Check out the frame strength. The gauge of steel is important. The lower the gauge, the thicker, heavier, and more expensive the frame will be. Eleven gauge or lower is plenty, even for the heaviest loads.
- How many pieces make up the frame? Multiple pieces with lots of joints that have to be bolted together can yield a rack that warps or moves at the joints. This can be corrected by bolting it to the floor, a platform, or a wall. Solid, one-piece racks are usually sturdier, but can be very expensive to ship. Find out what the shipping charges are before you commit to purchasing one, so you aren't surprised when the bill arrives.
- There should be holes every few inches along the uprights. Horizontal guide rods go through the holes. You can use these as range of motion limiters for partial squats, deadlifts, or presses. You can also use them as safety rods, where you set them slightly below where you intend to stop a given movement. Advanced lifters prefer that the holes be closer together because that allows them to progressively increase the range of motion.
- Make sure that the guide bars are heavy enough to handle some weight being dropped on them. They should be at least 1 inch in diameter.
- Attachments. A power rack is only as versatile as the gear that comes along with it. Don't assume power racks are only for squats; you can do all sorts of upper- and lower-body workouts as long as you have the right gear, such as chinup bars, adjustable dip bars, pulldown and row attachments, and so on.

How to Use a Power Rack

Power racks have so many potential features and attachments that it would almost take a separate book to describe them all. Assuming you're using the rack at the gym, or already have set one up in your garage or basement, here are some of the workouts you can design around it, and the key guidelines for doing so.

Get the full range of motion. Whether you're doing squats, deadlifts, pulls, or presses, take the extra minute to set the J hooks (or clamps) at the appropriate height for the bar to be unracked. While you're at it, set up the horizontal guide bars at the bottom position. They'll act as a safety catch in case you can't complete a repetition.

- For squats, set the bar at shoulder level. Set the safety rods about 2 inches below a safe bottom position. A safe bottom position means as deep as you can go without pain, and without compromising your mechanical position. You should squat to a point just before your lower back starts to round. A lot of men don't bother using the safety rods, and every year a lot of guys get hurt.

- For deadlifts, clean pulls, and snatch pulls, you can set the bar on the floor and just pull from there. Or set up the bar outside the rack at the top position. Unrack the weight, take two small steps back, and lower the bar to the floor, using proper back mechanics. This is a good approach for beginners because it helps get them used to the starting position. Advanced lifters also use this technique to reestablish their starting positions.

- Set the bar for presses about 2 inches short of full elbow extension. Set the safety rods about 2 inches below your clavicle for shoulder presses, or 2 inches below your chest for chest presses.

Take advantage of partial movements. Even though you usually want to move through your full range of motion, there are times when partial movements can pay off. When I was a teenager, I missed several attempts at 350 pounds in the squat. My coach recommended that I try partial squats. So I raised the cross bars in the power rack—and didn't have any trouble working up to 500 pounds. After

a while, I lowered the bar back down to allow a full squat—and made 350 pounds.

Many of today's power lifters come out of the bottom position in the squat very explosively. Then they seem to get stuck or stall out at the top part. This is probably due, in part, to all of the supportive equipment that athletes use today. Denim squat suits, knee wraps, and belts really help out the most on the bottom position of a squat. After a lifter comes up so far, the equipment is not as effective, and that's when the legs, hips, and back really have to work. Partial squats can address this issue.

It works for deadlifts, too. A lot of men start the deadlift with their lower back rounded. This can be addressed by setting the pins in the rack so that the bar is a few inches off the ground. This makes it easier to focus on your form. Later, you can progressively lower the bar and still maintain a flat or slightly arched back.

If you have a rack with technique trays, you can set them below the knee, above the knee, or just short of full knee extension. You can also do this with the safety rods, but be careful not to let the bar hit the rods too hard or you will wear out the knurling.

Work in some isometrics. Isometric workouts can be brutal. While performing a squat or a bench press, you might want to try getting a submaximal weight—say, 70 percent to 80 percent of your 1RM—into position, then having a training partner slide the cross bars into holes set at your "sticking" point. Push up against the cross bars for 3 to 5 seconds, have your partner remove the rods, and then complete the rep. This is tricky at first. But if done right, adding isometrics to your dynamic movements will add a lot of strength in a hurry.

If you train by yourself, you'll need to do more traditional isometric training. Unrack the bar and push up against the cross rods. You may want to have four rods set up at two levels. Unrack the weight off the first set, and push against the second set. This way you are protected when the weight comes back down. For deadlifts or pulls, you can start off the floor and just pull against pins set at your sticking point.

ADVANCED TRAINING CONCEPTS YOU CAN USE TODAY

If you've been lifting for any length of time, you have an instinctive sense of the workouts that give the best payoffs, and how long and heavy to lift. Instinct isn't a bad thing, but it can only take you so far. The men who show the most gains in size, strength, or definition don't depend on instinct, but *knowledge*. Sports physiologists have pretty much nailed down what you need to do to hit your optimal size. Most of that information, unfortunately, is buried in academic articles with titles like "The Effects of Muscle Overload on Male Cynomolgus Monkeys." Not exactly the kind of reading you can catch up on while waiting to get your teeth cleaned.

Whether you're a beginning lifter or have been doing it for years, you can use a lot of these principles today, *now*, to get the body you want.

Stay in the "rest window." The *only* way to make maximal gains in strength and size is to rest muscles between sets. But the window for resting is relatively short. Rest periods of 30 seconds to 60 seconds stimulate more growth hormone than longer rest periods.

Your best bet is to have a work-to-rest ratio of 1:1. Rest between sets for the same length of time that it takes you to perform the sets.

Superset opposing muscles. It's the best way to minimize the time spent working out while increasing muscle-building volume. The idea of supersetting, also known as "push-pull," is to alternate exercises that work opposing muscles. For example, bench presses followed by barbell rows, or leg extensions followed by leg curls, or biceps curls fol-lowed by triceps pushdowns. The time savings come from allowing one group of muscles to recover while you're working another group. You're not just standing around between sets.

Identify weak spots with balance training. This basically means using muscle strength for balance rather than holding on to something. For example, do single-leg squats without hanging on to the rack. Vary the position of your free leg for each set, putting it in front of you, beside you, behind you, and so on. This type of balance training increases body awareness and makes it easy to spot muscle weakness that can occur on either your right or left side.

You can incorporate all sorts of balance movements into your regular workout. For example, do single-leg squats while holding a dumbbell in each hand. Try squats on rockerboards or foam rolls. Challenge your upper body by putting your hands on a stability ball and do pushups. For the ultimate body-balance challenge, try kneeling or standing on a stability ball and pressing some weights overhead.

Shake up your tempo. Don't lock yourself in with the old-school rule about taking 2 seconds for the concentric (exertion) phase and 4 seconds for the eccentric (relaxation) phase. This is a good starting place, but you want to challenge your muscles by changing the tempo often. Do all of your reps very quickly or very slowly for a change. Do one quickly, and the next one slowly. Pause during the eccentric movements. Vary the number of pauses and hold times.

Suppose you're doing pullups. Pause three times during the lowering phase, and hold for 5 seconds at each pause. The next set, do something different. Or, during the eccentric portion of a bench press, pause the bar on your chest for 3 to 5 seconds, then explode it off your chest for the concentric movement.

Try the wave technique. Everyone gets stuck in

plateaus. If you find you're having trouble lifting a particular weight, or if you want to progress to a heavier weight more quickly, do exercise "waves."

Let's say that you've been squatting about 215 pounds for 5 reps, but can't quite make it to 225. Do your warmup sets, then perform a wave like this: 5 reps at 175 pounds, 5 reps at 195, and 5 reps at 215. Take a 3- to 5-minute rest between each set. Then, after resting for an additional 3 to 5 minutes after completing the first wave, perform the next one. This time, do 5 reps at slightly higher weights, say, 185, 205, and 225.

Double stimulate. For some real variety and cutting-edge training, try the Double Stimulation method. A Double Stimulation workout places a high demand on the neuromuscular system, which leads to great gains in strength, speed, and power. Perform 2 warmup sets of a movement. Next, perform 1 set of 5 reps. Rest, then perform a set with a heavier weight for 1 rep. Repeat this segment two more times.

It's not as confusing as it sounds. Once you've figured out your 1RM (see page 14) for a given exercise, you can use the following percentages and reps to maximize a Double Stimulation workout.

- Warmup: Five reps at 60 percent of your 1RM. Rest. Five reps at 70 percent. Rest.

- Segment 1: Five reps at 80 percent. Rest. One rep at 90 percent. Rest.

- Segment 2: Five reps at 80 percent. Rest. One rep at 90 percent. Rest.

- Segment 3: Five reps at 80 percent. Rest. One rep at 90 percent.

The rest periods should be 3 to 5 minutes. Lift the weights as quickly as possible.

Periodize your training. This is just a fancy way of saying you should *always* introduce variety into your workouts by changing the variables: the number of reps and sets; the length of rest periods; the tempo and intensity; adding supersets or eccentric training; and so on. Pick a workout and stick with it for a cycle of 4 to 12 weeks. Then change things around.

Periodization keeps muscles stimulated. It also reduces the risk of overtraining and injury. Lifters who stick to the same program month after month essentially stop making progress.

Allow plenty of downtime. Lifting weights for 2 hours at a pop, 6 days a week, is almost total overkill. It doesn't allow enough rest for muscle fibers to regrow. As a rule, split your workouts by movement patterns, keep them under an hour, and don't hesitate to take days off.

Stick to compound movements. Advanced bodybuilders do a lot of isolation exercises. It makes sense for athletes at this level because they already have a great deal of muscle mass, and only need to strengthen and build areas that need improvement. Recreational lifters don't require—and don't benefit from—this level of specialization. Stick with compound movements, exercises such as bench presses or pulldowns, which utilize more than a single muscle group. Compound movements cause the body to release more muscle-building hormones.

SAMPLE TOTAL-BODY WORKOUTS

Our goal with *Men's Health* Maximum Muscle Plan is to help you add on as much muscle as possible and to get as strong as possible. Subtle changes like grip width, stance position, toe angle, etc. can affect the specific muscle fibers utilized for the movement. Ultimately, this can help you take your physique to the next level. Throughout the rest of this chapter you'll see exercises with qualifiers like toes in or out, close grip or wide grip. These subtle changes can contribute to big results.

LEVEL 1 (FOCUS ON SIZE)
Level 1, Workout #1: Three Days a Week

The complete program is summarized in the chart below. Here are a few additional points to keep in mind.

- For each exercise, do 2 warmup sets. Use 50 percent and 75 percent of the weight you plan to lift for the exercise.

- Do 3 sets of each exercise, completing the specified number of repetitions.

- For each pair of exercises, perform them in an alternating fashion. On Day 1, for example, follow your dynamic warmup program (page 285) with a single warmup set for the barbell row, lifting 50 percent of your top weight. Then, do a warmup set on the bench press, again

WEEK 1

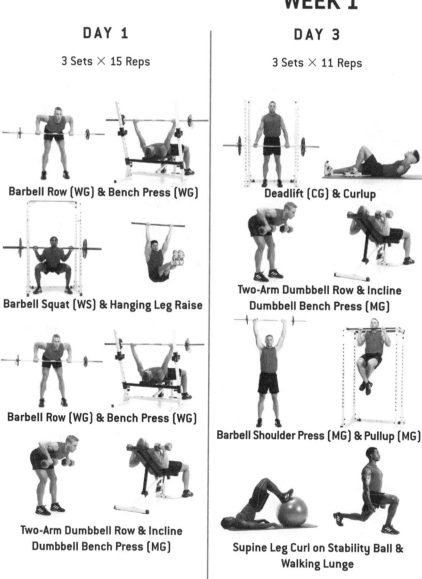
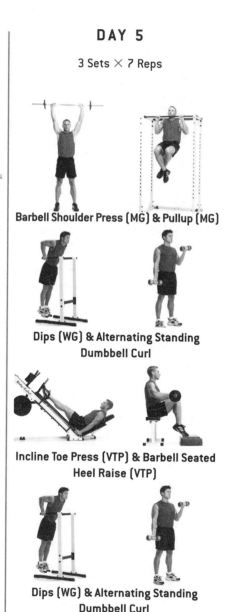

DAY 1
3 Sets × 15 Reps

Barbell Row (WG) & Bench Press (WG)

Barbell Squat (WS) & Hanging Leg Raise

Barbell Row (WG) & Bench Press (WG)

Two-Arm Dumbbell Row & Incline Dumbbell Bench Press (MG)

DAY 3
3 Sets × 11 Reps

Deadlift (CG) & Curlup

Two-Arm Dumbbell Row & Incline Dumbbell Bench Press (MG)

Barbell Shoulder Press (MG) & Pullup (MG)

Supine Leg Curl on Stability Ball & Walking Lunge

DAY 5
3 Sets × 7 Reps

Barbell Shoulder Press (MG) & Pullup (MG)

Dips (WG) & Alternating Standing Dumbbell Curl

Incline Toe Press (VTP) & Barbell Seated Heel Raise (VTP)

Dips (WG) & Alternating Standing Dumbbell Curl

lifting 50 percent of your top weight. Go back to the barbell row and do the second warmup set, with 75 percent of your top weight. Then do the same thing for the bench press. Finally, do "real" sets, alternating sets between the two exercises. Repeat this same strategy for all of the paired exercises.

- Note that you start with upper body workouts in Week 1. In Week 2, you start with lower body workouts.

- On days with lower rep counts, increase your top weight.

- Repeat this 2-week cycle for 12 weeks.

WEEK 2

DAY 1

3 Sets × 15 Reps

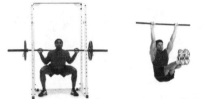

Barbell Squat (WS) & Hanging Leg Raise

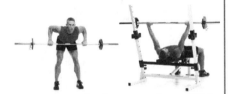

Barbell Row (WG) & Bench Press (WG)

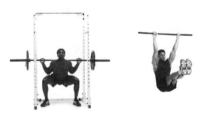

Barbell Squat (WS) & Hanging Leg Raise

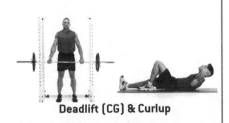

Deadlift (CG) & Curlup

DAY 3

3 Sets × 11 Reps

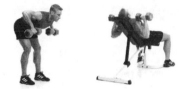

Two-Arm Dumbbell Row & Incline Dumbbell Bench Press (MG)

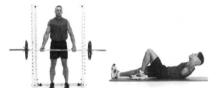

Deadlift (CG) & Curlup

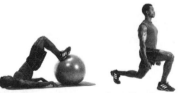

Supine Leg Curl on Stability Ball & Walking Lunge

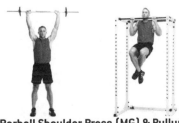

Barbell Shoulder Press (MG) & Pullup (MG)

DAY 5

3 Sets × 7 Reps

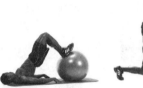

Supine Leg Curl on Stability Ball & Walking Lunge

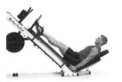

Incline Toe Press (VTP) & Barbell Seated Heel Raise (VTP)

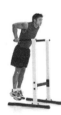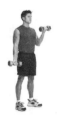

Dips (WG) & Alternating Standing Dumbbell Curl

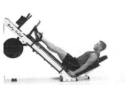

Incline Toe Press (VTP) & Barbell Seated Heel Raise (VTP)

CG = CLOSE GRIP; CS = CLOSE STANCE; MG = MEDIUM GRIP; MS = MEDIUM STANCE; VTP = VARY TOE POSITION EACH SET; WG = WIDE GRIP; WS = WIDE STANCE.

Level 1, Workout #2: Four Days a Week

The complete program is summarized in the chart below. Unlike Workout #1, this plan is based on a 3-week cycle.

- For each exercise, do 2 warmup sets. Use 50 percent and 75 percent of the weight you plan to lift for the exercise.

- Do 3 sets of each exercise, completing the specified number of repetitions.

- For each pair of exercises, perform them in an alternating fashion. On Day 1, for example, follow your dynamic warmup program (page 285) with

WEEK 1

Day 1
3 SETS × 15 REPS

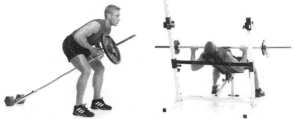

Barbell T-Bar Row (MG) & Incline Barbell Bench Press (MG)

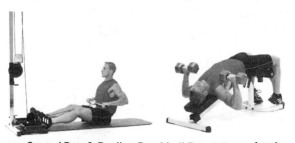

Seated Row & Decline Dumbbell Bench Press (WG)

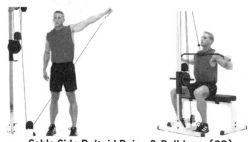

Cable Side Deltoid Raise & Pulldown (CG)

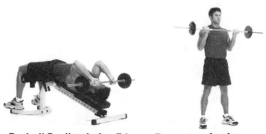

Barbell Decline Lying Triceps Extension (CG) & Narrow Grip Biceps Curl with Straight Bar

Day 2
3 SETS × 11 REPS

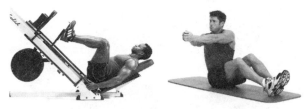

Incline Leg Press (CS) & Russian Twist

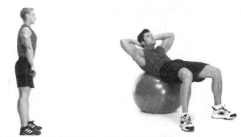

Romanian Deadlift & Stability Ball Crunch

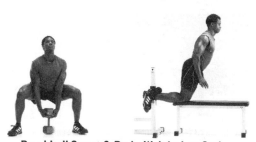

Dumbbell Squat & Body-Weight Leg Curl

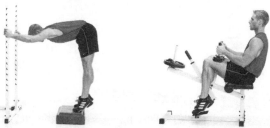

Body-Weight Donkey Calf Raise (VTP) & Machine Seated Heel Raise (VTP)

a single warmup set for the barbell T-bar row, lifting 50 percent of your top weight. Then, do a warmup set on the incline barbell bench press, again lifting 50 percent of your top weight. Go back to the barbell T-bar row and do the second warmup set, with 75 percent of your top weight. Then do the same thing for the incline barbell bench press. Finally, do "real" sets, alternating sets between the two exercises. Repeat this same strategy for all of the paired exercises.

- On days with lower rep counts, increase your top weight.
- Repeat this 3-week cycle for 12 weeks.

WEEK 1

Day 4	Day 5
3 SETS × 7 REPS	**3 SETS × 15 REPS**

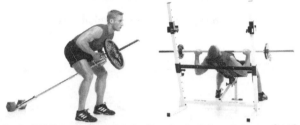

Barbell T-Bar Row (MG) & Incline Barbell Bench Press (MG)

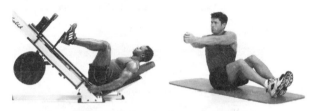

Incline Leg Press (CS) & Russian Twist

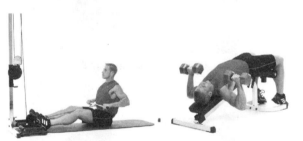

Seated Row & Decline Dumbbell Bench Press (WG)

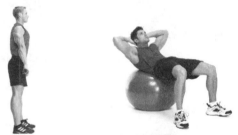

Romanian Deadlift & Stability Ball Crunch

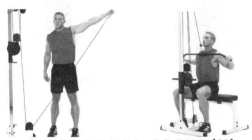

Cable Side Deltoid Raise & Pulldown (CG)

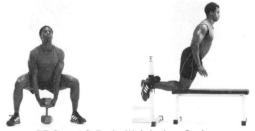

DB Squat & Body-Weight Leg Curl

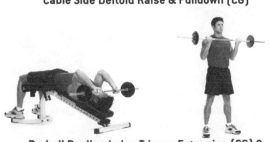

Barbell Decline Lying Triceps Extension (CG) & Biceps Curl with Straight Bar (CG)

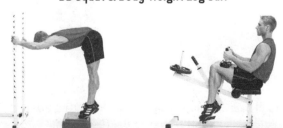

Body-Weight Donkey Calf Raise (VTP) & Machine Seated Heel Raise (VTP)

CG = CLOSE GRIP; CS = CLOSE STANCE; MG = MEDIUM GRIP; MS = MEDIUM STANCE; VTP = VARY TOE POSITION EACH SET; WG = WIDE GRIP; WS = WIDE STANCE.

WEEK 2

Day 1	Day 2
3 SETS × 11 REPS	**3 SETS × 7 REPS**

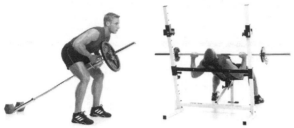

Barbell T-Bar Row (MG) & Incline Barbell Bench Press (MG)

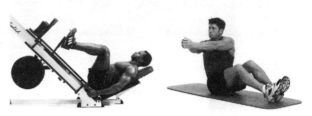

Incline Leg Press (CS) & Russian Twist

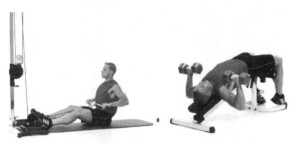

Seated Row & Decline Dumbbell Bench Press (WG)

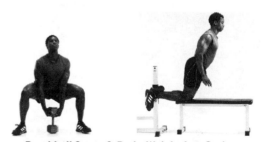

Romanian Deadlift & Stability Ball Crunch

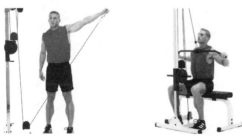

Cable Side Deltoid Raise & Pulldown (CG)

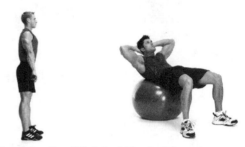

Dumbbell Squat & Body-Weight Leg Curl

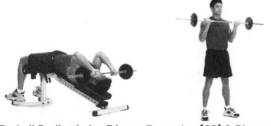

Barbell Decline Lying Triceps Extension (CG) & Biceps Curl with Straight Bar (CG)

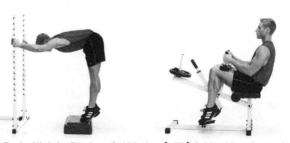

Body-Weight Donkey Calf Raise (VTP) & Machine Seated Heel Raise (VTP)

WEEK 2 (cont.)

Day 4
3 SETS × 15 REPS

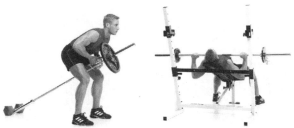

Barbell T-Bar Row (MG) & Incline Barbell Bench Press (MG)

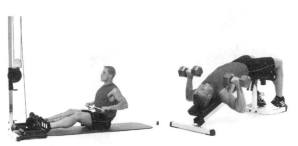

Seated Row & Decline Dumbbell Bench Press (WG)

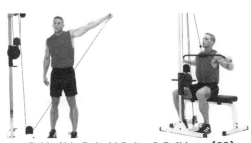

Cable Side Deltoid Raise & Pulldown (CG)

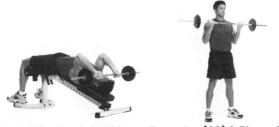

Barbell Decline Lying Triceps Extension (CG) & Biceps Curl
with Straight Bar (CG)

Day 5
3 SETS × 11 REPS

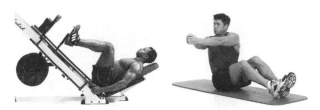

Incline Leg Press (CS) & Russian Twist

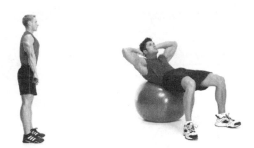

Romanian Deadlift & Stability Ball Crunch

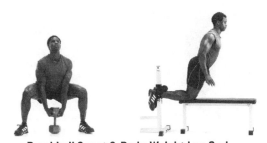

Dumbbell Squat & Body-Weight Leg Curl

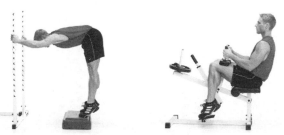

Body-Weight Donkey Calf Raise (VTP) & Machine Seated
Heel Raise (VTP)

CG = CLOSE GRIP; CS = CLOSE STANCE; MG = MEDIUM GRIP; MS = MEDIUM STANCE; VTP = VARY TOE
POSITION EACH SET; WG = WIDE GRIP; WS = WIDE STANCE.

WEEK 3

Day 1
3 SETS × 7 REPS

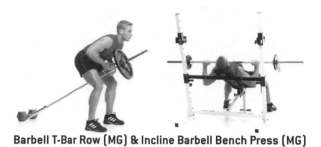

Barbell T-Bar Row (MG) & Incline Barbell Bench Press (MG)

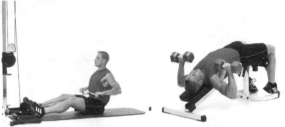

Seated Row & Decline Dumbbell Bench Press (WG)

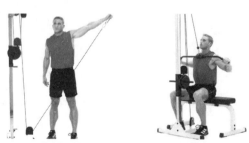

Cable Side Deltoid Raise & Pulldown

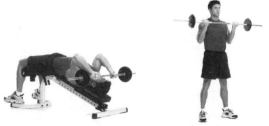

Barbell Decline Lying Triceps Extension (CG) & Biceps Curl with Straight Bar (CG)

Day 2
3 SETS × 15 REPS

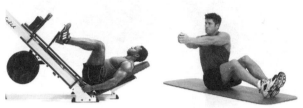

Incline Leg Press (CS) & Russian Twist

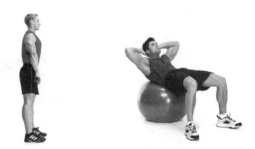

Romanian Deadlift & Stability Ball Crunch

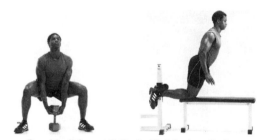

Dumbbell Squat & Body-Weight Leg Curl

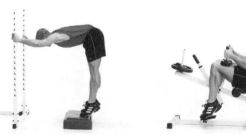

Body-Weight Donkey Calf Raise (VTP) & Machine Seated Heel Raise (VTP)

WEEK 3 (cont.)

Day 4
3 SETS × 11 REPS

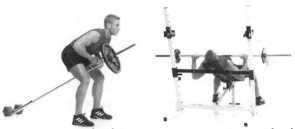

Barbell T-Bar Row (MG) & Incline Barbell Bench Press (MG)

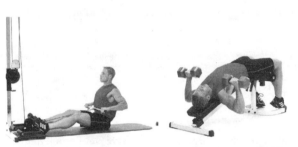

Seated Row & Decline Dumbbell Bench Press (WG)

Cable Side Deltoid Raise & Pulldown

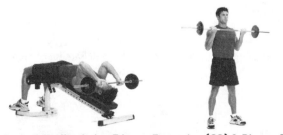

Barbell Decline Lying Triceps Extension (CG) & Biceps Curl
with Straight Bar (CG)

Day 5
3 SETS × 7 REPS

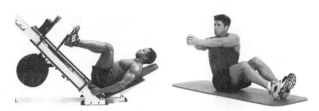

Incline Leg Press (CS) & Russian Twist

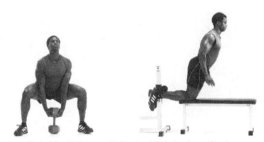

Romanian Deadlift & Stability Ball Crunch

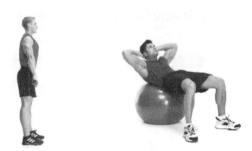

Dumbbell Squat & Body-Weight Leg Curl

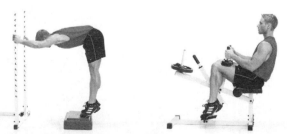

Body-Weight Donkey Calf Raise (VTP) & Machine Seated
Heel Raise (VTP)

CG = CLOSE GRIP; CS = CLOSE STANCE; MG = MEDIUM GRIP; MS = MEDIUM STANCE; VTP = VARY TOE
POSITION EACH SET; WG = WIDE GRIP; WS = WIDE STANCE.

LEVEL 2 (FOCUS ON STRENGTH)

Level 2, Workout #1: Three Days a Week

The complete program is summarized in the chart below. Here are a few additional points to keep in mind.

- For each exercise, do 2 warmup sets. Warm up with 50 percent to 75 percent of the weight you plan to lift during the "real" sets.

- For each pair of exercises, perform them in an alternating fashion. On Day 1, for example, follow your dynamic warmup program (page 285) with a single warmup set for the barbell row, lifting 50 percent of your top weight. Then perform a warmup set on the bench press, again lifting 50 percent of your top weight. Go back to the barbell row and do the second warmup set, with 75 percent of your top weight. Then do the same thing for the bench press. Finally, do "real" sets,

---

WEEK 1

DAY 1	DAY 3	DAY 5
3 Sets × 9 Reps	3 Sets × 6 Reps	3 Sets × 3 Reps

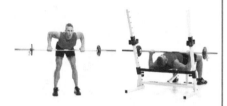

Barbell Row (MG) & Flat Barbell Bench Press (MG)

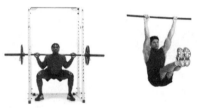

Barbell Squat (MS) & Hanging Leg Raise

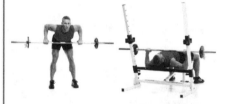

Barbell Row (MG) & Flat Barbell Bench Press (MG)

 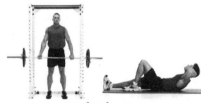

Two-Arm Dumbbell Row & Incline Dumbbell Bench Press (WG)

Deadlift (WG) & Curlup

Two-Arm Dumbbell Row & Incline Dumbbell Bench Press (WG)

 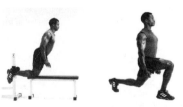 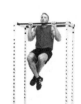

Pullup (WG) & Barbell Shoulder Press (Seated with WG)

Body-Weight Leg Curl & Walking Lunge

Pullup (WG) & Barbell Shoulder Press (Seated with WG)

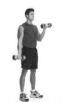   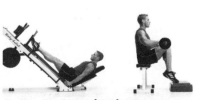 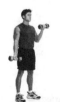 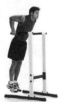

Alternating Standing Dumbbell Curl & Dips (MG)

Incline Toe Press (VTP) & Barbell Seated Heel Raise (VTP)

Alternating Standing Dumbbell Curl & Dips (MG)

---

alternating sets between the two exercises. Repeat this same strategy for all of the paired exercises.

- Note that you start with upper body workouts in Week 1. In Week 2, you start with lower body workouts.

- On days with lower rep counts, increase your top weight.

- Repeat this 2-week cycle for 12 weeks.

- Note that this program uses basically the same exercises as the program in Level 1, Workout #1. The difference here is that the reps are lower and the grip and stance widths are different. These subtle changes make the difference in targeting different muscle fibers.

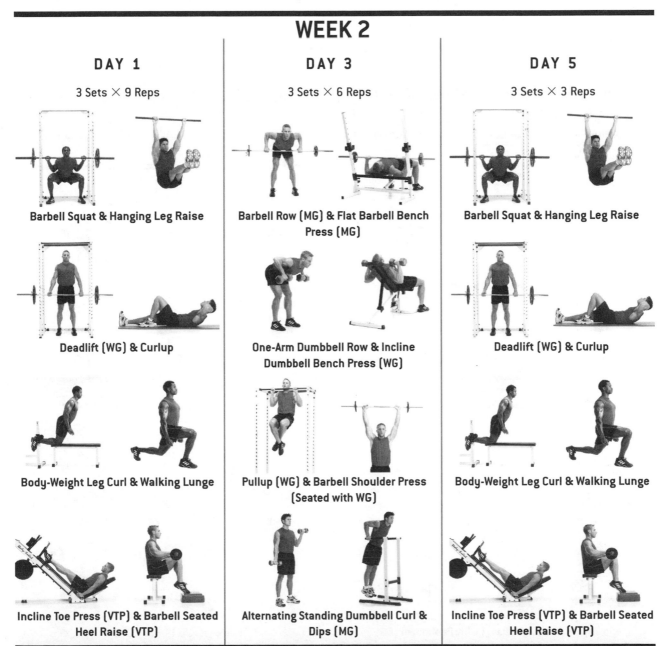

WEEK 2

DAY 1

3 Sets × 9 Reps

Barbell Squat & Hanging Leg Raise

Deadlift (WG) & Curlup

Body-Weight Leg Curl & Walking Lunge

Incline Toe Press (VTP) & Barbell Seated Heel Raise (VTP)

DAY 3

3 Sets × 6 Reps

Barbell Row (MG) & Flat Barbell Bench Press (MG)

One-Arm Dumbbell Row & Incline Dumbbell Bench Press (WG)

Pullup (WG) & Barbell Shoulder Press (Seated with WG)

Alternating Standing Dumbbell Curl & Dips (MG)

DAY 5

3 Sets × 3 Reps

Barbell Squat & Hanging Leg Raise

Deadlift (WG) & Curlup

Body-Weight Leg Curl & Walking Lunge

Incline Toe Press (VTP) & Barbell Seated Heel Raise (VTP)

CG = CLOSE GRIP; CS = CLOSE STANCE; MG = MEDIUM GRIP; MS = MEDIUM STANCE; VTP = VARY TOE POSITION EACH SET; WG = WIDE GRIP; WS = WIDE STANCE.

Level 2, Workout #2: Four Days a Week

This plan includes routines for maxing your bench press, squat, and deadlift. Round all weights to the nearest 5 pounds.

- For each of these routines, do 2 lighter sets to warm up. Use 50 percent and 75 percent of your 1RM for your warmup. Do only 5 reps each.

- Do 3 sets of each exercise, completing the specified number of repetitions.

- For each pair of exercises, perform them in an alternating fashion. On Day 1, for example, follow your dynamic warmup program (page 285) with a single warmup set for the seated row, lifting 50 percent of your top weight. Then, do a warmup set on the barbell bench press, again lifting 50 percent of your top weight. Go back to the cable row and do the second warmup set, with 75 percent of your top weight. Then do the same thing for the barbell bench press. Finally, do "real" sets, alternating sets between the two exercises. Repeat this same strategy for all of the paired exercises.

- On days with lower rep counts, increase your top weight.

- Repeat this program for 9 weeks.

Max Bench Press, Squat, and Deadlift Routine

On the first day of each week of the cycle, bench press 80 percent of your 1RM for 6 sets of 2 reps each.

Then, perform 3 sets of 9 reps for all other exer-

Day 1

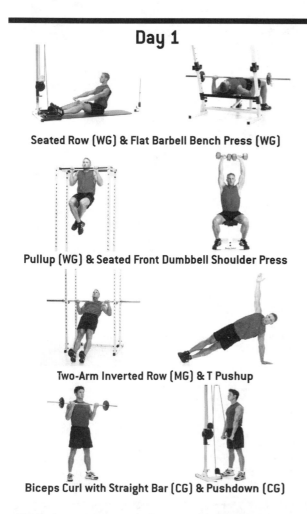

Seated Row (WG) & Flat Barbell Bench Press (WG)

Pullup (WG) & Seated Front Dumbbell Shoulder Press

Two-Arm Inverted Row (MG) & T Pushup

Biceps Curl with Straight Bar (CG) & Pushdown (CG)

Day 2

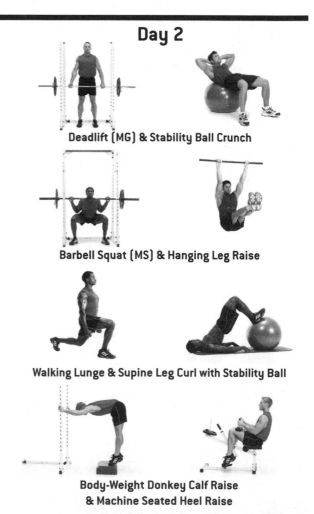

Deadlift (MG) & Stability Ball Crunch

Barbell Squat (MS) & Hanging Leg Raise

Walking Lunge & Supine Leg Curl with Stability Ball

Body-Weight Donkey Calf Raise
& Machine Seated Heel Raise

cises except seated rows. Those should follow the same rep and set scheme as the bench press.

On Day 2 of each week of the cycle, squat 80 percent of your 1RM for 6 sets of 2 reps each. Then, perform 3 sets of 9 reps for all other exercises except deadlifts and hanging leg raises. For the hanging leg raises, follow the same rep and set scheme as the squat. A separate program for deadlifts is given below.

Here's the "max" program for the deadlift (Day 2), bench press (Day 4), and squat (Day 5):

- In week one, lift 80 percent of your 1RM for 6 sets of 3 reps each.

- In week two, lift 80 percent of your 1RM for 6 sets of 4 reps each.

- In week three, lift 80 percent of your 1RM for 6 sets of 5 reps each.

- In week four, lift 80 percent of your 1RM for 6 sets of 6 reps each.

- In week five, lift 85 percent of your 1RM for 5 sets of 5 reps each.

- In week six, lift 90 percent of your 1RM for 4 sets of 4 reps each.

- In week seven, lift 95 percent of your 1RM for 3 sets of 3 reps each.

- In week eight, lift 100 percent of your 1RM for 2 sets of 2 reps each.

- In week nine, lift 105 percent of your 1RM for 2 sets of 1 rep each. After completing the 2 sets, keep doing single reps, allowing 2 minutes' rest between sets, increasing the weight 5 to 10 pounds each time. Keep going until you hit your new 1RM.

Day 4

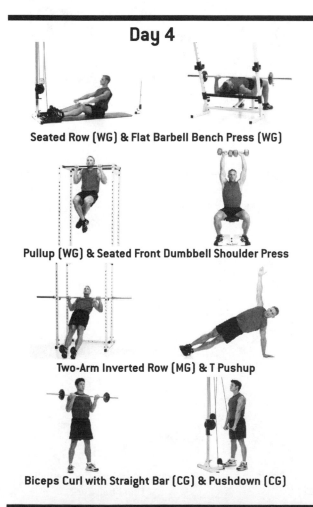

Seated Row (WG) & Flat Barbell Bench Press (WG)

Pullup (WG) & Seated Front Dumbbell Shoulder Press

Two-Arm Inverted Row (MG) & T Pushup

Biceps Curl with Straight Bar (CG) & Pushdown (CG)

Day 5

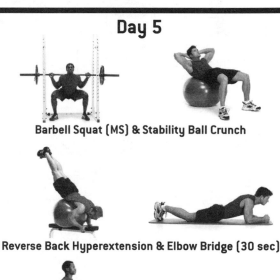

Barbell Squat (MS) & Stability Ball Crunch

Reverse Back Hyperextension & Elbow Bridge (30 sec)

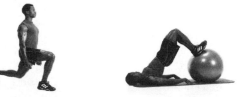

Walking Lunge & Supine Leg Curl with Stability Ball

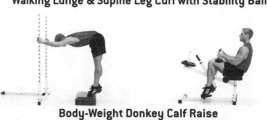

Body-Weight Donkey Calf Raise & Machine Seated Heel Raise

CG = CLOSE GRIP; CS = CLOSE STANCE; MG = MEDIUM GRIP; MS = MEDIUM STANCE; VTP = VARY TOE POSITION EACH SET; WG = WIDE GRIP; WS = WIDE STANCE.

LEVEL 3 (FOCUS ON SIZE AND STRENGTH)

Level 3, Workout #1: Three Days a Week

The complete program is summarized in the chart below. Here are a few additional points to keep in mind.

- For each exercise, do 2 warmup sets. Warm up with 50 percent to 75 percent of the weight you plan to lift during the "real" sets.

- For each pair of exercises, perform them in an alternating fashion. On Day 1, for example, follow your dynamic warmup program (page 285) with a single warmup set for the seated row, lifting 50 percent of your top weight. Then perform a warmup set on the decline bench press, again lifting 50 percent of your top weight. Go back to the seated row and do the second warmup set, with 75 percent of your top weight. Then do the same thing for the decline bench press. Finally, do

WEEK 1

DAY 1	DAY 3	DAY 5
3 Sets × 12 Reps	3 Sets × 6 Reps	3 Sets × 2 Reps

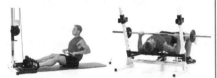

Seated Row (WG) & Decline Barbell Bench Press (WG)

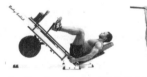

Incline Leg Press (MS) & Hanging Knee Raise Crossover

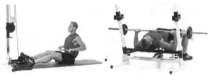

Seated Row (WG) & Decline Barbell Bench Press (WG)

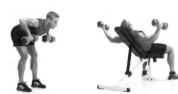

Two-Arm Dumbbell Row & Incline Dumbbell Fly (WG)

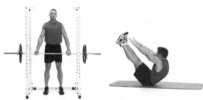

Deadlift (WG) & Jackknife Knee to Chest

Two-Arm Dumbbell Row & Incline Dumbbell Fly (WG)

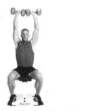

Seated Front Dumbbell Press (MG) & Alternating Grip Chinup (MG)

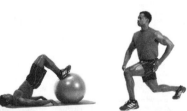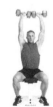

Supine Leg Curl with Stability Ball & Partial Split Squat

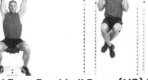

Seated Front Dumbbell Press (MG) & Alternating Grip Chinup (MG)

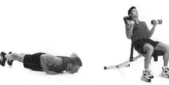

Floor Pushup (MG) & Double Incline Dumbbell Curl

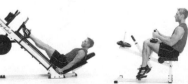

Incline Toe Press (VTP) & Machine Seated Heel Raise (VTP)

Floor Pushup (MG) & Double Incline Dumbbell Curl

"real" sets, alternating sets between the two exercises. Repeat this same strategy for all of the paired exercises.

- Note that you start with upper body workouts in Week 1. In Week 2, you start with lower body workouts.
- On days with lower rep counts, increase your top weight.

- Repeat this 2-week cycle for 12 weeks.
- Note that this program uses basically the same exercises as the program in Level 1, Workout #1. The difference here is that the reps are lower and the grip and stance widths are different. These subtle changes make the difference in targeting different muscle fibers.

WEEK 2

DAY 1	DAY 3	DAY 5
3 Sets × 12 Reps	3 Sets × 6 Reps	3 Sets × 3 Reps

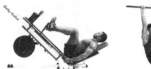

Incline Leg Press (MS) & Hanging Knee Raise Crossover

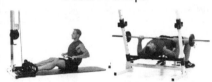

Seated Cable Row (WG) & Decline Barbell Bench Press (WG)

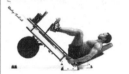

Incline Leg Press (MS) & Hanging Knee Raise Crossover

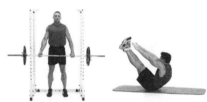

Deadlift (WG) & Jackknife Knee to Chest

 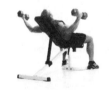

Two-Arm Dumbbell Row & Incline Dumbbell Fly (WG)

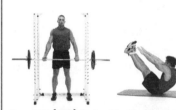

Deadlift (WG) & Jackknife Knee to Chest

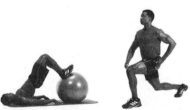

Supine Leg Curl with Stability Ball & Partial Split Squat

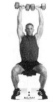 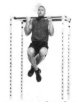

Seated Front Dumbbell Press (MG) & Alternating Grip Chinup (MG)

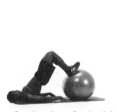 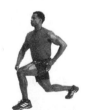

Supine Leg Curl with Stability Ball & Partial Split Squat

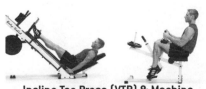

Incline Toe Press (VTP) & Machine Seated Heel Raise (VTP)

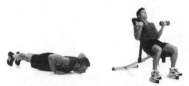

Floor Pushup (MG) & Double Incline Dumbbell Curl

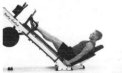

Incline Toe Press (VTP) & Machine Seated Heel Raise (VTP)

CG = CLOSE GRIP; CS = CLOSE STANCE; MG = MEDIUM GRIP; MS = MEDIUM STANCE; VTP = VARY TOE POSITION EACH SET; WG = WIDE GRIP; WS = WIDE STANCE

TOTAL HARD BODY 279

Level 3, Workout #2: Four Days a Week

- This plan includes heavy and light days each week, along with subtle changes in hand and foot positions. These changes stimulate different muscle fibers.

- For this routine, do 2 lighter sets to warm up. Use 50 percent and 75 percent of your top weight for

the workout for your warmups. Do only 5 reps each.

- For each pair of exercises, perform them in an alternating fashion. On Day 1, for example, follow your dynamic warmup program (page 285) with a single warmup set for the seated row, lifting 50 percent of your top weight. Then, do a warmup set on the barbell bench press, again lifting 50

Day 1

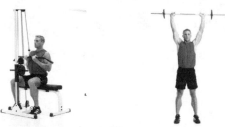

Seated Row (MG) & Flat Barbell Bench Press (MG)

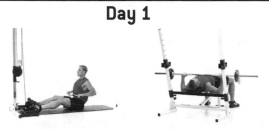

Reverse Grip Pulldown (WG) & Smith Machine Front Shoulder Press (WG) (Variation of Barbell Shoulder Press)

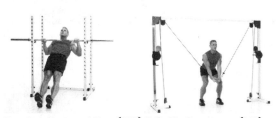

Two-Arm Inverted Row (WG) & Cable Crossover (LH)

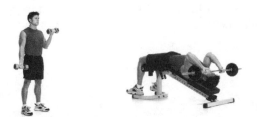

Alternating Standing Dumbbell Curl & Barbell Decline Lying Triceps Extension

Day 2

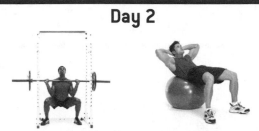

Front Squat (MS) & Stability Ball Crunch

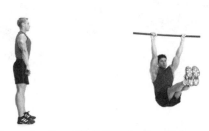

Romanian Deadlift & Hanging Leg Raise

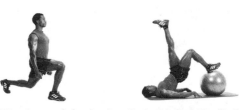

Walking Lunge & Supine Leg Curl with Stability Ball

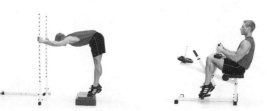

Body-Weight Donkey Calf Raise & Machine Seated Heel Raise

percent of your top weight. Go back to the seated row and do the second warmup set, with 75 percent of your top weight. Then do the same thing for the barbell bench press. Finally, do "real" sets, alternating sets between the two exercises. Repeat this same strategy for all of the paired exercises.

- On Days 1 and 2, do 3 sets of 4 reps of all exercises after your warmups.

- On Days 4 and 5, do 3 sets of 12 reps after warming up.

- When you can complete 3 sets at the desired rep count, increase your top weight on the following workout.

- Repeat this program for 12 weeks.

Day 4

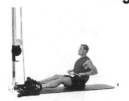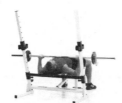

Seated Row (MG) & Flat Barbell Bench Press (MG)

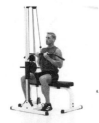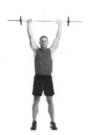

Reverse Grip Pulldown (WG) & Smith Machine Front Shoulder Press (WG) (Variation of Barbell Shoulder Press)

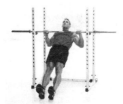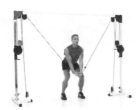

Two-Arm Inverted Row (CG) & Cable Crossover (HH)

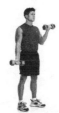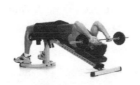

Alternating Standing Dumbbell Curl & Barbell Decline Lying Triceps Extension

Day 5

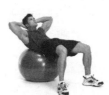

Front Squat (MS) & Stability Ball Crunch

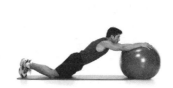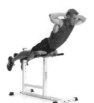

Back Hyperextension (WG) & Forward Ball Roll

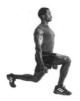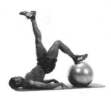

Walking Lunge & Supine Leg Curl with Stability Ball

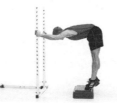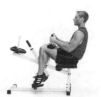

Body-Weight Donkey Calf Raise & Machine Seated Heel Raise

CG = CLOSE GRIP; CS = CLOSE STANCE; HH = HIGH HEIGHT; LH = LOW HEIGHT; MG = MEDIUM GRIP; MS = MEDIUM STANCE; VTP = VARY TOE POSITION EACH SET; WG = WIDE GRIP; WS = WIDE STANCE.

WHEN PAIN MEANS GAIN

Just about everyone knows by now that pain during lifting isn't a good thing. If you feel a "sharp" pain, or get a dull ache in a joint that persists after the workout, you're doing something wrong.

But there is an exception: the "burning" pain that you feel at the end of really tough sets. This kind of pain means that you're pushing muscle fibers to (and beyond) the point of breakdown. You want this kind of pain because it means you're pushing past the barriers—the key to getting bigger as well as stronger.

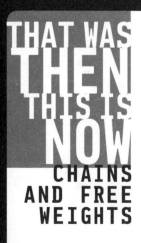

THAT WAS THEN THIS IS NOW
CHAINS AND FREE WEIGHTS

Traditionally, lifters only went to their absolute top, supramaximal weights during negative movements—lowering a heavy weight very slowly, for example, or lifting a heavy weight over a very short range of motion.

No more. Thanks to Louie Simmons, Dave Tate, and the Westside Barbell training methods, here's a more recent strategy to tap into the benefits of overloading.

Hang chains off your bar while you squat or bench press. As you descend, the weight gets *lighter* because more of the chain is in contact with the floor. As you ascend, the weight gets *heavier* because there's less chain on the floor. You can use this technique with many other exercises, including rows and deadlifts.

Use a chain with at least half-inch links. Using hooks or clamps, attach one end of the chain to the bar and the other end to something solid on the floor, such as around the legs of a heavy bench.

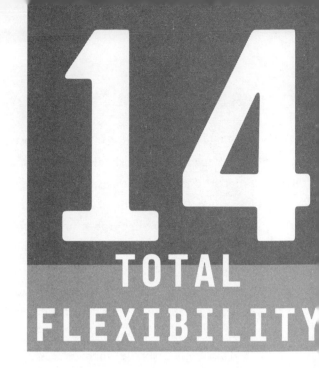

14

TOTAL
FLEXIBILITY

They say that the eyes are the first to go. Don't believe it. Unless you happen to be in the bloom of adolescence, your flexibility is already heading downhill.

After about age 15, your ability to stretch, turn, and twist starts the inexorable journey to flexlessness. As muscles shorten and resist going through their full range of motion, you'll find that it's harder to do all of the activities you always took for granted, such as getting out of bed in the morning.

It doesn't have to be this way. Age alone doesn't make stiffness happen. We do it to ourselves by constraining the types of movements we do over the years. Muscles are nothing if not efficient. If you don't force them to lengthen on a regular basis, they do the sensible thing and take the shorter, if stiffer, path of least resistance.

The real mystery is why we let it happen. Flexibility is one of those things that's easy to maintain with basic stretches. Stretching isn't complicated. It isn't difficult and it isn't painful. It's arguably the easiest part of any workout.

FLEXIBILITY EXPLAINED

Stretching means lengthening muscle fibers. It's the opposite of the contracting (shortening) phase, which occurs when muscles are active. Raise a dumbbell, your biceps shorten. Lower it, your biceps lengthen.

Stretching a muscle, then, means relaxing it. A key point is that in order to relax one muscle, you usually have to contract the opposite, or opposing, muscle. Trainers call this an agonist/antagonist relationship. To stretch your quadriceps, you contract the hamstrings. To stretch your chest, you contract your upper back.

This is an important concept—and it's the primary reason that an optimal, full-body workout combines both strength and flexibility exercises. The stronger you make one set of muscles with lifting, the better you'll be at using those muscles to promote relaxation in the opposing set.

Stretching doesn't mean that the muscles just passively sit there. Muscles don't like change. When you try to lengthen them beyond what they're used to, they resist and shorten. The so-called stretch reflex is a matter of self-protection; the muscles work against you to prevent overstretching. The only way to overcome this is to hold stretches for a certain period of time. This allows muscles to overcome the stretch reflex, relax more, and stretch a little farther.

THE TOTAL FLEXIBILITY WORKOUT

Very few of us are completely flexible or completely stiff. Your flexibility probably varies widely among different joints and muscles, or when doing different movements. Maybe you can touch your toes while standing, but you can't grab your foot and pull it toward your butt. This means you have flexible hamstrings, but tight quads. Do you feel a pull in the right hamstring when you bend over and touch the floor? It means your right hamstring is tighter than your left and needs extra work.

Every man should include a wide range of stretching exercises in his workout, but no one has to do *every* stretching exercise. Your program should hit all of the main muscle groups, while including extra stretches for areas that need the most work.

There are quite a few stretching techniques. In the following pages, we'll focus mainly on dynamic and static stretches.

- Dynamic stretch consists of movements that start out slowly and progressively increase in speed and range of motion. An example would be targeting a hamstring by raising an extended leg, lowering it, and then raising it again.

Dynamic stretches require repetitions; you don't hold the stretches for extended periods.

- Static stretch involves holding a muscle in a lengthened position for an extended period—anywhere from a few seconds to several minutes. As you hold the stretch and the muscles relax, you then attempt to lengthen the muscle fibers even more.

Stretching is partly a science and partly an art. There's surprisingly little research on "optimal" stretch techniques. Most of what's known about stretching is based on experience with top athletes, along with a little common sense. Here are the main points to keep in mind.

Start with dynamic, end with static. Trainers usually advise men to do dynamic stretches at the beginning of their workouts. You use them to warm your muscles and joints and prime them for movement. Static stretches, however, weaken muscles for up to 120 minutes. Use them as part of your cooldown, or on days you're not working out. Don't do static stretches before lifting.

Warm up before your warmup. There's some debate about whether this is necessary, but the reasoning is sound: If you engage in a few minutes of activity before stretching (enough to break a light

IS STRETCHING REALLY PROTECTIVE?

It's common knowledge that increasing muscle flexibility helps prevent injury, right? Well, maybe and maybe not.

A number of studies indicate that stretching increases the elasticity and energy-absorbing capacity of "muscle-tendon units"—important if you engage in sports that involve bouncing or jumping, such as soccer and football. On the other hand, lower-impact sports, such as cycling and swimming, put relatively little stress on muscles and tendons. Stretching will make you more flexible, but it won't necessarily keep you safer for lower-stress activities.

Stretching might not keep you out of traction, but it does increase range of motion, reduce joint pain, and improve performance at everything from swinging a driver on the front nine to hauling a case of beer out of the trunk. And it only takes a few minutes a day to do it right.

NO KIDDING?

sweat), your muscles will be warmer and more pliable.

Move gently into static stretches. You're not out to surprise your muscles. Move in slow, controlled movements, and never force the muscles past the point they want to go. Stretch until you feel a slight tug, then pause and hold the stretch.

Target dynamic stretches. By their nature, these stretches are done quickly, which can be dangerous should you propel your muscles too far beyond their customary range of motion. Most trainers advise men to only use dynamic stretches to prepare for specific sports or activities, such as sprinting or pitching.

Dynamic Stretching Instructions

- Warm up before stretching. Spend 5 to 10 minutes on a treadmill, stairclimber, or an elliptical device.

- Spend 10 to 15 minutes stretching.

- Do the stretches in a progressive fashion. With each repetition, try to increase the range of motion slightly. As you get more comfortable doing the movement, perform it a little more quickly. Your final repetition should have a greater range of motion and faster speed than your initial repetition.

- Always perform each movement with *total control*. Don't force the range of motion.

- Your movements should be performed at a cadence that you feel comfortable with. Don't worry about how fast or slow someone else is moving.

- If one side is tighter than the other, do extra reps for that side.

- Breathe out while stretching a muscle, and relax into the movement.

- Do 1 set of each stretch, with 5 to 10 repetitions per set.

HIP ROLL

A Lie on your back, with your arms extended out to the sides at shoulder height. Your palms should be against the floor. Bend your knees and bring your legs to a 90-degree angle. Your shins will be parallel to the floor.

B Twist all the way to one side, stopping either when your knees touch the floor or when your opposite shoulder leaves the floor. Lift the legs back to the starting position, then twist to the other side.

A

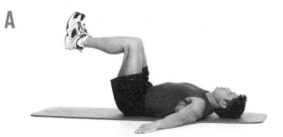

B

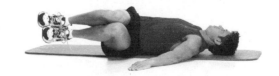

HAND WALK

A Start in a pushup position, with your hands shoulder width apart and extended slightly out in front of your shoulders. Your toes should be tucked under, and your heels pressing back.

B Without rounding your back, hinge at the hips and begin "walking" the hands back toward your feet. Bring them as close to your feet as you can; keep your heels and hands flat on the floor, your knees locked, and your legs engaged throughout the entire movement. Hold for a second, then walk the hands back out to the starting position.

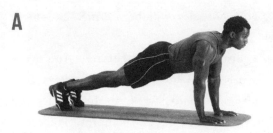

A

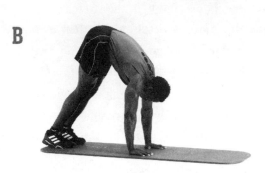

B

LUNGE WALK

A Stand straight, with your head in line with your spine and your feet shoulder width apart. Place your hands on your hips. Take a long step forward with one foot. Bend your leg until that thigh is parallel to the floor. Your other leg should extend back, with its knee slightly bent and almost touching the floor. Your step should be long enough so that your back leg becomes almost straight.

B From this position, push off of your front foot, raise your back leg, and step forward with it. Continue lunging until you reach the point that you planned on "walking" to.

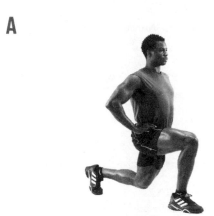

A

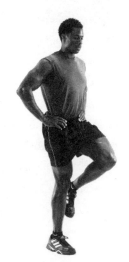

B

WALKING KNEE TUCK

A Stand with your feet no more than hip width apart. Step forward with the left foot.

B Using your hands to assist you, lift your right leg and squeeze the right knee up and into your chest. Hold briefly, then release and step forward with the right leg.

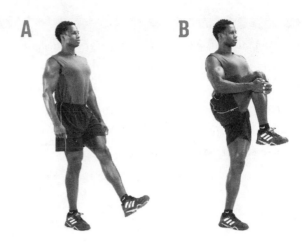

WALKING SIDE LUNGE

A Stand straight, with your feet more than shoulder width apart, toes pointing forward. Keep your head in line with your body, and your back straight.

B Lunge to the right, bringing your right leg to a 90-degree angle. Hold briefly, then shift your weight to the opposite side, keeping your hips low to the floor. Lunge with the left leg while straightening the right. Return to the starting position, bring the feet back together, and stand upright.

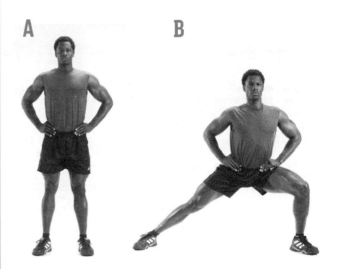

LEG SWING

A Stand straight, with your right side facing a wall. Place your left hand on the wall for balance. Raise your right leg straight in front of you. Don't swing the leg, but use the thigh muscle to steadily lift it.

B Lower the leg and let it fall back. Then, using the hip and butt muscles, raise the leg behind you, going as high as is comfortable. You will need to lean forward a bit to keep your balance, but keep your back as straight as you can. Lower the leg and repeat, moving it forward and back in a slow, rhythmic pace. Repeat with the other leg.

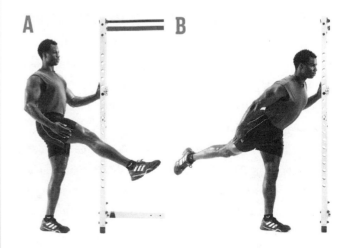

ARM CIRCLE

A Stand straight, with your feet shoulder width apart. Extend your arms until they are parallel to the floor, palms facing down.

B Trace small circles in the air with both arms moving in the same direction. Gradually increase the size of the circles until you're at your maximum range of motion.

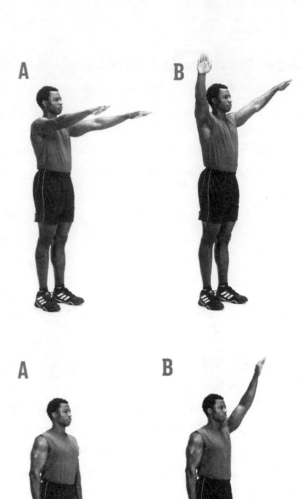

ARM SWING

A Stand straight, with your feet shoulder width apart. Let your arms hang at your sides, palms facing behind you.

B Raise your right arm in front of you. Move it in a semi-circular motion until it is directly overhead. As you begin to lower your right arm, raise your left arm. Swing the arms gently, alternating them up and down in a steady, controlled manner. Do not swing them past the point of mild tension.

NECK ROLL

A Stand straight, with your feet shoulder width apart, knees and shoulders relaxed. Allow your head to drop toward your chest, going as far as you comfortably can. Slowly roll your head to the left until your ear almost touches your shoulder. Pause for a moment.

B Roll your head slowly backward. Don't force the movement or let your head hang so far back that it rests on your shoulder. Pause for a moment, then roll your head to the right. Pause, then roll it forward. Repeat the movement, rolling your head to the right.

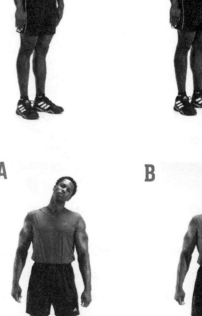

Static Stretching Instructions

- Warm up before stretching. Spend 5 to 10 minutes on the treadmill, stairclimber, or an elliptical device.

- Spend 10 to 15 minutes stretching.

- Perform all stretches in a slow, controlled fashion.

- Always perform each movement with *total control*. Don't force the range of motion.

- If one side is tighter than the other, do extra reps for that side.

- Breathe out while stretching a muscle, and relax into the movement.

- Do 1 set of each stretch, with 3 repetitions per set.

- Hold each stretch for 10 seconds. After each workout, add 5 seconds to your "hold" time. Aim for a 1-minute hold for each repetition.

PRETZEL

A Sit on the floor, with your legs straight. Place your left foot on the floor on the outside of the right knee. Turn your torso toward the left side, while extending your left arm behind you for support. Place your right elbow on the outside of the bent knee.

B Turn your torso farther around by pushing your right elbow against your left knee. Hold for 10 seconds, then slowly return to the starting position. Repeat to the opposite side.

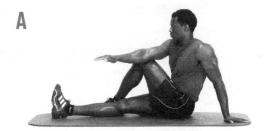

LYING KNEE-TO-CHEST

A Lie flat on your back, with your legs extended and your feet flexed.

B Pull your right knee toward your chest by clasping your hands behind the thigh or around your shin. Use your biceps to pull the leg in. Keep your lower back pressed to the floor. Hold for 30 seconds, then slowly return to the starting position. Repeat with the left leg.

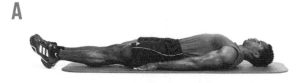

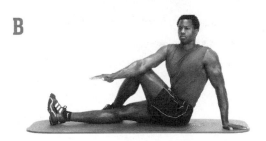

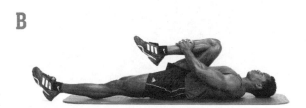

LYING LEG PULL

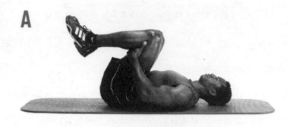

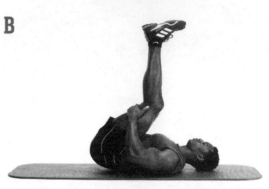

A Lie on your back, with your hands and arms under your thighs. Pull your knees as close to your chest as they will comfortably go. This part of the movement works the lower back.

B Keeping your knees against your chest, extend your legs over your head. This extends the stretch to include the hamstrings and butt muscles. Hold for 15 seconds, then return to the starting position. As you get more comfortable with the stretch, increase the hold time to about 30 seconds.

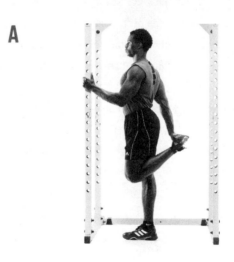

THIGH PULL

A Facing a rack or wall, stand with your feet hip width apart. Place your left hand on the rack or wall for support. Bend your left leg behind you, and grab the top of your foot with your right hand.

B Gently pull your heel toward your butt. Hold for 30 seconds, then relax and switch legs.

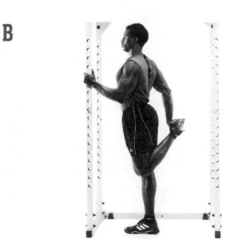

HAMSTRING STRETCH

A Stand with your left leg bent and your toes pointing straight ahead. Space your feet more than shoulder width apart. Extend your right leg behind you. Your toes should point at a slight angle to the right. Place your hands in the middle of your left thigh and lean into the leg, keeping your back straight.

B Push your hips back and down, bending your back leg slightly. Lower your torso until it is parallel to the floor, or as close to parallel as you can get. Extend your left leg and raise the ball of your foot off the floor; maintain pressure on your front heel. Hold for 30 seconds, then switch legs.

CALF STRETCH

A Kneel on your right knee, resting your left forearm on your left thigh. Lean forward slightly at the waist, keeping your back straight.

B Shift your weight to the front knee, bending it as far as it will comfortably go. Keep your front heel on the floor. Shift your weight onto your kneeling leg. As you externally rotate the hip of the rear leg, bring the inside of the knee and lower leg to the floor. Hold for 30 seconds, then switch legs.

A   **B**

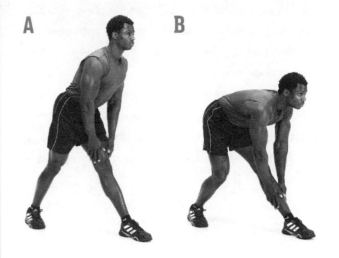

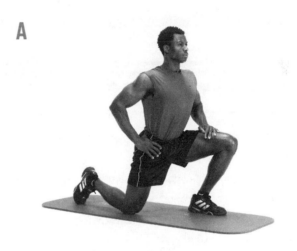

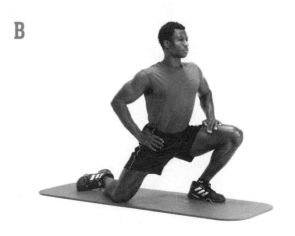

BEHIND-NECK STRETCH

A Stand straight, with your feet shoulder width apart and your knees slightly bent. Bring both arms up overhead. Hold your left elbow with your right hand.

B Let your left hand drop toward the center of your back. Slowly pull your left elbow toward your right arm. You should feel a stretch along the outside of the upper arm and shoulder. Hold for 10 seconds, then repeat on the other side.

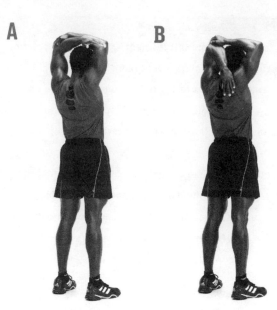

HANDS BEHIND BACK

A Stand straight, with your feet hip width apart. Interlock your fingers behind your back, with your elbows bent. Your neck should be straight and relaxed.

B Tuck in your chin slightly, and gently straighten your elbows and stretch the fronts of the shoulders inward. Hold for 30 seconds, then slowly release. Don't try to get out of the position quickly.

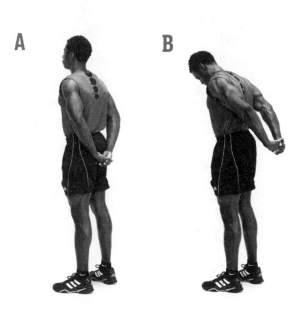

"NO" STRETCH

A Stand with your legs shoulder width apart and your knees slightly bent. Make a fist with your right hand, and place it on the right side of your chin, keeping your elbow and forearm parallel to the floor.

B Using your fist for resistance, rotate your head to the right until your chin touches your right shoulder. When your chin reaches your shoulder, return to the starting position. Repeat on the other side.

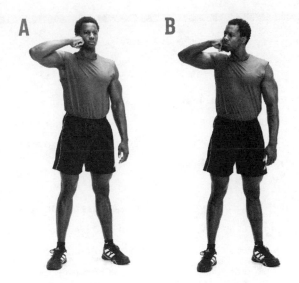

"YES" STRETCH

A Stand with your legs shoulder width apart, your back and neck straight, and your shoulders relaxed. Without bending your upper body, tuck your chin to your chest until you feel a mild pull in the back of your neck. Hold for 10 seconds.

B Slowly tilt your head back until you are looking straight up. Don't go so far back that your head rests on your shoulders. Hold for 10 seconds, then relax

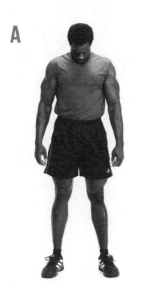
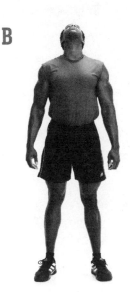

ANOTHER WAY TO WORK OUT THE KINKS

Studies show that massage is more effective than simple rest at optimizing recovery. It improves the circulation of bodily fluids. With increased circulation, tissues are better able to receive nutrients and other substances that are vital for optimal functioning. Massage also flushes out lactic acid and other metabolic by-products that trigger muscle swelling and soreness.

If you can get a massage on a regular basis, go for it. You'll be amazed how much better, and stronger, you'll feel before, during, and after workouts. Just be sure you get the right kind of massage. A massage therapist who specializes in sports massage is your best bet. Avoid getting a deep-tissue massage the day before a hard-core workout or event: You might be too sore to hit your peak performance.

At $60 or so a pop, massage isn't something most of us can afford every day. Fortunately, you can take matters into your own hands. Self-massage is easy, effective, and of course affordable.

Shoulders

- Stroke your right shoulder with your left hand. Mold your hand to the natural shape of your muscles. Starting at the base of your skull, stroke down the side of your neck, over your shoulder, and down your arm to the elbow. Glide back to your neck, and repeat at least three times. Then repeat this process on the other side.

- Press on either side of the spine, making small, firm circles with your fingertips. Work up the neck and around the base of the skull. Then knead each shoulder. Squeeze and release the flesh on your shoulders and at the top of your arms.

- Loosely clench your left hand into a fist, and gently pound your right shoulder. Keep your wrist flexible. This springy movement improves the circulation and can be very invigorating. Repeat on the other side.

- Finish by stroking softly and smoothly with both hands. Start with your hands on the sides of your face, and glide them gently down under your chin. Slide your hands past each other at the front of the neck, so that each hand is on the opposite shoulder. Stroke gently over your shoulders, down your arms, then down past the fingertips. Repeat as often as you like. This hypnotic stroke is relaxing, and can relieve muscle (and emotional) tension.

Legs

- Start with your foot flat on the floor, with one knee bent up. Mold your hands to the shape of your leg. Start by stroking your whole leg, going from the ankle to the thigh, with one hand on either side of the leg. Repeat five times.

- Knead the whole thigh, paying attention to the front and outside. With alternate hands, rhythmically squeeze and release the muscles.

- Gently stroke the entire thigh, moving upward from the knee, with one hand following the other.

- Gently pound the front and outside of your thigh with loosely clenched fists. This bouncy movement brings blood to the surface and relieves stiffness.

- Massage all around your knee. Stroke the area gently, then apply circular pressure with your fingertips around the kneecap. Finish by stroking softly behind your knee, moving upward toward the body.

- Knead your calf with both hands, alternating squeezing the muscle away from the bone, and then releasing it. Then gently soothe the area by stroking upward on the back of the leg, with one hand following the other.

Feet

- Put one hand on top of your foot, and the other hand under the sole. Stroke smoothly from your toes to your ankles. Glide your hands back to your toes, and repeat.

- Support your foot with one hand. With the other hand, squeeze and gently stretch each toe.

- With one thumb on top of the other, press firmly along the sole. Then, with one thumb, press firmly and trace small circles on the arch and ball of the foot.

- Support your foot with one hand. Make a loose fist with the other hand, and "knuckle" all over the sole in circular movements.

- While still holding the foot with one hand, hack the sole with the side of your other hand. Keep the effect light and springy.

- Stroke around the ankle with your fingertips. Stroke up toward the leg, then glide back. Finish by stroking smoothly from the toes to the ankle.

Hands

- Stroke the back of your hand, pushing firmly up toward the wrist, and gliding back gently. Squeeze the hand all over, pressing it between your palm and fingers.

- Squeeze each finger all over. Press firmly with your thumb and make circular movements over the joints. Then, hold each finger at the base and pull gently to stretch it, sliding your grip up the finger and then off the tip.

- Stroke between the tendons on the back of the hand with your thumb. Stroke in the furrows all the way to the wrist, doing four strokes in each furrow.

- Turn your hand over and support the back of it with your fingers. Use your thumb, pressing firmly, to trace small circles. Work all over the palm and around the wrist.

- Finish the massage by stroking the palm of your hand, moving from the fingers to the wrist. Push into it with the heel of your hand, then glide gently back, and repeat. Finish by applying hand lotion.

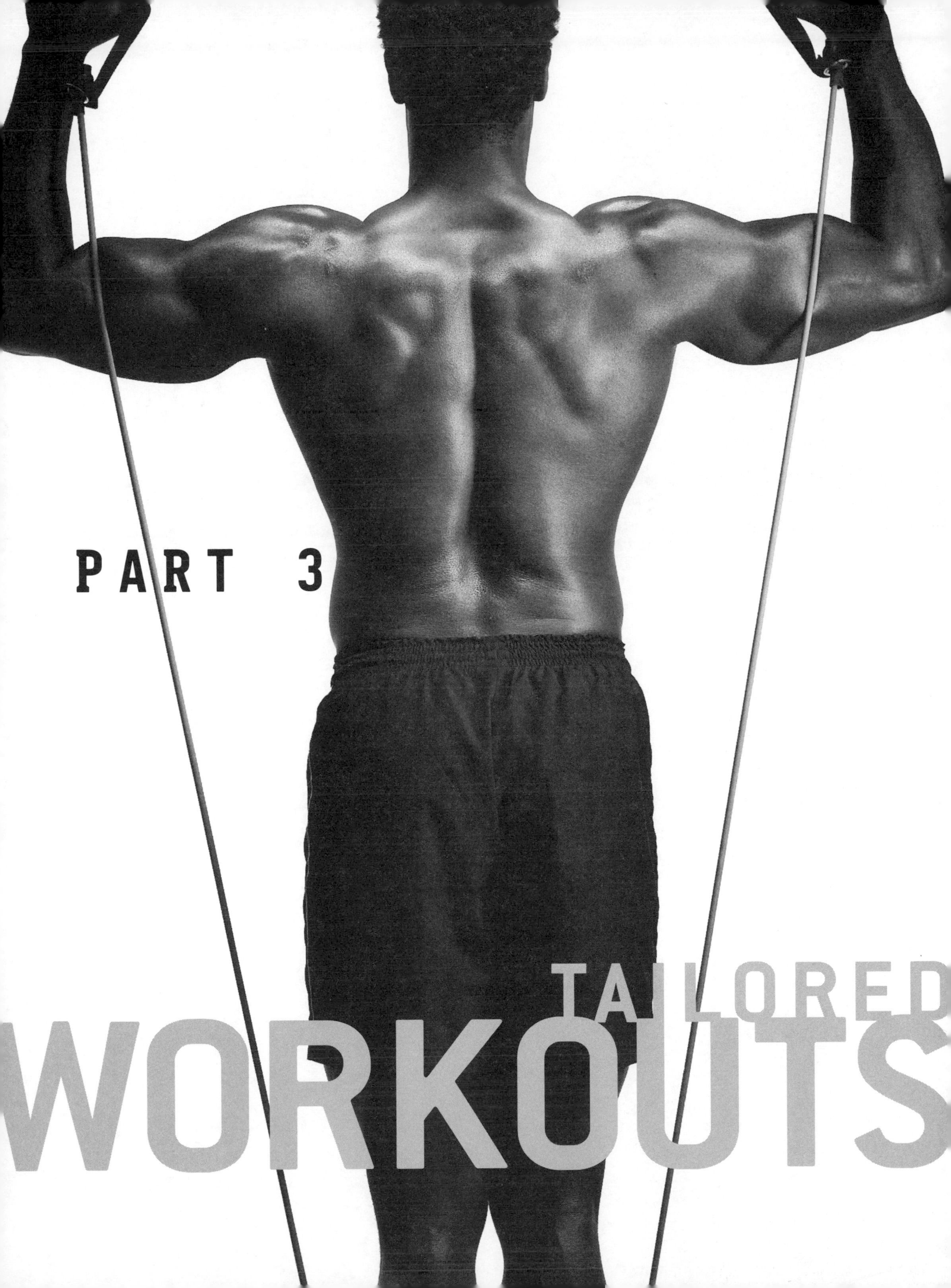

PART 3

TAILORED
WORKOUTS

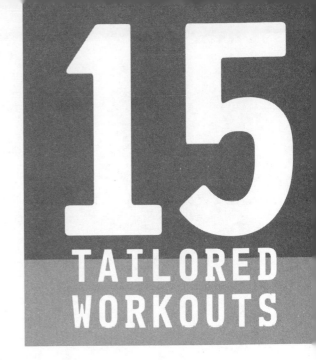

15

TAILORED WORKOUTS

The problem with traditional exercise plans is that they're based on the premise that all men can benefit equally. Not true. Men have different body types, accident histories, and genetic makeups—and different goals that they want to achieve. They require individualized plans.

Most men basically walk into the gym and just start lifting. Some exercise is always better than none, but that's a pretty shaky way to hit specific target points—gaining X amount of muscle in Y weeks, say, or working around bad joints or a back injury. You can save a lot

of time and effort by clarifying what you really want to achieve. Maybe you want to rehab a knee injury. Drop 10 pounds of fat. Reduce pain from arthritis. Get stronger for a specific sport.

Then there are things like your basic body type and disease history—as well as the very practical issue of how much time you have to spend. A good trainer will take all of this into account. The specific exercises you wind up doing, and the way you do them, should be different from the guy next to you. That's the whole idea behind tailored workouts.

In the following pages, we've provided core plans that take into account the most common issues men face, among them back pain, joint pain, obesity, and cardiovascular disease. They won't be specifically targeted to you, of course, but they provide a solid foundation that you can build on later. Work with a trainer if you can. He or she can tweak your workouts so that they

build on your strengths while allowing for current weaknesses.

No matter what program you wind up doing, there are a few points to always keep in mind.

Learn the exercises well. That sounds pretty obvious, but it's amazing how many men do the same workouts *wrong* for years. Form is everything. You can't build solid muscle without moving a certain amount of weight, but the weight itself is less critical than practicing the precise movement mechanics that target specific muscle fibers, break them down, and allow them to build back up to greater size.

Check out the Web site www.thomasincledon.com. You'll find hundreds of step-by-step instructions for basic as well as more advanced techniques.

Practice light. Too many guys spend their gym time heaving weights around without paying much attention to either body mechanics or the re-

BALL SIZE COUNTS

A lot of superb exercises call for a stability ball. If you belong to a well-equipped gym, there are probably quite a few different sizes rolling around. Does it matter which one you use?

Absolutely. Stability balls have different diameters to accommodate men of different heights. Using a ball that's too large or small for your size is going to cause all sorts of problems with basic exercise mechanics. You can use the chart below to pick the ball diameter that's right for you.

YOUR HEIGHT	BALL DIAMETER
Under 4'6"	30 cm (11.8")
4'6" to 5'0"	45 cm (17.7")
5'1" to 5'7"	55 cm (21.6")
5'8" to 6'1"	65 cm (25.5")
6'2" to 6'7"	75 cm (29.5")
6'7" and up	85 cm (33.5")

quirements of the equipment itself—and then they wonder why their joints hurt. If you don't have much experience with various gym paraphernalia—resistance tubes, cable weight stacks, balance boards, stability balls, and so on—practice with light weights at first. Notice how the equipment and movements make your body feel. Don't bump up the weight until you're comfortable with the gear.

Work in cycles. Never stick with the same program for more than 4 to 12 weeks. (The wide time range reflects the fact that the body adapts to different movement patterns at different rates.) Your muscles adapt surprisingly quickly to exercise move-

ments. The more experienced you are, the quicker the rate of adaptation.

You *never* want the body to adapt completely. That's the point at which progress dramatically slows. You always want to introduce variety in your routine: changes in exercises, the order of exercises, and the number of sets and reps. Variety is the quickest way to gain size and strength.

Work with a pro. There are a lot of mediocre trainers out there, but almost every gym has a few folks who are really good at what they do. Work with them. Studies show that men who work with trainers work harder, and see faster gains, than guys who do the solo act.

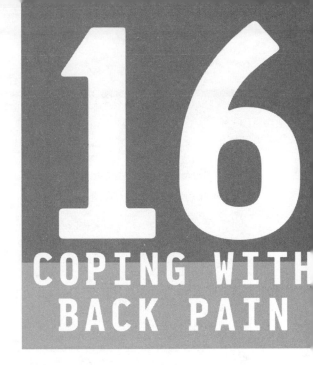

16 COPING WITH BACK PAIN

From an evolutionary point of view, we're not that far removed from our knuckle-dragging ancestors. Sure, we take delicate bites of filet mignon instead of tearing our meat in slabs, and we spend more time burning disks than lighting fires. But our bodies haven't completely adapted to the modern requirements of standing upright or, for that matter, spending long hours with our butts planted in office chairs.

In the early years of human development, we had to walk and hunt and gather food. Today, we're more likely to spend our days cooped up in cubicles, then get in the car to pick up some fast food that we'll eat while sitting on the couch in front of the TV. Our muscles have become so deconditioned that they struggle just to hold us up against gravity.

That's where a lot of back pain originates. The muscles surrounding the spine often aren't as strong as they should be. Weak muscles, combined with an upright posture and highly flexible spine, make the back highly vulnerable to injury. The ironic thing is that relatively few back injuries are caused by heavy lifting. They're more likely to occur when you bend over to pick up a sock.

BACK FROM THE BRINK

Back problems tend to feel a lot worse than they really are. More than 90 percent of cases are due to nothing more than spasms or overloaded muscles. That doesn't make them any less painful, though.

Back pain can put you out of commission for days—if you're lucky. It's not uncommon for back pain to last months or years, even when the underlying problems are relatively minor.

A back injury doesn't mean you should quit exercising. It doesn't even mean you should quit temporarily. You obviously don't want to push yourself hard when you're hurting. You don't want to engage in sports that involve twisting or jolting. But keeping up with your weight program makes sense because you can precisely control all the movements while keeping the muscles strong and limber.

Whether you have a history of back problems or just want to make sure it doesn't happen to you, here are some points to keep in mind.

Stretch and keep stretching. Everything in the body is connected in a kinetic chain. When one part of your body moves, it affects the adjoining segment. Which means that it's not enough just to focus on your back when you're in pain. You have to keep your whole body flexible.

Consider the large leg and hip muscles. They attach to the pelvis, and the pelvis is attached to the spine. If your back is tight or sore, it could be because these other muscles are tight and sore. The hamstrings are often to blame. Suppose you're standing up from a heavy deadlift. If your hamstrings are tight, they'll transfer the stress to the lower back. The muscles in the lower back are relatively small and can't withstand a lot of stress. You might feel fine during the lift—but be unable to move when you try to get out of bed the next morning.

Most men don't like to stretch. Most men don't like back pain, either. Take your pick—it's one or the other. If you incorporate some stretches into your workout, you'll be less likely to find yourself in bed counting ceiling tiles, or, in the worst case, booking an appointment with a back surgeon.

Watch your form outside of the gym. The reason that relatively few men get hurt lifting weights is that they're consciously aware of what they're doing. They squat with perfect form: head up, shoulders back, abs tight, and back arched. But what happens when you reach down to pick up your gym bag? Your legs are as straight as sticks and you round your back like a turtle—which is about the time your back seizes up.

It's not enough just to have great form when lifting large loads. You want to maintain good form all the time. The next time you pick up a sack of groceries, imagine you're doing a full-fledged squat. Take the movement seriously. It's those lapses of attention that can really cause injury.

Brace, don't belt. Competitive lifters routinely use lifting belts. The rest of us? Forget it: They don't work.

Lifting belts don't prevent injuries. They can actually cause lower-back problems. Studies have shown that men who wear belts during squats get more activation of the lower-back and ab muscles. That's fine during the squat, but doesn't help outside the gym. If your body is accustomed to wearing a belt at the gym, it's less likely to brace the abdominals and prepare the trunk for heavy lifting in other situations.

Want to protect your back? Get rid of the leather belt and spend more time working your back and ab muscles. They'll act like a natural belt and stabilize the lumbar spine both inside and outside the gym.

Don't fight fatigue. Studies have shown that gym injuries tend to occur toward the end of workouts. That's when your concentration is starting to slip. It's also when your muscles are reaching the point of pure fatigue. It's good to push yourself. It's good to keep going even when your natural instinct is to collapse to the floor. It isn't smart to push yourself too hard for too long, or to sacrifice perfect form in the quest for one more set.

When you're getting too tired to focus, or your muscles are so tired that just standing upright seems like a chore, it's time to call it a day.

KEEP YOUR LOWER BACK STRONG

A lot of back injuries could be prevented if men would take the time to add more lower-back exercises to their workouts. At the same time, we can all benefit by bumping up the ab portions of our workouts. The two together—lower back and abs—strengthen your core, or trunk muscles. A strong trunk is what protects you from injury, whether you're deadlifting a toddler or lifting weights at the gym.

Check out the ab workouts in Chapter 6, the back exercises in Chapter 10, and the hip exercises in Chapter 11. Some of the best exercises for preventing back pain include back extensions and back hyperextensions; reverse back hyperextensions; twisting reverse back hyperextension; hip and forward ball rolls; elbow bridge; forward ball roll; hip roll; side-lying leg lifts; and double leg supine hip lifts.

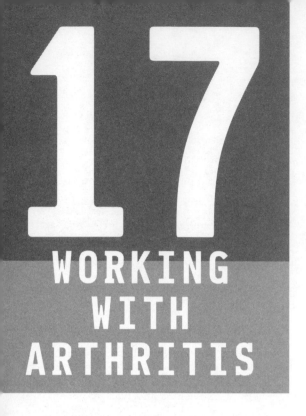

17

WORKING WITH ARTHRITIS

Nothing can suck the steam out of your workouts like an arthritis flare-up. Good luck finishing a set of bench presses when your shoulders are rusted in place or spending a half hour on the stairclimber when your knees feel like they're held together with nails.

If you're over 30, there's a good chance you have some degree of osteoarthritis, the most common form. You might feel fine for months at a time, then wake up one morning with joints that feel as creaky as an old barn door. The pain will probably diminish once you get up and move around, but you still won't feel 100 percent.

There isn't a cure for osteoarthritis. If you've got it now, you're going to have it 10 years from now. You've got a few choices to make. A lot of men essentially give up the physical parts of their lives. They pop pain pills, sit on the couch, and get real handy at punching buttons on the remote control. Then there's the smart choice: You keep working out. Men who exercise have less pain. Regular workouts protect and lubricate the joints and build the muscle that you need to keep them stable and strong.

You'll probably have to tweak your workouts when you're dealing with arthritis. You'll still be able to do most of the same exercises that you did before. You'll still progress to heavier and heavier weights. The only difference is that you'll have to lift a little smarter.

JOINT EFFORTS

Osteoarthritis means that the cartilage on the ends of bones has started to break down. Without that spongy, shock-absorbing coating, bone starts rubbing against bone. That's what causes inflammation and pain—and, if you aren't careful, increasing damage over time.

You do want to rest when you have a particularly severe flare-up of arthritis. A day spent in the company of ice packs and aspirin makes sense. In the long run, though, you want to spend more time in the gym. Exercise exerts compressive forces on the joints—forces that wash the joints with lubricating, synovial fluid and distribute the nutrients that cartilage needs to rebuild and repair.

Exercise has been called the most effective (and least expensive) treatment for osteoarthritis. One study, for example, found that people with arthritis who did nothing more vigorous than walking and aquatic exercise for 12 weeks had significant improvements in aerobic capacity, along with less tangible benefits, such as decreased anxiety and depression.

Admittedly, this study involved pretty light-weight exercise. A lot of men—and, unfortunately, the doctors who treat them—are still convinced that serious lifting has the potential to make things worse. Not true. When sports scientists compare men with arthritis who weight-train, endurance-train, or do some combination of the two, they find no difference in arthritis symptoms.

The Arthritis Foundation recommends the same types of exercise that we've talked about throughout this book: range-of-motion flexibility exercise, endurance exercise, and weight training. If you have arthritis, you might want to shift your focus just slightly to the first two. Endurance and range-of-motion workouts are superb for strengthening and protecting joints. But don't give up the weight training. It's good for your joints—and, more important, it's good for motivation because you'll feel, and look, a whole lot better.

JOINT-PROTECTING WORKOUTS

An arthritis-specific workout is basically the same as any other hard-core plan. You want to increase strength, build muscle size, improve your range of motion, and boost endurance. At the same time, of course, you need to ensure that you achieve these goals without causing more pain or joint damage. This is actually easy enough. Here's the best approach.

Follow isometric with isotonic movements. In other words, do your usual workouts, but start with serious static contractions, also known as isometric exercises. No one should walk into the gym and immediately start pushing serious iron. You have to give the muscles and joints a chance to warm up. This is especially true if you already have joint pain or weakness because of arthritis.

Suppose you're planning to work your legs. You might start out with isometrics, exercises in which the joint doesn't move, but muscles around the joint are tightened and held for about 10 seconds and then relaxed. Quadsetting is a good example of an isometric. You simply extend your leg on a flat surface, tighten the quads on top of the thigh, then relax. Do this a few times, then go into your regular, isotonic routine. An isotonic movement is simply one in which you contract a muscle through its full range of movement—weight lifting, in other words.

Time your workouts. Most men with arthritis have more pain and stiffness in the morning—though everyone is different. It doesn't make sense to go to the gym at your "bad" times. Even if you've always done your workouts first thing in the morning (or whenever), you have to be flexible and shift things around if you need to. You won't come close to moving your max weight if you do it when your joints are screaming. Listen to your body. Work out when *it* wants to.

Combine surf and turf. Water workouts are superb if you're dealing with arthritis. Whether you're doing water aerobics or swimming laps, working out in water greatly reduces joint pressure while building impressive strength and endurance. Water workouts alone aren't enough, though. You need to keep your feet on solid ground to get the weight-bearing benefits. So mix up your workouts. Spend a few hours a week in the pool, and do your regular weight workouts on the other days.

Get serious about stretching. It's typically the least popular part of any workout, yet it's arguably the most important. You need to pump blood to your muscles and joints before you put them to serious work. See Chapter 14.

For normal, pain-free joints, you generally want to do dynamic movements at the beginning of weight-training sessions. Follow your workout with static stretches. If you have arthritis, you'll want to modify your strategy. Precede your regular workouts by stretching the muscles you plan to use during that session. Do each stretch two or three times, holding each for 30 to 60 seconds.

After your workout, take 3 to 5 minutes to cool down with additional flexibility exercises.

Wake up to walking. Okay, it's not the most glamorous exercise. It won't build massive muscle or improve your appearance in a T-shirt. But it's among the best ways to keep joints flexible and improve aerobic capacity and endurance. These core gains will pay off when you're looking for the *oomph* to do some serious lifting.

No complicated formulas here. All you have to do is walk at a good clip for 20 to 30 minutes at least three times a week. Actually, any aerobic exercise, such as swimming or biking, provides the same benefits as fast walking.

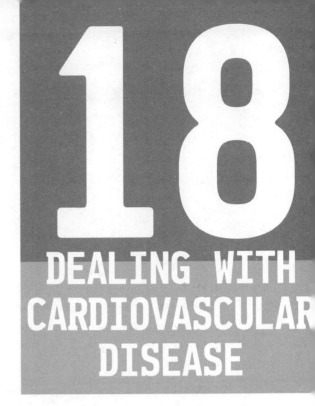

18
DEALING WITH CARDIOVASCULAR DISEASE

Unless you've been living in your recliner for the last 23 years, you already know that regular workouts protect the heart. They reduce your risk of dying from a heart attack or stroke. They lower the risk of developing diabetes—and make it easier to control if you already have it. They lower cholesterol, trim fat, and help lower blood pressure into the safety zone.

That's all on the prevention side. What if, like millions of Americans, you already have cardiovascular disease or have even had a heart attack?

The answers are exactly the same. Exercise is vital for just about every heart problem you can name. If you've already had a heart attack, or you've had angioplasty or other procedures to clear gunk from the pipes that supply the heart, regular workouts can, quite literally, save your life.

Heart patients of all ages who start workout programs and stick with them have less stress and depression than those who are sedentary. They have more energy. They have better blood flow and lower blood pressure. They live longer.

Anyone who's been sedentary for a long time (we're talking years, not a few weeks) obviously needs to check with a doctor before launching a hard-core workout plan. This is especially true if you've been diagnosed with heart problems, or have risk factors for heart disease, such as obesity or sky-high cholesterol. Your doctor will almost certainly give you the thumbs-up, but you'll get some extra suggestions for easing into workouts without putting too much stress on the heart.

LIFT AND PROSPER

Doctors talk a lot about aerobic exercise. Anything that kicks your lungs and heart in the direction of the red zone will help control cholesterol and blood pressure and will improve the ability of the heart to push more blood. But aerobics is just one corner of a solid workout. It's crazy to neglect flexibility exercises or weight training just because you've had a little bit of ticker shock. All exercise is good exercise—and a combination of the three is the best way to whip all your muscles, including the heart, into top shape.

Don't worry that you'll have a heart attack during your workout. Sure, it could happen. The risk of a heart attack is slightly higher during exer-

EXERCISE CLOBBERS CALORIES
FOR HEART HEALTH

Obesity is one of the main risk factors for heart disease, but the actual calories that you consume may be less important than doctors previously thought.

A national research project that studied data from nearly 10,000 adults compared the effects of physical activity, body mass index, and calorie intake on heart disease deaths. To no one's surprise, those who were overweight and exercised less had higher death rates from heart disease.

What was surprising was that calorie intake by itself had little to do with keeling over. Subjects who took in a lot of calories, but also exercised a lot, had less than half the cardiovascular disease mortality than those who exercised less and ate less.

You should certainly watch your weight if you want to protect your heart. But don't obsess over calories. You're better off focusing your attention on energy expenditure. Regular workouts beat calorie counting, hands down.

cise than during rest. But it's a *lot* higher when you don't exercise at all.

When you do start working out, pay attention to how you feel. If you notice symptoms such as pain or pressure anywhere between your neck and navel, or you experience dizziness, nausea, shortness of breath, or a strange heart rhythm, stop immediately and call your doctor.

That caveat aside, here are some smart ways to get started.

Slowly accelerate your heart rate. It's never a good idea to jump into an aerobic or weight-training workout. You want to give your heart, along with your muscles, a chance to warm up. Start with slow walking or easy stretches. You want to raise your heart rate to within 20 beats a minute of the rate recommended for aerobic conditioning—say, a minimum of 50 percent of your max heart rate. Hold it there for 10 to 15 minutes. Then go all out into your workout, allowing time for a 5-minute cooldown at the end.

You'll get optimal cardiovascular gains when you exercise 30 to 60 minutes at least 5 days a week.

Start out with less than that. You can divide your aerobic workouts into sessions—say, 15 minutes on a treadmill in the morning, followed by a fast walk later in the day.

You should be sweating and pleasantly tired at the end of your workout. If you're totally whipped and feel like you're about to cough up your lungs, take it down a notch. Work out at a slower pace until you get in better shape.

Lift light. Strength training is superb for men with heart problems. Apart from the fact that you'll feel stronger and better, pushing iron reduces both heart rate and blood pressure. But don't go crazy with it. Pushing too much weight puts a lot of stress on the heart.

Unless your doctor tells you otherwise, stick with weights that allow you to complete at least 10 to 15 reps. You'll probably do better with single-set workouts initially. Once you're in better shape, you can increase the sets as long as you don't overdo it.

Lift fast. For a long time, doctors were all aboard the cardio train because early studies showed that aerobic workouts promoted better cardiovascular fitness than weight training. As it turns out, however, the early studies looked only at people doing low-intensity weight training. Later studies that looked at men pumping serious iron came to a totally different conclusion.

The men in these studies had very high levels of cardiovascular fitness, even though they weren't doing "formal" aerobic workouts. What they were doing was moving from weight exercise to weight exercise without letting their heart rates come down to baseline. They kept their heart rates elevated for extended periods, and their heart function improved.

Plug in "real-life workouts." This means riding a stationary bike when you watch TV. Taking stairs instead of elevators. Walking your dog at the end of a long day. Increasing daily activity strengthens the heart, improves blood flow, and makes it easier to progress in your gym workouts.

Don't hold your breath. Make sure you breathe properly when lifting. Breathe in while lowering or doing the negative part of a repetition, and breathe out when lifting or doing the positive part of the repetition. Holding your breath can cause blood pressure to skyrocket—the last thing you need if you already have cardiovascular problems.

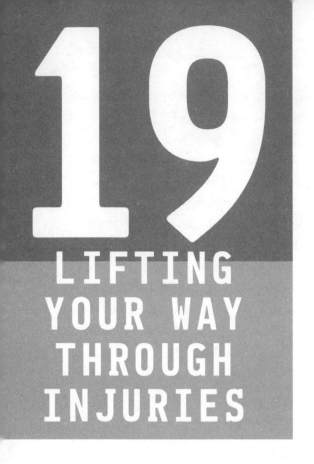

19

LIFTING YOUR WAY THROUGH INJURIES

No one gets through this life without pain. If you're a human and live long enough, sooner or later your hinges will get a little creaky. It's no fun to lift when your joints feel like they're tied together with barbed wire.

Then there are the everyday pulls, strains, and sprains. Common sense says that taking a few days off from your regular routine is the smart thing to do. But what about after a few weeks? Or a few months? Skip your workouts long enough and you can watch all your hard-won gains disappear like a puff of smoke. It happens a lot quicker than you might think.

Sports docs usually give the same advice: *Keep moving.* That doesn't mean working out hard during the most painful phase of an injury or joint flare-up. The idea is to stay comparatively active—to "train around" the injury while it takes its own sweet time to heal. If you do this, you'll experience very little loss in conditioning and will return to normal training faster than men who basically give up and hang an "occupied" sign on the sofa.

FIRST RESPONSE

The injuries that can put you out of commission may be either minor (muscle strain) or major (torn ligament). You can't always tell which is which from the pain level: They can all hurt like crazy.

Obviously, if you can't move a particular limb,

you would classify that as major. As for those minor, dull aches—ignore them at your peril. Even when they aren't all that painful initially, they can quickly get worse. So check with your doctor. Same goes for persistent joint pain. If you normally hurt a little, and then suddenly you hurt a lot, talk to a pro.

In the meantime, here are the main things you need to do in the initial stages of hurt.

Treat it quickly. Swelling and inflammation are your enemies when you have a sprain or strain. The longer you take to treat inflammation, the worse the damage will be, and the longer your recovery time— and the greater your loss of conditioning.

The first-line treatment for a lifting or sports injury is R.I.C.E.: rest, ice, compression, and elevation. Rest means to stop doing whatever caused the injury. Apply ice for about 20 to 30 minutes every hour or

WHEN TO SEE A DOC

There are a few tip-offs that tell you when an injury is more than just an annoyance—that you really need to see a doctor.

- Joint pain that lasts more than 48 hours. Remember, some joints—the knee, ankle, elbow, and wrist—aren't covered by muscle. Pain in these areas can't be dismissed as "just a strain."

- Tender points. If it really hurts when you press your finger into a specific point over a bone, muscle, or joint, you may have a significant injury.

- Clicking sounds within a joint. This typically occurs when tendons snap over one another after they've been pushed into a new position by swelling. Underlying swelling and inflammation are potentially serious.

- Comparative weakness. Lift or press the same weight with your right and left sides. If you're significantly weaker on one side than the other following an injury, you could have done real damage.

- Numbness and tingling. They're often caused by nerve compression. Anything affecting the nerves is risky. See a doctor immediately.

so. Compress the area by wrapping it with an elastic bandage. This will help reduce swelling. Finally, elevate the hurt area above the area of your heart.

Never apply heat to an injury in the first day or two. It will increase swelling.

Pamper pain—and keep training. Maybe your shoulder's screaming with a bursitis flare-up, or you've pulled a muscle in your hip or groin. There's probably inflammation in there, and some tissue damage. Let the area heal for awhile. Don't work it. In the meantime, keep training the parts of your body that aren't hurt.

Take that shoulder injury. You might not be able to train your upper body for a few days, but you can still work your legs. Or you can modify your workouts—doing exercises seated or lying down instead of standing, for example—so that you put less pressure on the injured joint or muscle. This is a good time to take advantage of tubing, cables, or machines. They're usually easier to use than free weights when you have an injury.

Work the opposite limb. Studies show that you can reduce conditioning loss in an injured arm or leg by working the "good" arm or leg. Can't do curls with your right arm? Go ahead and work the left. While you're at it, try to *gently* work the right arm, even if you can only move it a few inches through your normal range of motion. If you feel pain, you've gone too far. Short of pain, any movement will help prevent loss of conditioning and will speed recovery.

Get a massage. It can dramatically speed the healing of muscle injuries. Wait a few days after the injury before getting a massage. Doing it too soon will increase circulation and inflammation.

INJURY-SPECIFIC WORKOUTS

After you've wrapped up the initial order of business—icing the area, resting it, and talking with a doctor if you need to—get back in the gym. This isn't the time

HOW MUCH DO YOU LOSE?

Suppose you've really wrecked your shoulder, knee, or some other part of your anatomy. It hurts. You can barely move. You feel a little sorry for yourself. So you do the usual thing: blow off your workouts. In fact, you blow off anything more strenuous than compressing couch cushions. How fast will your muscles go downhill?

If you quit virtually all physical activity for a week, you'll only lose about 5 percent of your overall fitness level. Not too bad, right? But each week after that, you lose another 5 percent. Which means, after a few months, you'll almost be back at beginner level.

It takes roughly twice the number of weeks that you were "down" to gradually build yourself back up to pre-injury levels. So don't fall into the do-nothing trap. You might not be able to exercise a specific body part, but you *can* keep working out.

to sacrifice months of work. Depending on the injury, there's probably quite a bit you can do to keep the area moving.

Elbow tendonitis. It's frequently caused by overuse. Definitely reduce the intensity of training while it heals. Consider using a soft-sleeve elbow brace, which will keep the area warm while you work out.

You may notice some discomfort when you use your usual grip for doing pullups or other pulling movements. Play around with hand spacing and grip positions. There's probably one that feels better. Use it until you're fully healed.

Postsurgical knee pain. Keep training the healthy knee to maintain strength and decrease atrophy (muscle loss) of the bad knee. Use machine or cable exercises for upper body workouts; free weights force the body to brace itself and put too much pressure on a bad knee. Gradually introduce light cycling and free-weight training.

For leg workouts, begin with reverse stepups and gradually increase the step height. Then progress to relatively light squats and deadlifts.

Lower-back strain. Your immediate line of de-

fense is to prevent additional muscle spasms. Take aspirin or ibuprofen, for starters. Greatly reduce your weight loads—or, if you need to, go through the exercise motions without using any weight at all.

This is a good time to identify and correct any weakness you have in your core muscles—the abdominals and obliques as well as the lower back. Most back injuries occur in part because these core muscles aren't strong enough. As soon as you can, start building all of these groups with additional exercises. While you're at it, incorporate more strengthening and stretching exercises for the entire *posterior chain*—the muscles on the back of the body.

Patellofemoral dysfunction. It's an injury that occurs where the patella (kneecap) meets the underlying femur. It probably happens when the two bones don't fit together as precisely as they should, leading to increased friction and cartilage breakdown.

After you've done the usual—ice, rest, and anti-inflammatory drugs—start working the entire leg, from the hip to the foot. Safe and effective exercises include backward walking or running; backward stairclimbing; lateral stepups and stepdowns; and bicycling at low tension with the seat set higher than usual.

Leg presses and squats are helpful because they activate the quadriceps, which in turn can help alter the contact areas between the patella and femur and reduce pressure. However, limit your range of motion initially to about 30 degrees. If you can get more range of motion with *no* pain, go for it. You get the best quad workouts when the angle is between 88 and 102 degrees.

Shoulder impingement. It occurs when the rotator cuff tendons get trapped by the biceps tendons or other structures. It's often caused by overuse or overtraining; this is one case where you might want to rest the area for a few weeks. After that, focus on strengthening and flexibility exercises that target the rotator cuffs. In some cases, this is all you have to do to prevent future problems.

Strained finger tendon. If you spend much time wall- or rock climbing, you've probably strained a finger tendon at some point. Until you're totally healed, stick with mantel and stem (pressing) movements—or pick a course that mainly requires footwork. After that, incorporate more grip-strengthening exercises into your workouts, especially those that target the forearms and fingers.

Strained hamstring. These take longer to heal than other muscle groups, especially if you keep re-injuring them. One of the best things you can do is maintain *perfect* form on lower-body exercises, especially heavy-load or higher velocity exercises, such as squats, deadlifts, stiff-legged deadlifts, snatches, cleans, lunges, dips, and jumps of any kind. Include more dynamic stretches in your warmup routine. Leg exercises that improve balance, such as one-legged squats, can also help.

Foot or toe fracture. You'll probably need to wear a walking boot for a couple of weeks, but you can start working out again in a few days. It's fine to include aggressive strength training in your rehab plan—doing squats and deadlifts, for example—but don't do exercises that require you to stand on one leg. It will overload the injured area.

Wrist fracture. Even if you have to wear a cast, there's no reason for the rest of your body to atrophy and suffer. Good training options include walking, jogging, stationary biking, and strength training with machines rather than free weights. In fact, you can probably do wrist exercises, as well, as long as they don't require gripping.

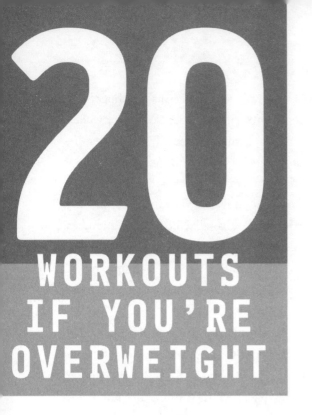

20 WORKOUTS IF YOU'RE OVERWEIGHT

Take a look at the men (and women) working out on the treadmills, stationary bikes, and other cardio gear. You'll notice a common theme: Most of them are either skinny or fat. You won't see a whole lot of muscle. In the free-weight area, by contrast, you'll see men who are built *and* lean.

It takes time for old scientific theories to die. Until fairly recently, the medical establishment was hooked on aerobic training. The consensus of the time was that the only way to strip body fat was to spend countless hours on step machines, treadmills, bikes, and running tracks. A generation of Americans, fitness enthusiasts and overweight hopefuls alike, took it all to heart. They spent the next decade or so locked in the mind-numbing tedium of endless stepping and cycling.

For most of them, of course, it didn't work. Aerobics made them healthier, but it sure didn't make them leaner.

LIFT AND LOSE

The fastest way to lose weight is to spend a lot more time in the weight room. Aerobic workouts are fine; every smart exercise plan includes them. But aerobic exercise mainly affects the expenditure of calories. Pumping iron, on the other hand, literally changes your body's composition. It builds lean muscle, kicks you to a higher metabolic rate, and burns fat faster and more efficiently than anything else. As a bonus, you can design your weight workouts to get an aerobic burn at the same time—which means you don't necessarily have to set aside 3 or 4 hours a week for aerobic-only sessions.

Scientists divide your total body mass, or composition, into three categories. Fat-free mass (FFM) consists of the portions of muscle, bones, and organs that contain zero fat. Fat mass (FM) is your total fat—the stuff that hangs off your hips as well as the internal fat that you need to survive. Then there's lean body mass (LBM), which you can think of as a healthful combination of FFM and, to a lesser degree, FM.

When you get your body composition checked with skinfold calipers, the results are percentages of FM and LBM. When FM is low and LBM is high, you look good. Your body has a harder, more muscular appearance, with little flab.

How do you get to this point? The key word is

LIFT MORE, BURN MORE

You will burn more calories during a typical endurance-training session than you will during a comparable weight workout. But there's a limit to the amount of calories you can burn at one time. At some point, if you mainly do aerobics, you're going to have to get serious about restricting calories, as well. "Dieting," for most of us, is an ugly word.

Resistance training helps get you off the hook. The muscle that you build lifting weights burns additional calories in all those daily hours when you're *not* exercising. You get a 24-hour burn, in other words.

A recent study compared calorie expenditure on *nontraining* days in a group of men who regularly exercised at moderate to high levels. Those who had significantly higher levels of lean body mass—the kind of muscle that you get from weight training—burned between 8 and 14 percent more calories on their "off" days.

The bottom line: Build more muscle, burn more calories.

"metabolism." Fat isn't a biologically active tissue; it doesn't do much of anything except keep you warm. Muscle, on the other hand, is constantly working, even when you're not. It's constantly sucking calories and generating heat. The more muscle you have, the more energy you use, even when you're doing nothing more active than tying your shoes.

Which takes us back to weight training. It has a direct effect on weight loss because it burns a tremendous amount of calories while you're doing it. At the same time, the muscle you build with lifting jacks up your resting metabolic rate, the calories you burn every minute of every day.

A 14-week study at North Dakota State University compared the effects of different workouts on resting metabolic rates and fat loss. Some people in the study only did aerobic training. Others only lifted weights, and some did both. The study showed that those who combined aerobic exercise (swimming and biking) with weight training lost an average of 10 pounds of fat and gained 13 pounds of fat-free mass. In addition, their resting metabolic rate increased about 380 calories a day.

Weight training alone can increase muscular strength and your basic metabolic rate. Aerobic workouts build your cardiovascular system and decrease body fat. Doing both together will put you on the fast track to a leaner, tighter body.

MIX IT UP

There are all sorts of formulas for maximizing weight loss and pumping up muscle. Don't bother with them. The basic premise couldn't be simpler: Don't spend all of your time in the weight room, and don't count entirely on running, biking, or other endurance activities. Every week, set aside time for both lifting and aerobic workouts.

If you have infinite time to spend at the gym, you could conceivably combine lifting and aerobic sessions in a single workout. This isn't practical for most men because it can add 30 to 60 minutes to each workout. It isn't even optimal because you won't get anywhere near your top weights if you've already spent 30 minutes blowing out your lungs on the treadmill.

A better choice is to alternate cardio and weight

days. Two or 3 days a week, spend all your time lifting. If you really want to blast your body and your heart, use the supersetting technique (page 19). You alternate exercises that work opposing muscle groups—say, a chest exercise followed by one for the back, or a quad exercise followed by one for the hamstrings—without resting in between. Do this long enough, and your heart will be pounding like a drum. You get an aerobic blast while you're building muscle.

On the purely aerobic side of things, you can shave quite a bit of time from your sessions by increasing the intensity. For example, instead of running or stepping for 45 minutes at a steady clip, push yourself harder and cut the session to 20 to 30 minutes. More intensity means a faster workout.

Better yet, do interval training. If you're running on a treadmill, say, run at a moderate pace for 1 minute, then sprint for 10 to 15 seconds. You can do the same thing with any aerobic workout. In the pool, maintain a steady pace for a minute, then really put on the speed for 10 to 15 seconds. Interval training is superb for the cardiovascular system, and you can burn a tremendous amount of calories in a relatively short time.

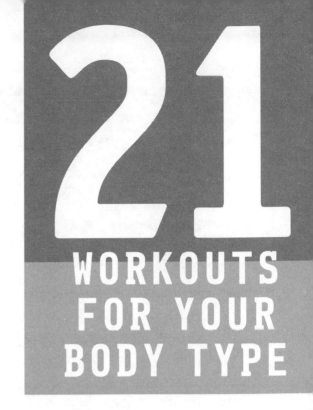

21

WORKOUTS FOR YOUR BODY TYPE

We've talked quite a bit about the fallacy that all workouts are more or less the same, no matter who's doing them. You know that something is wrong when a trainer recommends the same exercises, sets, reps, and intensity for a 50-year-old overweight woman as he does for a 25-year-old athlete. Yet this cookie-cutter approach is employed at most gyms, even though the men who walk in the door come with vastly different bodies, levels of strength, and experience.

It doesn't make sense for a guy who's low to the ground and built like a tank to do the same workouts as the tall drink of water without any bulk. Even when you strip out all of the individual variations from man to man, the very fact that there are three distinct body types—endomorph, ectomorph, and mesomorph—means that workouts need to be tailored to the guy who's doing them.

ENDOMORPH TRAINING

If you had to describe the endomorph body in one word, it would probably be "curvy." The body fat in an endomorph tends to settle in the lower abdomen, hips, and thighs. Keep in mind, though, that relatively few endomorphs (or other body types) possess all of the classic features; most men have a blend of different body types. Still, endomorphs do tend to lean in the bottom-heavy direction.

An endomorph typically has the capacity for high fat accumulation and storage. The shape is usu-

ally pearlike: more weight in the lower regions and less in the upper body. More is involved in fat distribution than aesthetics. Many research studies have shown that the fat deposits in the abdominal area are much more dangerous than fat in the legs or butt. Specifically, endomorphs with the classic fat pattern have a higher risk of heart disease, diabetes, stroke, hypertension, and some cancers. So the major concern of any endomorph is maintaining a healthful weight.

Endomorphs also tend to have limbs that are short in relation to the trunk and musculature that isn't all that well defined. They generally have a large bone structure. This is good because it means they can hoist relatively heavy weight. But because they have a slower metabolism than other body types, it can be a challenge to lose fat, which can conceal their hard-earned muscle gains.

Eat smart. Since endomorphs metabolize calories slowly and accumulate quite a bit of bulk, they should eat a relatively low-fat diet and keep carbo-

COMBINATION BODY TYPES

You may be a combination of the three basic body types —and may require a slightly different workout than classic endos, ectos, or mesos. Here are some possible combos and recommended workouts.

The Hourglass

The waist is quite a bit smaller than the chest and hips. The upper and lower bodies tend to have more strength than endurance. Men with this shape gain and lose weight easily.

- Plenty of cardio, such as low-impact aerobics, cycling at low to medium tension, and high-speed walking, preferably on a treadmill set to a slight incline.

- Moderate to high repetitions—say, 12 to 15 reps—in weight training. Periodically introduce very high-rep, low-weight workouts—say, up to 25 reps.

- A combination of compound and isolation exercises.

The Ruler

The waist, chest, and hips are all about the same size. Men with this shape tend to accumulate fat in the middle, and have a hard time increasing muscle mass. They're naturals at endurance workouts, but struggle with strength training.

- A lot of cardiovascular exercise to aid in weight loss. Good choices include biking with high tension, uphill walking, using steppers or stairclimbers with moderate resistance.

- More strength training. Specifically, they should use moderate to heavy weights, going for reps in the 20+ range. They should focus on basic and compound movements, and use isolation exercises only as a "finishing" exercise.

The Cone

The upper body is quite a bit larger than the lower half. The stomach often protrudes a bit. The arms and chest bulk up easily. Adding muscle to the lower body is more of a challenge.

- Bicycling at moderate to high tension, along with fast walking on a treadmill set to a moderate incline.

- For the upper body, lift relatively light weights, going for higher repetitions. For the lower body, move moderate to heavy weights, keeping reps in the 12 to 15 range.

- Use compound as well as isolation movements for the upper and lower body.

The Spoon

The lower body is distinctly larger than the upper half. Men with this build have thick upper thighs, bulky inner thighs, dense calves, and thick ankles. The upper body and the lower abdominals are usually on the weak side.

- Bicycle at a high speed with relatively little tension. Brisk walking is good. So is walking on a treadmill without an incline. Avoid steppers, stairclimbers, or high-impact aerobics, which will add unwanted bulk to the lower body.

- For the upper body, stick with compound movements, using moderate to heavy weights and relatively low reps. For the lower body, do both compound and isolation exercises, using lighter weights and higher reps.

hydrate intake in the low to medium range, but not dropping below 100 grams of carbs daily.

Get the aerobic burn. More than most body types, endomorphs absolutely have to include plenty of cardio routines in their workouts. Apart from protecting the heart, it helps accelerate fat loss. The American College of Sports Medicine recommends at least 30 minutes of aerobic exercise *daily,* hitting the target heart rate of 60 percent to 75 percent of their top capacity.

Lift for endurance. Since endomorphs put on bulk easily, they should focus on lifting routines that build endurance rather than size. This usually means picking a weight that's light enough that they can complete at least 15 repetitions per set and take relatively short rest breaks between sets.

To get the best workouts for this body type:

- Include both compound and isolation movements in weight training.

- To avoid plateaus, change the exercise mix often. Add new exercises and subtract old ones. Frequently change the exercise order, as well.

- Avoid training too heavy, too often.

- Do a few more sets than usual—up to 12 sets for larger muscle groups, and 8 to 10 for smaller ones.

- Keep reps high even on "heavy" days: Try for 12, at a minimum, or go as high as 25.

A word of caution: Endomorphs have a high risk of lower-body joint damage because they tend to carry quite a bit of weight higher up. They need to be especially careful to maintain perfect form when lifting, and to allow themselves plenty of warmup and cooldown time, to protect the ankles, knees, and hips.

ECTOMORPH TRAINING

A one-word description for the ectomorph is "slim." If you're an ecto, mesomorphs and endomorphs usually don't want to stand next to you. It's not that ectomorphs aren't personable. It's just that they're usually the tall, skinny individuals who have trouble gaining weight.

The classic ectomorph has a delicate build, narrow hips and pelvis, and long arms and legs. They usually don't have a lot of muscle bulk, but they do tend to have good muscle definition because there's so little fat padding. Their light structure comes with a price. They tend to have small joints and bones that are easily injured during sporting activities.

A man with this body type isn't likely to be a star on the football team or the next champion gladiator. This body type is naturally suited for endurance sports: swimming, running, biking, and so on. These men perform so well in endurance activities, however, that they tend to stick with what they do best and neglect muscle training. They have to work harder than men with other body types to get good results.

Be patient. Because ectomorphs have very high metabolic rates, they make slow gains when it comes to adding bulk. The gains will come, but slowly. Men with an ectomorph body have to remind themselves not to get frustrated.

Go for intensity. The only way an ectomorph will gain significant muscle is in the basic, hypertrophy stage of training. In other words, stay in the 8- to 12-rep range. Fewer reps means going heavy; lift the top weights you can manage safely to get a solid, high-intensity workout. Allow plenty of rest between sets. When you're lifting heavy, you need extra rest time to allow muscles to recuperate.

Limit cardiovascular routines. The ectomorph already has a metabolism like a hummingbird and a relatively low risk of obesity or cardiovascular disease. He should limit high-intensity cardio to about 20 minutes, three times a week.

Hit the major muscle groups. Ectomorphs should avoid isolation-type movements, and stick with the basic, mass-building movements that work major muscle groups and deep muscle fibers. Good examples include squats, presses, and deadlifts.

Because ectomorphs have to move heavy weight to gain size, they also have to be cautious of overtraining. If you don't seem to be making gains, adjust the workout intensity and take in more calories. Don't increase the frequency of your workouts.

Other workout tips:

- Do up to 10 sets for larger muscle groups. Drop to 6 to 8 sets for smaller muscle groups.

- When doing warmup sets, stop before the point of muscle failure.

- Choose weights that are heavy enough that you can only complete 6 to 10 reps. This is the ideal range for putting on size.

MESOMORPH TRAINING

These guys are muscular. Mesomorphs are the envy of their workout partners because they can increase muscle size quickly and with little effort. They have thick bones and muscles, which is what gives them their well-developed shapes. The classic mesomorph has a well-defined chest, a taut abdomen, and shoulders that are larger and broader than the waist. The hips are generally the same width as the shoulders, and the buttocks, thighs, and calves tend to be toned and defined.

Sound like a perfect body? It almost is, by the usual standards of how men are supposed to look. Yet mesomorphs tend to be less flexible than other guys, which can lead to all sorts of joint and muscle injuries. Unlike endomorphs, they tend to store fat evenly all over their bodies. Overweight can be a real concern if the mesomorph loses his typical energy and gets more sedentary than usual, or takes in too many calories.

Cardiovascular disease is a threat to the overweight meso. Men in this category need to always maintain a healthful diet and exercise compulsively.

They also need to pay more attention to cardio routines.

Guys with this body type struggle with endurance activities, but excel at muscle building. They saunter into the gym and stay for a relatively short time. Even if they don't have a clue what they're doing, they make tremendous gains. They can basically get away with doing less and achieving more. Yet there are a few things they need to be aware of.

Endurance is a must. Cardiovascular disease can kill the overweight meso. Men with this kind of body have to stay serious about eating nutritiously and exercising regularly. Although aerobic activities are a struggle for these guys, and they tend to dislike it, that's what they should focus on for at least 30 minutes, 4 days a week.

Don't get stuck in a rut. A lot of mesomorphs do the same routine over and over because they're so satisfied with the results. They could do a lot better. Men with this body type should change their routines often. They should also include pyramid training because it gives the greatest gains in size and strength. At the same time, they'll probably need to increase their calorie load to get appreciable gains in size.

Beware of damage. Mesomorphs are more prone to overtraining than men with other body types—again, because they get such good results that they start to feel nothing can hurt them. As a rule, they should do fewer sets, and fewer exercises per body part.

Other workout tips for mesomorphs:

- Start with compound exercises, followed by single-joint isolation exercises.

- Choose weights that force workouts into the 10-rep range.

- Cycle periods of heavy lifting with periods of lighter weights and lower reps.

- Plan on 3 to 4 sets of each exercise, with 2 to 4 exercises per body part.

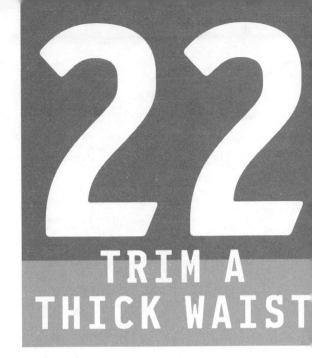

22

TRIM A THICK WAIST

If your waist is thicker than you'd like, you have to focus on exercises that encourage the body to burn more fat for energy. You can do this indirectly, by increasing calorie-burning lean body mass with weight training, or directly, by increasing the burning of fat with aerobic workouts. Ideally, you'll do both.

Cardiovascular exercise is always a good choice. Your body burns energy through a variety of pathways, including the aerobic pathway. You don't have to burn like an acetylene torch to get the benefits. In fact, as the intensity of aerobic exercise increases,

you mainly burn short-term energy stores, such as carbohydrates and ATP. At lower intensity levels, however, you burn more energy from fat. Exercises that are relatively low in effort and performed for a long time, such as swimming, rowing, and fast walking, cause the body to switch into an efficient, fat-burning gear.

True, they won't target your waist directly. But they burn fat all over the body, including the hips and waist. Make aerobic workouts part of your life, and you will lose inches where it counts.

WAIST-FRIENDLY WORKOUTS

Even though your body can't glean all of the energy that it needs from one area alone—the reason that spot reducing is a myth—you can combine whole-

body, calorie-burning efforts with gut-specific workouts to get faster results.

Abdominals consist of three layers of muscle that slide over each other. If you have poor muscular tone, your internal organs will actually distend the abdominal wall, making you look heavier than you really are. When you strengthen the abs, the muscles get flatter and tauter. Your innards stay where they're supposed to, and your waist *looks* smaller, even if you didn't burn a shred of fat. It's like what happens when you straighten your torso and sit upright rather than slouching. It makes you look leaner, regardless of how much weight you're carrying.

It's still worth incorporating plenty of ab routines in your workouts. They don't burn much fat because they're done relatively quickly; they provide only an anaerobic (without oxygen) workout, which mainly burns carbs. But the standard ab exercises, such as torso twists, side bends, and hip extensions, do tighten and firm the gut. Toning this area, and also taking some of the air out of the spare tire with whole-body workouts, is the secret to getting that washboard look.

Side bends are probably the best choice for toning the love handles because they put a lot of stress on the external obliques. To do side bends:

- Stand straight with your knees slightly bent and your feet about a foot apart.

- Slowly lower your trunk a few inches to the left. Return to center, then lower it a few inches to the right.

- To get the most "burn," keep your body and legs in line. Don't bend forward or backward when doing the movements.

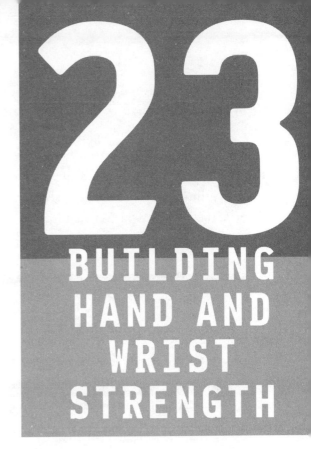

23
BUILDING HAND AND WRIST STRENGTH

Lots of men have weak grips. This is due in part to anatomy. The hands contain a vast array of ligaments, bones, and joints. There isn't a lot of room for muscle. If you're a politician and can't keep up with the hand-shaking part of the job, this is obviously a problem. More practically, a weak grip can really set you back in the gym.

You may have seen some guy deadlifting a huge amount of weight—then stand there with his mouth open because the bar dropped right out of his hands. You'll never deadlift serious weight, or manage a respectable number of pullups, if you can't hold on to the bar.

Even if your arms and back are strong enough to lift heavy weight, a weak grip can hold you back. You can compensate to some degree with assistive straps or wraps, but why not train your hand and forearm muscles so that you lift the way nature intended?

IMPROVE YOUR GRIP

To strengthen your grip, try these simple but unusual exercises and techniques.

Pad the bar. One of the best techniques for improving grip strength is to wrap a towel around any handle that you have to grip. The towel makes the bar thicker, which forces you to grip harder. As your grip strength increases, use a thicker towel.

While you're at it, get in the habit of using the thick rope attachment on pullups and cable pushdowns. It does the same thing as the towel. It forces the muscles to work harder. Also, the thick rope is inherently unstable, which challenges the neuromuscular system and greatly improves grip strength.

Blast your grip with Rolling Thunder. If you're serious about improving your grip, look online for IronMind Rolling Thunder handles. They attach to cable machines like regular handle attachments, but with a difference: The handles are about 2½ inches around. That might not sound like much, but it really challenges your grip—so much so that you may find you have to reduce the weight you move by as much as half.

If you use the handles for a few workouts—for exercises such as one-arm cable rows or cable curls—you'll notice a significant improvement in your grip. Then, when you go back to regular handles, the weights will feel significantly easier, and you should be able to lift more.

Do the Farmer's Walk. A standard exercise in strong-man competitions, it involves nothing more than walking around with a dumbbell in each hand. Most men can't walk very far with even a 60-pound set. Yet you'll see these behemoths on ESPN literally *running* with 300 pounds, or more, in each hand.

The Farmer's Walk isn't that hard to do.

GRIP STRENGTH WORKOUT

If you're serious about training your grip, set aside 2 days a week to work it. Do the exercises at the end of your workout; otherwise, fatigue will interfere with your other exercises. You'll notice that the starting weights and volumes are at the low end. This will allow you to develop good technique before taking on more weight.

GRIP STRENGTH CYCLE

Wk	Workout	Exercise	Wt (lb)	Distance/Time	Reps	Sets
1	1	Bar hanging	BW	30 sec	1	2
	2	Farmer's walk	60	100 ft	1	2
2	1	Bar hanging	25	30 sec	1	3
	2	Farmer's walk	60	150 ft	1	3
3	1	Bar hanging	50	30 sec	1	3
	2	Farmer's walk	60	200 ft	1	3
4	1	Bar hanging	75	30 sec	1	3
	2	Farmer's walk	70	100 ft	1	3
5	1	Deadlift holds	80% MDL	30 sec	1	3
	2	Farmer's walk	80	100 ft	1	3
6	1	Deadlift holds	90% MDL	30 sec	1	3
	2	Farmer's walk	90	100 ft	1	3
7	1	Deadlift holds	95% MDL	30 sec	1	3
	2	Farmer's walk	100	100 ft	1	3
8	1	Deadlift holds	100% MDL	30 sec	1	3
	2	Farmer's walk	110	100 ft	1	3

* BW = BODY WEIGHT; MDL = MAX DEADLIFT

Naturally, you'll start with much lighter weights. The trick is to learn how to walk fast without oscillating from side to side.

- Keep your lats (upper back muscles) flared so that the dumbbells hang farther out from your sides.
- Push off with your back foot while essentially pawing the floor with your front foot—the foot that pulls you forward.
- Start light at first. Work on your form before piling on the weight.

With a little practice, you'll find that you can develop amazing speed, even when you're holding massive weights.

Grip and hang. It's a good move for the end of your workout.

Hang from a chinup bar for about 30 seconds. Just use your body weight at first.

When that gets easy, hold a dumbbell between your legs. If you can hang and hold a 100-pound dumbbell, challenge yourself more by hanging by one hand.

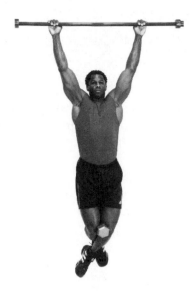

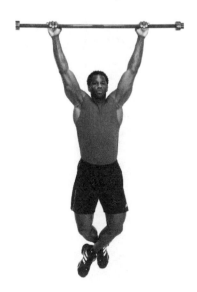

The key to this move is to learn how to *relax* your grip. You don't want a death grip, just enough force so that you can hold on to the bar. If you squeeze too tightly, you'll fatigue prematurely.

Strap into a deadlift. Another grip-trainer is to hold a weighted barbell in both hands in front of your thighs.

Set up the bar in a power rack above knee height. Unrack the barbell by gripping it and extending your hips and back. Use the same grip with both hands. Hold the bar in front of you, the same way you'd maintain the top position of the deadlift. Hold the bar for 30 seconds.

You can make the move more effective by using straps, but still gripping the bar as tightly as you can. The straps allow your grip to continue past the point at which it would normally fatigue. This technique mimics the effects of performing forced reps, which can really power up your grip.

Do the clean hold. This exercise is superb for improving your grip for deadlifts, Farmer's Walks, or other exercises that require holding the weight at thigh level. It isometrically strengthens your hand—especially the finger flexors—as well as the shoulders and neck.

Set a barbell in a rack so that it's just above your knees. Grip the bar with an overhand grip, placing your hands slightly wider than shoulder width. Your knees should be slightly bent, your back flat, your abs tight, and your chest and head up.

Extend your knees to lift the bar from the rack to lockout. Hold for 30 to 60 seconds. Try not to rest the bar on your thighs or lean backward.

Return the bar to the rack. Rest for 1 to 2 minutes, then repeat. Try to complete 5 reps, resting between each rep.

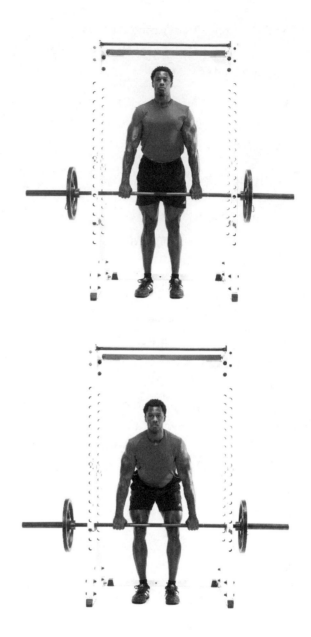

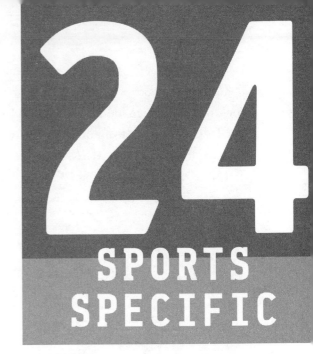

24

SPORTS SPECIFIC

Even if the main reason you go to the gym is to put a little more muscle on your frame, chances are, you have some additional motivations. Millions of men these days participate in at least a few sports or weekend activities, such as taking the occasional weekend hike or diving at the municipal pool. Maybe you need short surges of strength for pulling ahead with the oars, or better stamina and side strength for the tennis court. Whatever your sport of choice, you need a workout that complements it.

Every sport-specific workout has a few similar components:

- Sports-needs analysis. What does the sport require? More strength? More speed? More endurance? Other variables might include balance, flexibility, agility, reaction time, and coordination.

- Self-needs analysis. What are you good at—and what are your weaknesses? These are the things you'll want to focus on first.

- Specificity. Pick strengthening movements that target the specific muscles your sport requires.

In the following pages, we've provided basic workouts for the most popular sports and activities. Just don't forget the basics. Once you're set up in the gym, remind yourself to start at easier-than-usual weights. As you progress, increase the intensity or volume—but only at a pace you feel you can handle. Allow plenty of down days. Muscle recovery is just as important as exertion for developing size and strength.

BASEBALL

You don't need huge forearms to pound 'em into the stands, but you do need decent muscle strength along with speed, agility, hip and shoulder flexibility, and superb eye-hand coordination. You'll want to focus on building the hips, legs, forearms, wrists, calves, and the back.

Unless otherwise noted, do 3 sets of 8 to 10 repetitions for each of the following exercises, allowing 2 minutes' rest between each set. Repeat the workouts three times a week, with at least 1 day of rest between workouts.

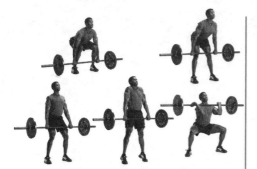

Power Clean (page 199)

Plan on doing 2 to 4 sets, with 2 to 4 reps per set.

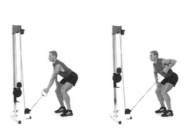

One-Arm Cable Row (page 167)

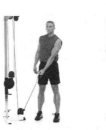

Cable Side Deltoid Raise (page 140)

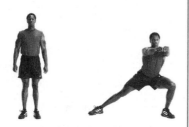

Lateral Lunge (page 204)

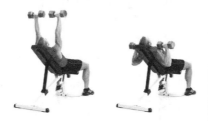

Incline Dumbbell Bench Press (page 125)

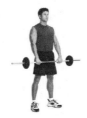
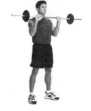

Barbell Reverse-Grip Curl (page 89)

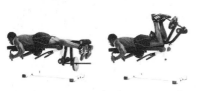

Machine Leg Curl (Lying Leg Curl) (page 236)

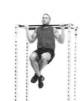

Wide-Grip Chinup (page 169) (Variation on Chinup)

Single-Arm Dumbbell Lying Cross-Shoulder Triceps Extension (page 94)

BASKETBALL

More than most sports, basketball requires a tremendous amount of speed, along with the ability to jump and twist. The main muscles to work, apart from the legs, are the shoulders, triceps, hands and wrists, and the back.

Unless otherwise noted, do 3 sets of 8 to 10 repetitions for each of the following exercises, allowing 2 minutes' rest between each set. Repeat the workouts three times a week, with at least 1 day of rest between workouts.

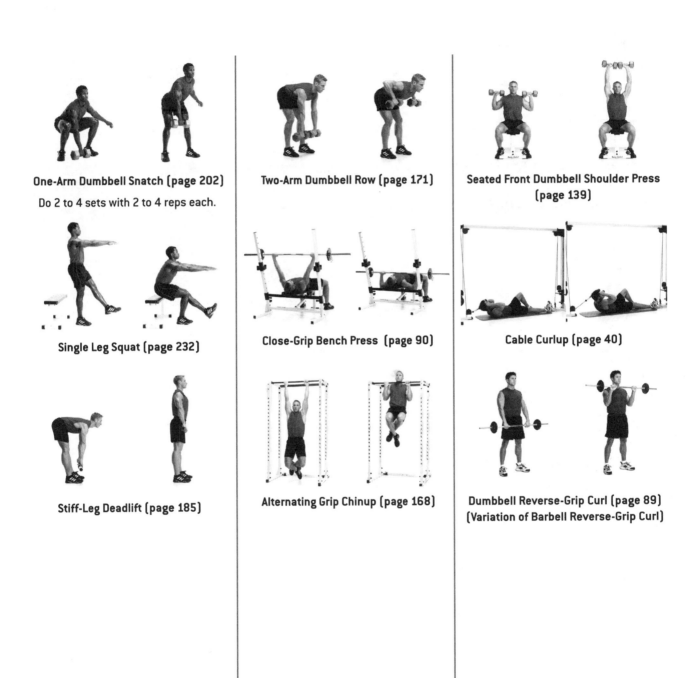

One-Arm Dumbbell Snatch (page 202)

Do 2 to 4 sets with 2 to 4 reps each.

Two-Arm Dumbbell Row (page 171)

Seated Front Dumbbell Shoulder Press (page 139)

Single Leg Squat (page 232)

Close-Grip Bench Press (page 90)

Cable Curlup (page 40)

Stiff-Leg Deadlift (page 185)

Alternating Grip Chinup (page 168)

Dumbbell Reverse-Grip Curl (page 89) (Variation of Barbell Reverse-Grip Curl)

BOWLING

The secret to bowling, apart from the ability to drink a tremendous amount of beer and still remain standing, is to strengthen your grip strength, along with muscles in the hips, thighs, back, and arms.

Unless otherwise noted, do 3 sets of 8 to 10 repetitions for each of the following exercises, allowing 2 minutes' rest between each set. Repeat the workouts three times a week, with at least 1 day of rest between workouts.

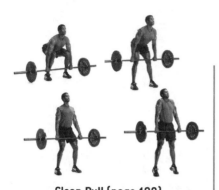

Clean Pull (page 198)

Do 2 to 4 sets with 2 to 4 reps per set.

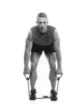

Wide Grip Row with Tubing (page 178)

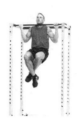

Wide Grip Chinup (page 169)
(Variation of Chinup)

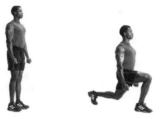

Walking Lunge (page 206)

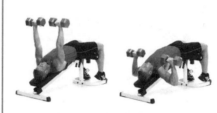

Decline Dumbbell Bench Press (page 119)

BOXING

First of all, it helps to be big. Failing that, you'd better be fast—real fast. Main muscles to work: the triceps, forearms, wrists, calves, and the back.

Unless otherwise noted, do 3 sets of 8 to 10 repetitions for each of the following exercises, allowing 2 minutes' rest between each set. Repeat the workouts three times a week, with at least 1 day of rest between workouts.

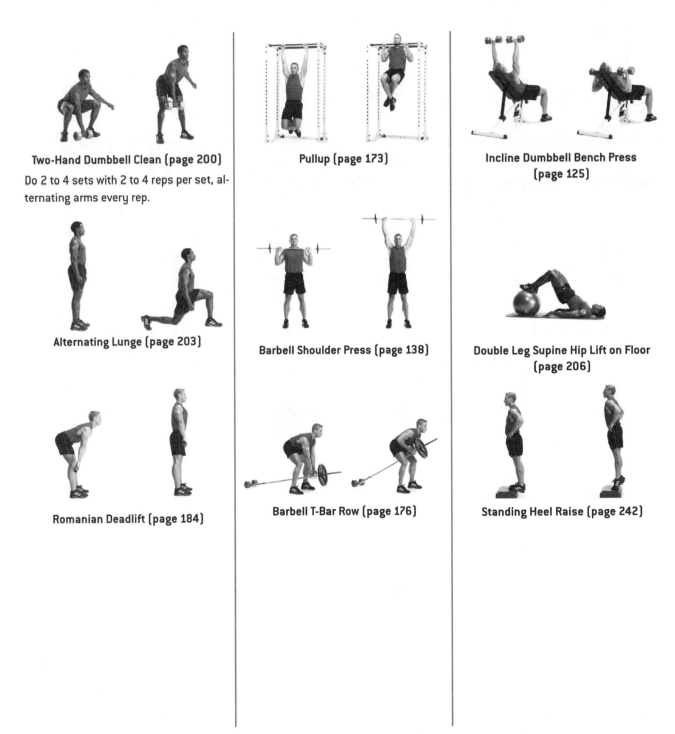

Two-Hand Dumbbell Clean (page 200)

Do 2 to 4 sets with 2 to 4 reps per set, alternating arms every rep.

Pullup (page 173)

Incline Dumbbell Bench Press (page 125)

Alternating Lunge (page 203)

Barbell Shoulder Press (page 138)

Double Leg Supine Hip Lift on Floor (page 206)

Romanian Deadlift (page 184)

Barbell T-Bar Row (page 176)

Standing Heel Raise (page 242)

FOOTBALL

Depending on your position, football can require either more speed or more strength. Agility, muscular endurance, and coordination are important for every position. Focus on working the hips, legs, back, and shoulders.

Unless otherwise noted, do 3 sets of 8 to 10 repetitions for each of the following exercises, allowing 2 minutes' rest between each set. Repeat the workouts three times a week, with at least 1 day of rest between workouts.

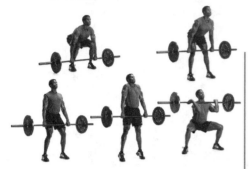

Power Clean (page 199)

Do 2 to 4 sets with 2 to 4 reps per set.

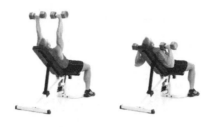

Incline Dumbbell Bench Press (page 125)

Seated Front Dumbbell Shoulder Press (page 139)

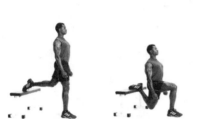

Bulgarian Split Squat (page 222)

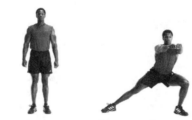

Lateral Lunge (page 204)

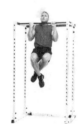

Alternating Grip Chinup (page 168)

Two-Arm Dumbbell Row (page 171)

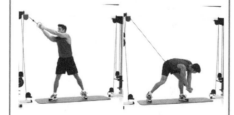

Wood Chop (page 66)

GOLF

Want to get beyond the duffer stage? You'll need a lot of rotational power, decent muscle strength, good hand-eye coordination, and flexibility in the spine, hips, and shoulders. These exercises will work the abdominals, lower back, forearms, and wrists.

Do 3 sets of 8 to 10 repetitions for each of the following exercises, allowing 2 minutes' rest between each set. Repeat the workouts three times a week, with at least 1 day of rest between workouts.

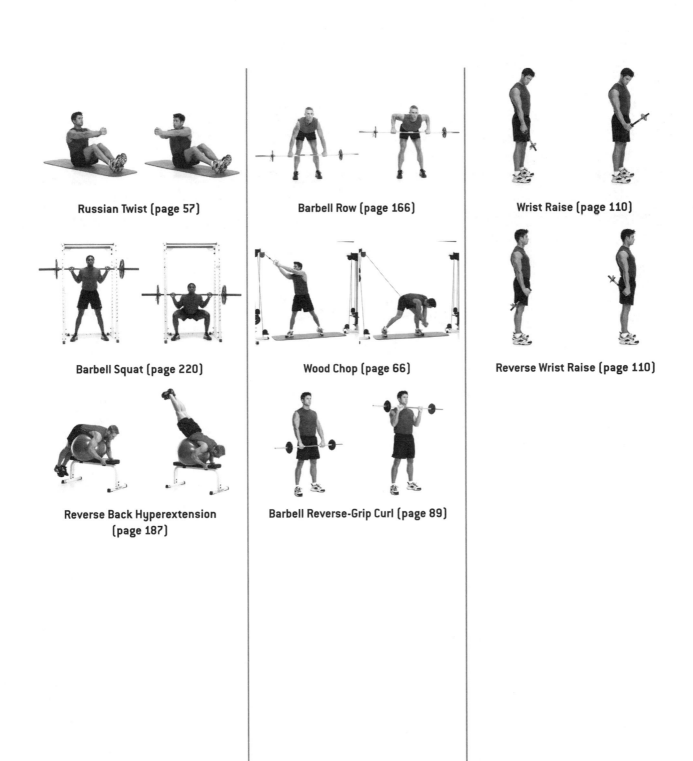

Russian Twist (page 57)

Barbell Row (page 166)

Wrist Raise (page 110)

Barbell Squat (page 220)

Wood Chop (page 66)

Reverse Wrist Raise (page 110)

Reverse Back Hyperextension (page 187)

Barbell Reverse-Grip Curl (page 89)

HIKING

You obviously need good endurance if you're planning to hike farther than the mailbox. Apart from that, you'll want to concentrate on your legs as well as your back. Climbing up hills, and more so going down, can totally thrash your back if you don't keep it strong.

Do 3 sets of 8 to 10 repetitions for each of the following exercises, allowing 2 minutes' rest between each set. Repeat the workouts three times a week, with at least 1 day of rest between workouts.

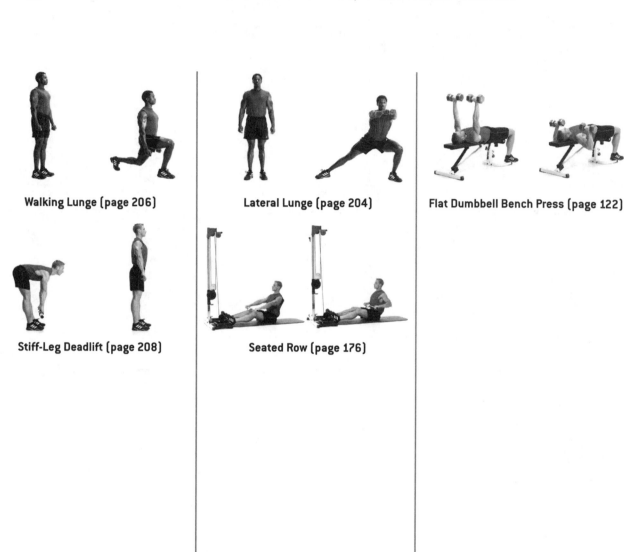

Walking Lunge (page 206)

Lateral Lunge (page 204)

Flat Dumbbell Bench Press (page 122)

Stiff-Leg Deadlift (page 208)

Seated Row (page 176)

HOCKEY

Hockey requires a lot of speed, agility, muscle strength, muscle endurance, cardiovascular conditioning, hand-eye coordination, and hip flexibility. You'll want to strengthen the legs, abdominals, and shoulders.

Do 3 sets of 8 to 10 repetitions for each of the following exercises, allowing 2 minutes' rest between each set. Repeat the workouts three times a week, with at least 1 day of rest between workouts.

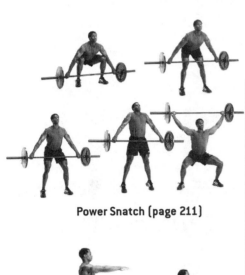
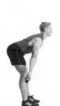

Power Snatch (page 211)

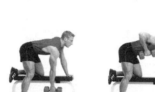

Romanian Deadlift (page 184)

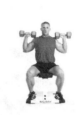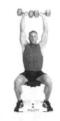

Seated Front Dumbbell Shoulder Press (page 139)

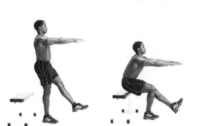
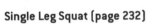

Single Leg Squat (page 232)

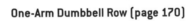

One-Arm Dumbbell Row (page 170)

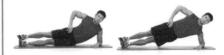

Side-Lying Hip Lift (page 58)

RACQUETBALL AND SQUASH

Unlike tennis, these are racquet sports that you play on an area roughly the size of a postage stamp. The combination of a tight playing area and a high-speed ball means that you're constantly lunging, twisting, and reversing direction. The only way to survive an hour on the court is to build up good shoulder flexibility, along with strength in the legs, chest, arms, and wrists.

Do 3 sets of 8 to 10 repetitions for each of the following exercises, allowing 2 minutes' rest between each set. Repeat the workouts three times a week, with at least 1 day of rest between workouts.

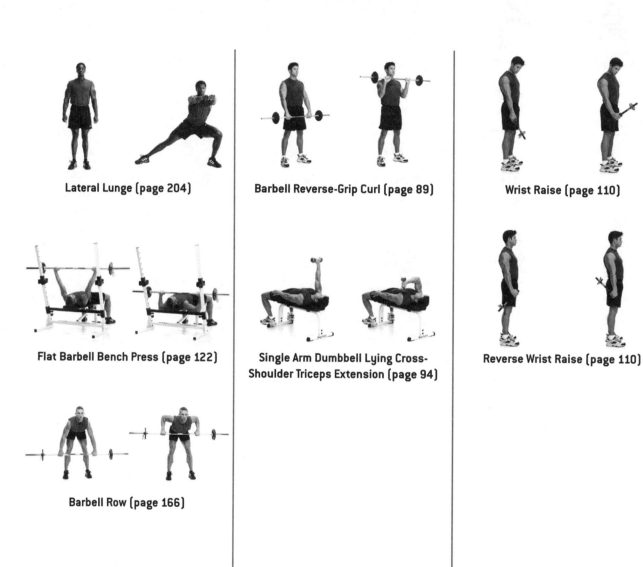

Lateral Lunge (page 204)

Barbell Reverse-Grip Curl (page 89)

Wrist Raise (page 110)

Flat Barbell Bench Press (page 122)

Single Arm Dumbbell Lying Cross-Shoulder Triceps Extension (page 94)

Reverse Wrist Raise (page 110)

Barbell Row (page 166)

ROCK CLIMBING

It won't give you much of a cardiovascular workout unless you happen to look down and realize that the only toehold is out of reach. But rock climbing is one of the best workouts for building muscular strength and endurance. If you hope to live long enough to earn bragging rights, you'd better spend some time building grip strength, along with muscles in the arms, legs, and back.

Do 3 sets of 8 to 10 repetitions for each of the following exercises, allowing 2 minutes' rest between each set. Repeat the workouts three times a week, with at least 1 day of rest between workouts.

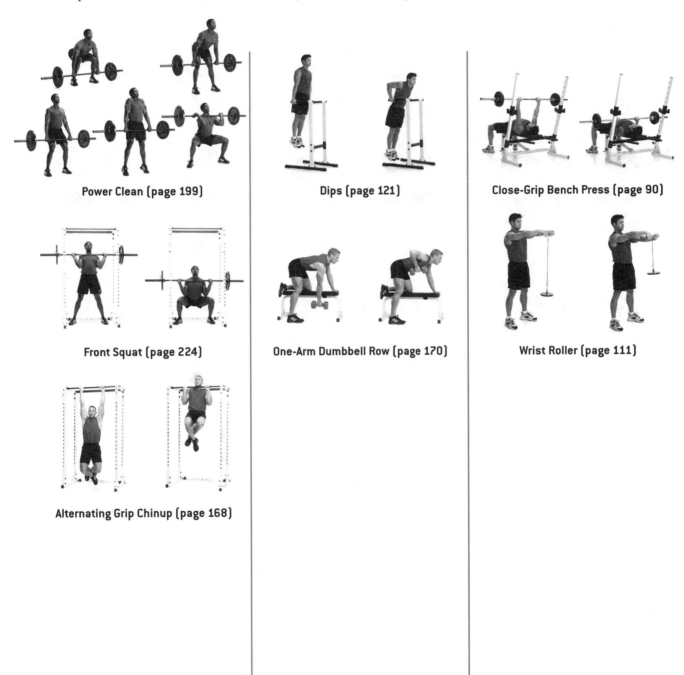

Power Clean (page 199)

Dips (page 121)

Close-Grip Bench Press (page 90)

Front Squat (page 224)

One-Arm Dumbbell Row (page 170)

Wrist Roller (page 111)

Alternating Grip Chinup (page 168)

RUNNING

Forget the mythical "high" of running: While some runners claim to experience a near orgasmic buzz, others admit that they have to force themselves to put step in front of tedious step. Either way, running can either give you a great workout or kick you in the butt with debilitating injuries. The most important thing is always to stay below the threshold of total fatigue and soreness. You'll do a lot better if you combine running with gym workouts that focus on the lower back and upper and lower legs.

Perform the following exercises in a circuit. Complete 50 to 100 reps each for the first three exercises and 10 to 20 reps for the last two.

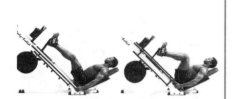

Incline Leg Press (page 226)

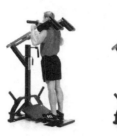

Machine Standing Heel Raise (page 244)

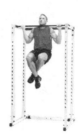

Wide-Grip Chinup (page 169) (Variation of Chinup)

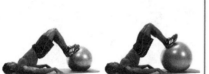

Supine Leg Curl on Stability Ball (page 238)

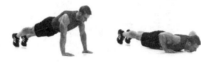

Floor Pushup (page 127)

SKIING

If you've spent any time on a cross-country or downhill ski trail, you're probably way too familiar with next-day pain. Skiing requires constant balance, which means that virtually every muscle in your body is called into play. The only way to minimize muscle burn—and retain the ability to walk back to your car unassisted—is to prepare by working the back, abs, legs, and shoulders.

Do 3 sets of 8 to 10 repetitions for each of the following exercises, allowing 2 minutes' rest between each set. Repeat the workouts three times a week, with at least 1 day of rest between workouts.

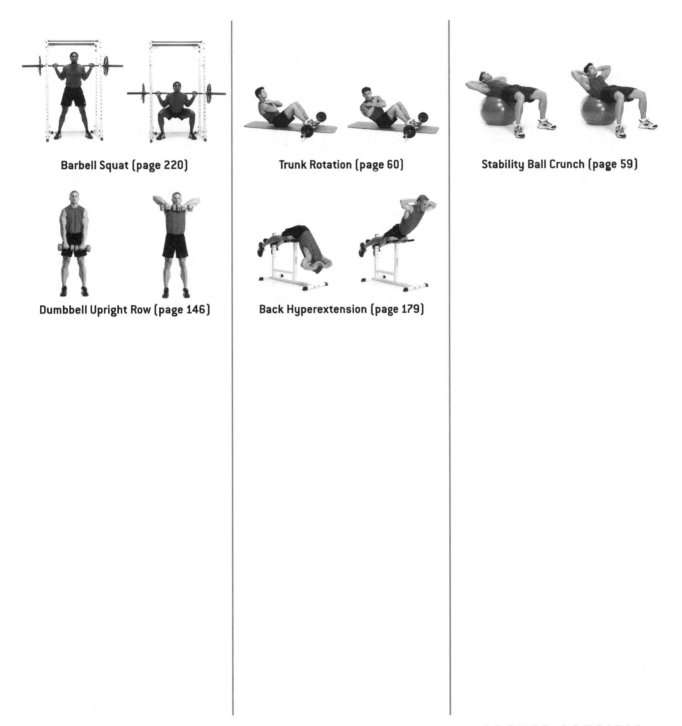

Barbell Squat (page 220)

Trunk Rotation (page 60)

Stability Ball Crunch (page 59)

Dumbbell Upright Row (page 146)

Back Hyperextension (page 179)

SOCCER

Soccer is a fast game that never lets up. You block, twist, turn, skip, jump, kick, and head the ball. But mostly you run—and keep running. You'll need superb cardiovascular conditioning if you expect to finish a match without spitting up your lungs. At the same time you'll want to power up your hips and legs.

Do 3 sets of 8 to 10 repetitions for each of the following exercises, allowing 2 minutes' rest between each set. Repeat the workouts three times a week, with at least 1 day of rest between workouts.

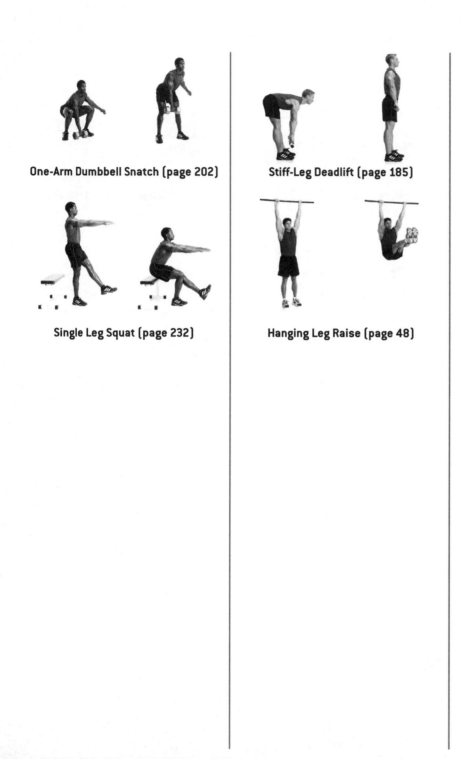

One-Arm Dumbbell Snatch (page 202)

Stiff-Leg Deadlift (page 185)

Single Leg Squat (page 232)

Hanging Leg Raise (page 48)

THE CARDIO
EDGE

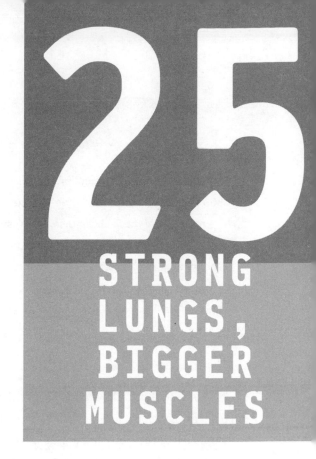

I f you want to see "slow" in action, take a look at some of the behemoths hulking around the weight racks—the guys with tats on their necks and biceps the size of basketballs. They're too big to stride. They can't swing their arms. They sort of *cruise* when they walk, like Mack trucks coasting to a light. It can take them a good 3 minutes just to get from the bench press to the lat pulldown machine.

Are they well developed? Certainly. Are they in good shape? Not even close. Aerobic workouts are the only way to get the kind of endurance that you need to push hard—at work or at play.

Aerobic exercise, also called endurance training, is effort that requires an enhanced flow of oxygen to supply energy. The oxygen spills from your lungs into your blood. Your heart pumps it to the muscles. There, it's used to break down carbohydrate, fat, and protein, and supply the energy that the muscles need to move. Weight lifting requires plenty of oxygen, but it isn't aerobic because the muscles mainly rely on the oxygen and glucose that's already present. For an exercise to be aerobic, it has to put continuous demands on muscles, enough to force the heart and lungs to deliver a heightened stream of oxygen.

An effective aerobic workout requires exercising at roughly 40 to 80 percent of your maximum effort, and keeping it up for a minimum of 20 minutes. A lot of this is intuitive; you'll know when your heart and lungs are pounding. For a little more precision, you can use a relatively simple formula:

- Subtract your age from 220. This tells you, roughly, your maximum heart rate (MHR).

- Multiply your max heart rate by the amount you want to increase it. If you want to exercise at 60 percent of that, just do the math: MHR × 0.60 = your target beats per minute.

Of course, not every 40-year-old man has the same maximum heart rate. You might get a solid aerobic workout at a heart rate of 100, or 120. Unless you're an elite athlete, you don't have to track the numbers too closely.

What you will want to do, though, is come up with a smart way to integrate endurance workouts into your weight-training program. A lot of men simply get on the treadmill for 20 or 30 minutes before starting their "real" workouts. That's not

SHOULD I TRAIN ON AN EMPTY STOMACH?

Trainers keep telling men that they should go to the gym hungry, as though a stomach that growls like a sackful of ferrets is somehow conducive to better lifting.

This is one of those old myths that refuse to die. The thinking, apparently, is that men burn more fat calories when they work out on an empty stomach. Not true. In fact, you'll burn *less* fat because your muscle cells won't have the energy to work very hard.

A smarter approach is to eat a normal meal about 1 hour before your workout, or drink a "liquid meal" 30 minutes before. That will supply your muscles with sufficient glycogen for the duration of any normal workout.

smart. For one thing, they tend to treat the aerobic portion as more of a time filler than a serious workout. Also, the body adapts quickly to any exercise, which means that the gains essentially stop after a few weeks unless you incorporate some variety.

You have to shake things up—say, by pushing hard on the endurance component for 3 to 6 weeks, and going a little easy on the weights. After that, flip it around and push harder on the strength training. Do this for a few months, and you'll find that you've made significant progress in both phases of your training.

A TOTAL ENDURANCE-RESISTANCE PLAN

Running, biking, and swimming used to be the main endurance workouts. These days, there are a lot more options: elliptical machines, stationary bikes and treadmills, outdoor obstacle courses, and plenty more. Take advantage of them. A long run or bike ride is great for endurance fitness, but it won't do much when you're trying to build size at the same time. The best endurance program pounds your heart and lungs *and* hammers the muscles you're trying to build.

Take the "talk test." Men who push themselves on the weight floor tend to do the same thing in endurance sports. That's fine if you're already in good shape and know what you're doing. Otherwise, plan on a few days of excruciating soreness.

Don't be a maniac. The best cardio workouts are when you're moving fast enough that you are breathing harder but have enough wind left over to talk almost normally. If you're pushing so hard that your lungs feel like they're roasting on a spit, back off a notch or two. The extra exertion isn't worth it.

Start with the 6-week plan. If you're totally new to cardio workouts, set up a 6-week schedule, in which you exercise 3 days a week. For the first day or two, for example, run for 10 minutes at a pace that allows you to talk. Every day after that, add 1 minute to the run. At the end of the first week, you'll be running for about 12 minutes. Keep it up, and you'll be running for 30 minutes straight at the end of 6 weeks—and you didn't have to kill yourself to get there.

Alternate fast and slow. There's nothing wrong with slow-moving (and time-consuming) endurance workouts. If you love distance running, go for it. But to build size, faster is better. Interval training is a good bet. When you're on a run, incorporate quick, hard sprints. For example, blast uphill for about 30 seconds, *walk* back down, then blast up again.

Interval training is tough—so tough, in fact, that you'll need some recovery time. Don't do it the day before your usual leg-training workouts.

Watch out for overtraining. For a long time, trainers were convinced that men should do either endurance activities or weight training, but not both. Early studies showed than men who combined the two didn't excel at either. Scientists have since learned, however, that the real problem was overtraining: Pushing too hard made progress slower.

When you're combining the two, a good rule of thumb is to limit the resistance phase of your training to about an hour. Keep your endurance workouts under 30 minutes. If you're already in good shape, it's fine to do both workouts on the same day. Most men, however, will do better if they lift and do endurance activities on alternating days.

Lift early, run late. This is important if your main goal is putting on size. If you fatigue your muscles with sprints or other endurance activities, you won't have enough residual power to complete a tough weight workout on the same day. Start with the weights. Then, later in the day, knock off the cardio component.

Do circuit training. It's a great strategy when you're trying to boost endurance without sacrificing muscle. Pick a compound exercise for each muscle group—say, bench presses for the chest, lat pulldowns for the back, and so on. Choose a total of six or eight exercises. For each, load up enough weight that you have to work, but not so much that you can't complete about 20 reps. You won't actually do that many repetitions, though. Do 1 set of 10 reps for the first exercise, then immediately move on to the next. Don't rest in between. Go through all the exercises to complete one circuit. Then go back to the beginning and finish up two or three more circuits.

Get the cross-training edge. Variety, remember, is the key to building muscle as well as endurance. On your cardio days, mix up a variety of activities. For example, use an elliptical machine for 10 minutes, then immediately switch to the rowing machine and do another 10 minutes. From a mental perspective, cross-training is ideal because it helps prevent the boredom that tends to set in when you do any long, repetitive activity.

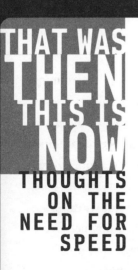

THAT WAS THEN THIS IS NOW
THOUGHTS ON THE NEED FOR SPEED

In the early days of the cardio craze, it was thought that men who wanted to lose weight needed to focus on long, slow workouts, such as running or biking. This approach never worked very well. For one thing, it failed to take tedium into account. Most men got bored and started looking for other, more stimulating things to do, like lawn darts. More important, the science didn't support the theory. It's true that moving slowly burns a higher percentage of fat calories than fast-moving workouts. Sleeping, in fact, burns a higher percentage of fat calories than anything else. You don't have to be a dues-paying member of Mensa to know that sleeping isn't a very effective fitness tool.

Go for a long run if you want to solve the mysteries of the universe or figure out what to say after forgetting your fifth wedding anniversary. If your main goals are size, strength, and endurance, kick in the after-burner. Exercise as hard and fast as you comfortably can.

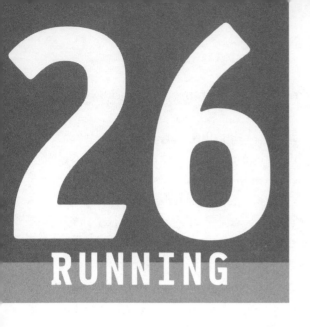

26 RUNNING

Running is the easiest sport to get into, and the hardest to continue. A lot of men try it because it requires little more than a modicum of coordination and balance and a good pair of running shoes. Look down the road a few months, and most of these guys have probably given it up. Running is a weight-bearing, repetitive sport. It can totally trash your joints if you aren't careful. It's hard to stay motivated when your knees and ankles feel like they're filled with chipped ice.

But if you do it correctly, running doesn't hurt. More important, it provides impressive fitness gains. For example, running an 8-minute mile will burn about 15 calories a minute—600 in a 40-minute run.

Ignore the conventional wisdom that you won't get significant benefits unless you're spitting up your lungs. More than most sports, running requires a healthy dose of moderation, along with a little common sense.

Walk before you run. Starting out with a 5-mile run almost guarantees you'll spend the next few days in serious pain. You don't load the big plates when you're new to lifting, and you don't run a marathon when you're new to running. Start by walking for about 10 to 15 minutes a day. Pick up the speed and distance as it gets more comfortable.

In the first few months of training, alternate walking with slow jogging. Run at a slow pace for 1 to 2 minutes. Drop down to a fast walk for 2 to 4 minutes, then kick up the pace again. Repeat the cycle for about 30 minutes at least 3 days a week.

Go for time or go for distance. Don't try to do both initially because you'll force your muscles and joints to perform at a level they're not prepared for. In the first few months of your program, decide which approach suits you best, then stick with it. Trainers usually recommend running for time—say, 20 or 30 minutes—and sticking with a pace that feels right.

Take advantage of treadmills. Indoor running has several advantages. You can do it in any weather. You can stay entertained by setting up in front of the TV. And you can set a speed that automatically keeps you in a smart training zone. Treadmill running also makes it easy to change conditions and progressively intensify your workouts—by increasing the incline, ramping up the speed, wearing a weighted vest, or holding a couple of light dumbbells and keeping your arms moving.

Pay attention to pain. When you run, your feet

HOW GOOD IS RUNNING FOR WEIGHT LOSS?

If you're serious about running, you'll burn some serious fat. Notice the word "serious." Jogging at a moderate pace for 15 minutes or so won't burn an impressive number of calories. But if you keep your feet moving for 30 to 45 minutes—or less, if you hit a good clip—you'll turn into a calorie-torching furnace.

Here's the formula. First, multiply your weight in kilograms by your running distance in kilometers. Then, multiply that by 1.036. So, a man who weighs 185 pounds (84.09 kilograms) and runs 10 kilometers will burn roughly 871 calories—the equivalent of about a quarter-pound of fat—in one run.

hit the ground with a force that's equal to three or four times your body weight. Runners who ignore this fact and "push through" the pain are facing a future filled with orthopedic bills.

Listen to your body. If you hurt, you're pushing too hard. Take a few days off. Ice the area, prop your feet up, and pop a few aspirin or ibuprofen. Wait until the pain is completely gone before lacing up your running shoes again.

BASIC TRAINING

Running, like any other workout, should be customized to your current level of fitness, as well as where you want to be a few months from now. Here are a couple of programs to get started.

Beginning Workout

- Start with 15-minute sessions. Run for 5 minutes, then turn around and take about 10 minutes to walk back.

- Every day, add 1 minute to your run time (and 2 minutes to your walk time). Keep doing it until you're running 15 minutes and walking 30 minutes.

- Three days a week, jog at a moderate pace for 30 minutes. The other 4 days, walk for 30 minutes.

- Gradually increase the distance you cover in 30 minutes. If you're running on a treadmill, increase the speed by $\frac{1}{10}$ mile per hour for each workout.

- Cool down with a 5-minute walk, followed by 10 to 15 minutes of static stretches.

If you follow this program for a month or two, you'll easily cover 5 miles in a 30-minute run.

Advanced Training for Speed

- Warm up with a 5-minute jog.

- Sprint 100 yards. Walk back to the starting point, then repeat. Complete the cycle 10 times. Bring a stopwatch so you can time yourself.

- Every time you run, try to shave $\frac{1}{10}$ of a second off your average time for the 10 sprints. Don't try to hit your top speed on the first few sprints. Allow time to warm up before going all out.

- Cool down with 5 minutes of light walking, followed by 10 to15 minutes of static stretches.

Do this program every day that you aren't lifting weights. At a minimum, do it 2 to 3 days a week.

Advanced Training for Endurance

- Warm up with a 5-minute jog.

- Alternate distance runs with shorter, fast runs. For example, run 30 minutes at the fastest pace you can comfortably handle. On the next workout, run for distance—say, 5 or 10 miles. Don't worry about speed, just hit the distance. Every workout, add a little more distance.

- Once you reach your distance goal, gradually increase your speed. You should be able to cover 7 to 10 miles in an hour.

- After your run, cool down with 5 minutes of light walking, followed by 10 to 15 minutes of static stretches.

Do this program every day that you aren't lifting weights. At a minimum, do it 2 to 3 days a week.

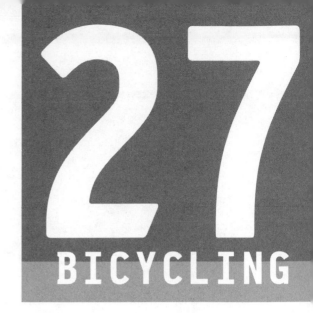

Anyone who has bought a bike in the last 10 years knows that the market has split into two camps: road cycling and mountain biking. Different mentalities, different bikes, different styles, different pleasures. Road riders cover the miles, get into a rhythm, and stay locked in, often for hours. They're like long-distance runners. Mountain bikers are into the thrill, the risk, the bursts of power. They're like sprinters.

Whichever style works for you—on the road, off-road, or even in the gym—biking is a serious fat burner. You'll use up close to 50 calories in 10 minutes if you pedal at a sedate, 5.5-mile-per-hour pace. Boost the speed to race pace,

and you'll burn up to 130 calories in those same 10 minutes. A Tufts University study found that gym riders lost 19 pounds and added about 3 pounds of muscle by riding regularly for 3 months.

Cycling is a non-weight-bearing activity. This makes it great for burning calories and conditioning the legs without stressing the joints the way, say, running does. It won't give the same muscle-building benefits that you get from weight training, but it will tighten and tone your muscles while giving your cardiovascular system one heck of a kick.

To get a great workout, here are a few points to keep in mind.

Keep the wheels spinning. Beginning bikers tend to ride in too high a gear, as though the mere act of shifting upward confers superior benefits. Give your shifting hand a rest. You want to find a gear that lets you spin at 80 to 90 revolutions a minute. This is the pace that gives your heart and lungs a top-flight workout, while maximizing the efficiency of your pedaling—and reducing the risk of knee damage.

Skip cruise control. Even off-roaders have a tendency to slip into a comfortable speed and just stay there. That's fine for pleasure, but not for fitness. If you want to burn fat and feel the burn—the increase of muscle metabolites that result in greater growth—you have to push hard and fast. Better yet, change your pace often. Cruise at a steady pace for a while, then turn up the heat for brief bursts.

Stay in the safety zone. Even though higher speeds or greater intensities are optimal for building muscle, you don't want to go flat out too long or too often—and you definitely don't want to exceed your physical capabilities or consistently push your muscles to pure fatigue. Sports scientists call this overtraining, and it can grind your progress to a halt.

Keep your rides between 60 percent and 90 per-

TRAIN FOR ENDURANCE

Like any workforce, the heart, lungs, and muscles do best when they specialize. If you're doing some serious road cycling, you need to work on endurance more than speed. Here's a simple program that works.

- Plan on riding at least 2 to 3 days a week. Start out with 5 minutes of light pedaling.

- Alternate distance rides with shorter, faster rides. For example, pedal for 30 minutes at a fast pace on one day. On the next, pedal for distance—say, 20 nonstop miles.

- Keep pushing speed as well as distance. Don't settle for the status quo. On every ride, cover a little more distance or move with a little more speed.

- Once you've reached your distance goals, bump up the speed. If you're in decent shape, you should be able to average 14 to 20 miles an hour.

- After every ride, cool down with 5 minutes of light pedaling, followed by 10 to 15 minutes of static stretching.

cent of your maximum effort. This will give you all of the fitness gains, without running yourself into the ground.

BASIC TRAINING

You can get in good shape just by "freestyling," but you'll increase muscle gain, cardiovascular conditioning, and calorie burn by following a more formal workout now and then. Here are a few ways to get started.

Beginning Workout

- Start out with a short, 20-minute ride (including the return trip).

- Every day, add 1 minute to your riding time. Keep adding time until you're riding for 30 minutes straight.

- Three days a week, stick with the 30-minute ride, but pick up the pace as much as you can comfortably handle. On the other 4 days, ride for 30 minutes or more at a more leisurely pace.

- Gradually increase the distance you cover in 30 minutes—say, by increasing your riding speed by about $\frac{1}{10}$ mile per hour in each workout.

- Cool down with 5 minutes of light pedaling at the ends of your rides, followed by 10 to 15 minutes of static stretching.

Advanced Speed Training

- Warm up with 5 minutes of light pedaling.

- Do a 1-mile sprint. Pedal lightly for 1 mile, then do another sprint. Repeat the cycle 10 times.

- Don't try to hit your top speed immediately. Do one or two sprint cycles first, then go all out. Your goal should be to shave $\frac{1}{10}$ of a second off your average time for the 10 sprints.

- Cool down with 5 minutes of light pedaling, followed by 10 to 15 minutes of static stretching.

- Repeat the program at least 2 or 3 days a week. Do it on your non-weight-training days so you don't compromise your regular leg workouts.

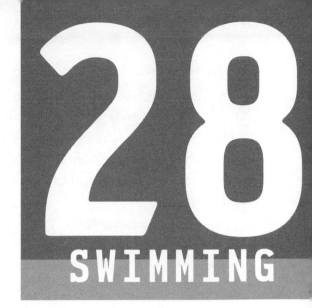

Swimming looks easy, especially when you watch experienced swimmers glide through the water. But swimming is an extremely demanding sport. For beginners, it can be a fight just to get to the other end of the pool.

It's worth getting the hang of it. Swimming uses just about all of the major muscle groups—the legs, hips, abdominals, chest, shoulders, and upper back. It can get the heart and lungs pounding like a drum. And it's superb for men with arthritis or other joint problems because the water supports the body and minimizes the kinds of joint compressions that can leave you hobbling around like someone twice your age.

Swimming, it needs to be said, is not a sport that comes naturally. Here's the usual scenario: Man goes to pool. Man dons suit and goggles. Man pushes off the wall and makes for the other end. Man gives self and lifeguard a serious scare.

Take a look around any recreational pool, and you'll see a lot of guys who look like they're more concerned with self-preservation than getting any kind of a workout. Here are a few tips to make it easier.

Get qualified instruction. True, the average man is more likely to stop and ask for directions than sign up for swimming classes. Do it anyway. Good technique isn't something you can learn on your own. Even men in masters swim classes undergo a barrage of stroke technique drills before they even think about working on fitness. The basic strokes aren't hard, but you have to learn to do them right if you're going to get any kind of serious workout.

Go for distance. You'll get a solid water workout by swimming three to four times a week, logging between 2,000 and 3,000 yards each time. Most swimmers can get that kind of yardage in about an hour.

If you're new to swimming, don't go for that kind of distance initially. Stick with shorter swims—say, between 500 and 1,000 yards each workout. Then slowly build up from there. You'll be using a lot of new muscles, and it's easy to stress them. Shoulder injuries are especially common among overzealous swimmers.

Work up to intervals. You can get an excellent workout by swimming "straight time"—doing the same stroke at the same pace for a half hour or more—but you'll burn a lot more calories by doing an interval workout: a series of swims separated by a specific amount of rest (the interval).

For example, you might do ten 50-yard freestyle

swims, leaving the wall every minute. Or you might do five 100-yard freestyle swims, leaving the wall every 2 minutes. A typical workout consists of several sets, with roughly 10- to 30-second intervals between each swim of the set, then several minutes' rest between each set.

Mix your speeds. Rather than plodding through the water at the same steady speed, work in some variety. Alternate slow, steady swimming with sprints. Fast swimming brings more muscle fibers into play, taxes the heart and lungs more, and can burn as much as twice the calories.

Mix your strokes. Many swimmers swim nothing but freestyle. If you're one of them, you're missing out. Adding other strokes to your workouts will help you hit more muscles and improve your flexibility by bringing different motions into play.

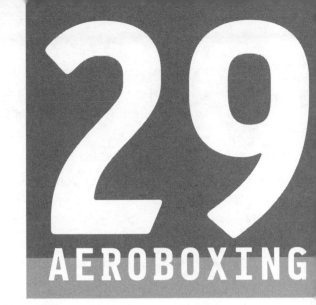

29

AEROBOXING

Exercise physiologists have measured boxing's caloric burn, and it's impressive—up to 1,400 calories an hour in the middle of a round, roughly twice the burn of hard running. That probably explains why you rarely see a fat boxer.

The idea of boxing as a fitness and weight-loss tool escaped the public for years, possibly because the public wasn't keen on having its face caved in. But these days, you can get all of the benefits of boxing—and take advantage of boxing's proven tools, such as hitting the heavy bag, jumping rope, and shadow boxing—without risking your bridgework.

Most clubs offer classes in aeroboxing (also called boxercise, boxerobics, and executive boxing). Don't be put off by the cute names. While these activities involve no real boxing—that is, there's no glove-to-face contact—they take advantage of all of boxing's moves. Do it for a few months and you'll muscle up your shoulders, stomach, legs, and back, while shifting your cardiovascular system into overdrive.

For a lot of men, aeroboxing is a superb stress reducer, as well as a workout that sharpens reflexes and agility and greatly increases muscular endurance and power. You'll definitely want to pick a class that's geared to your fitness level. Even if you're in decent shape, you'll probably want to start at the beginner level. That's challenging enough.

GETTING STARTED

Boxing is not a complex sport. There are four punches—jab, cross, hook, and uppercut. The ex-

ercises and equipment are simple. Unlike certain exercise machines that require physics training to operate, heavy bags and jump ropes are easy to use.

Still, when you take up aeroboxing or other boxing-related workouts, you do need to know what you're doing. Hit the heavy bag with a poorly thrown punch, and you could hurt your shoulder or break your wrist. More important, you need to remember what you're not doing: learning to be a fighter. Fancy legwork and jumping rope will get you in great shape. It won't help you survive in the ring against Mike Tyson.

To get the most from your sessions, here are a few points to keep in mind.

Work into it slowly. Boxing workouts, even the "lite" aeroboxing workouts taught at some gyms, are ruthlessly efficient conditioners and calorie burners for a simple reason: You expend a huge amount of energy while getting very little rest. If you push yourself too hard, you aren't going to get fit. You're going to get hurt. It's not worth it.

Do three-on, one-off. A professional boxing bout consists of 3-minute rounds, with a minute of rest between each round. Aeroboxing workouts are often patterned on this rigorous model. For instance, you might go three 3-minute rounds on the heavy bag, with a minute of rest between each round. This cycle—hard exercise followed by rest—will keep your heart rate up and the calories burning.

Check your pulse. Throwing punches for 3 full minutes, whether you're hitting a heavy bag or jabbing at air, will make your arms feel like noodles. A minute's rest in between rounds might not give you enough time to recover fully. You need this recovery time. Without it, your muscles will quickly build up lactic acid and get sore and heavy. It's hard to throw punches when your arms have turned to stone.

On the other hand, you don't want too much rest because that will slow your training. This is where taking your pulse comes in handy. When your pulse drops to 120 to 130 beats a minute, it's time to get moving again.

Watch your form. There's a tendency, especially when you get tired, to begin flailing away. That's hard on your joints—and sloppy punches, if you happen to be hitting the heavy bag, are more likely to break your wrist than dent the bag.

Push hard. There are as many boxing workouts as there are personal injury lawyers. If you're new to aeroboxing (or boxing), but are still fairly fit, here's a good workout:

- Start with 1 to 2 miles of running.
- Do three 3-minute rounds of jumping rope, 2 sets of 30 situps, 3 sets of 15 pushups, 3 sets of 8 pullups, and three 3-minute rounds of shadow boxing.
- Then do two 3-minute rounds on the heavy bag. Follow that with one (or more) 3-minute rounds of jumping rope.

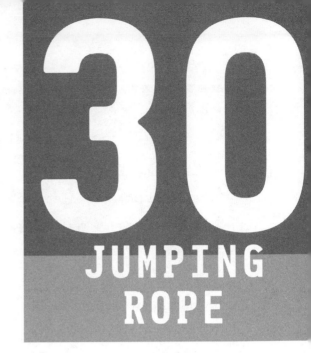

If you want to power up your heart and lungs and rev your internal machinery so that it burns calories hotter than a furnace, you should definitely get into the swing of things. Jumping rope can burn upward of 17 calories a minute. It strengthens your legs, butt, forearms, upper arms, and shoulders. It develops coordination and balance as well as or better than any other workout. About the only drawback is that it's hard on the knees, which isn't likely to be a problem if you do it on a padded surface.

Jumping rope looks simple—and it is, if you're 10 years old and chanting rhymes in a schoolyard. Otherwise, it takes a little practice to nail the rhythm and timing. Here are a couple of additional points to get you started.

Get the right rope. They aren't all the same length, for obvious reasons. The best way to tell if you're getting the right rope for your physique is to step on the middle and hold up the ends. They should reach to about the middle of your chest.

Step, don't jump. Don't bounce up and down like a beach ball. You want to lift your feet just high enough off the floor for the rope to pass underneath. Jumping higher throws off your timing and makes it impossible to achieve any sort of speed.

It's all in the wrists. You don't want to rotate your entire shoulders when spinning the rope. The action should all be in your wrists.

Land softly. Jumping rope is an impact sport; it can wreck your knees or ankles the same way running can. Always jump on a soft or padded surface.

Also, land on the balls of your feet to cushion impact and protect your knees.

BASIC MOVES

There are probably dozens of moves you can do when jumping rope. Stick with the basic, garden-variety jump at first. Here's how it works.

- Start with a warmup. Jog in place for a few minutes, then do some dynamic stretches. Jumping rope is more work than it looks. You have to prime your muscles first.

- Stand with your feet shoulder width apart. Rest the rope behind your calves.

- Keep your torso relaxed. Hold your head high and look straight ahead to establish balance.

- Grip the handles with a comfortable but firm grip. Make small circles with your wrists to get the rope going.

- Start your jump when the rope passes over your

JUMP VARIATIONS

Is regular jumping getting too monotonous? Here are some additional moves to try.

- Double foot jump: Jump and land with both feet, instead of moving one foot at a time.

- Alternate foot jump: Jump first with your right foot, then with your left. Keep alternating with each rope revolution.

- Running step: You incorporate a jogging pace while jumping. It increases the intensity of the workout.

- High step: You lift your feet several inches off the ground. The higher knee lift increases the intensity.

- Cross step: While you're in the air during the jump phase, cross your lower legs slightly, and land with them crossed.

- Side to side: Alternate landing areas between your left and right sides.

head. Jump or step only high enough for the rope to clear your feet; an inch is enough. The rope should touch the floor lightly as it passes underneath.

As with lifting or any other workout, jumping rope will yield less-than-optimal results unless you maintain good form and also follow a program that gradually boosts the duration and intensity of the workout. Here's a basic program to get started.

WEEK 1. Practice about 5 minutes a day. You can do it all at once or break it up into sessions. If you're a novice, you might want to limit yourself to a couple of jumps at a time. Rest, then jump again for awhile. You want a jump-to-rest ratio of 1:2. If you jump for 1 minute, say, rest for 2 minutes. Then go again.

WEEK 2. As your technique and jumping capacity improve, add 10 or 20 jumps to whatever you're currently doing. Reduce the rest time so that you're jumping and resting for the same amount of time. By the end of the second week, you'll probably be able to do 100 to 300 continuous jumps without a miss.

WEEK 3. Work up to 5 minutes of continuous jumping. Try to do 120 turns a minute. Repeat the workout three to five times a week. Increase the duration of the workout each time. You want to get up to 10 minutes of continuous jumping, moving the rope at 140 to 180 turns a minute. It might take 3 to 6 weeks to get to this point.

FOLLOW-THROUGH PHASE. Once you've reached this level, continue jumping three to five times a week. When you're able to jump for 10 minutes straight, vary the intensity of the workout by changing the rope speed now and then. Go from 140 turns a minute up to 180, or drop down from 180 to 140. Variety is the key to keeping your muscles challenged.

PART 5

HARD-BODY EATING

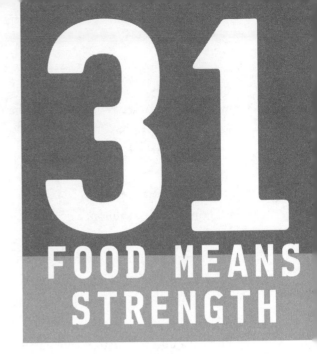

31 FOOD MEANS STRENGTH

The *only* way to get significant gains in size and strength is to pay attention to what you eat as well as to when you eat it. Once you control the nutrition variables, such as the number of calories, meal timing, and the optimal levels of fat, protein, and carbohydrates, you'll be primed to take your body to the next level. That means more muscle more quickly.

We take it for granted that men who are serious about working out already know the nutritional basics and a little bit about how nutrients work in the body. They know they should eat plenty of plant foods, relatively little red meat, and so on. What they may not know is how to incorporate all of this information into their daily lives.

If there's just one message that you should take away from all of the nutrition talk that comes your way, let it be this one: Include a lot of variety. It's the only way to get all of the nutrients you need for peak power. Definitely avoid any dietary strategy that requires giving up entire classes of foods, such as dairy or fruit. You'll miss out on a lot of the components that you need to stay healthy—and your workouts will pay the price.

What should go on your plate?

• Lean meats: beef, fish, chicken, turkey, and pork
• Vegetables: broccoli, cauliflower, spinach, asparagus, onions
• Fruit: blueberries, strawberries, grapes, oranges
• Nuts: almonds, walnuts, pecans, cashews
• Dairy: skim milk, low-fat cheese
• Whole grains: oats, rye, wheat, barley
• Fresh or frozen instead of canned foods
• Foods as unprocessed as possible

This list seems pretty basic. Yet a lot of men out there eat the same foods day after day. Their bodies take in only limited amounts and varieties of nutrients. Even if they aren't malnourished in any classic sense, they're still suffering (even if they don't know it yet) from nutritional inadequacies. That means that their cells aren't getting the specific molecules that are needed for specific biochemical reactions. The short-term result may be a diminished level of strength or endurance. In the long run, they're looking at cell damage that's the genesis of all sorts of diseases. You don't want that to happen.

Good nutrition doesn't mean being a fanatic. For the most part, it just means being *prepared*.

Plan ahead. If you don't know what you're planning to eat—today, tomorrow, or the day after that—how will you have it available? Even if you aren't the type to write out meal plans for the entire week, at least take the time to figure out, roughly, what sorts of things to have in the house: salad fixings, frozen salmon, a couple of vegetables, plenty of onions and garlic, and so on.

If you're as busy as most of us, get in the habit of batch-cooking. On the nights you're in the kitchen anyway, make extras so you'll have something to keep in the freezer.

Pack a cooler. What do you eat when you're hungry? You eat what's available—and that usually means something that comes out of a vending machine or a fast-food drive-up window. If you want to get in top shape, you'd better get in the habit of packing up a lunch and popping it in a cooler. You'll save a fortune, and you'll also be in control of what goes into your body. When you're putting together a total fitness plan, that step alone can make a huge difference because you'll be able to control the amount of calories you take in, the optimal mix of carbs and protein, and even when you eat so it makes the most difference in the weight room.

Drink shakes. They're faster to make than a sandwich. Need another reason? If you're smart about the ingredients you use, you can get almost a day's worth of some nutrients—including the protein you need for putting on muscle—just by pounding one down. For example, pour low-fat or soy milk in a blender, add frozen berries, a banana, or other fruit, then splash in some olive oil. For pure muscle fuel, add a few scoops of whey protein, as well.

Get the right mix. The optimal mix of nutrients for maximizing muscle size and strength is 40 to 60 percent carbohydrates, 25 to 30 percent protein, and 15 to 30 percent fat. If you stay in this range, you'll notice quite a few changes: more energy, more strength, and, if you keep lifting, significant increases in muscle size.

WHEN TO EAT

We don't have the luxury of knowing exactly which vitamin, mineral, amino acid, fatty acid, or other nutrients our bodies need each instant. When you're

CALORIES: WHAT'S RIGHT FOR YOU?

You need a minimum number of calories simply to survive. At the same time, you don't want to exceed the calorie "ceiling" because you'll start putting on weight. Since every man requires a different number of calories, how do you figure out what's right for you?

- Multiply your current (or desired) weight by 11. This number represents your *resting* calorie needs.

- Identify your activity level. Give yourself a 1.2 if you're mainly sedentary; 1.3 if you walk less than 2 miles a day; 1.4 if you're somewhat active (you work in the yard, take exercise classes, and so on); or 1.5 if you exercise a lot or work at a hard, physical job.

- Multiply your activity score by your resting calorie needs. This number represents your *activity* calorie needs.

- To get the calories you need to maintain your current weight (or reach your desired weight), multiply your activity calorie needs by 1.1.

going for maximum size and strength, your best bet is to make sure that *all* of the nutrients enter your bloodstream every few hours. Sound impossible? It's not. In the last few years, sports scientists have spelled out an effective and realistic dietary strategy for adding muscle.

Eat often. It doesn't matter if you're a thin guy trying to bulk up or a big guy trying to get bigger: frequency counts. Plan on eating five to seven times a day in order to gain weight. If you want to add muscle, but have a little extra baggage around your midsection, plan on four to six meals daily.

Don't skip breakfast. You need those morning calories to get your muscle-glycogen levels back where they should be. Glycogen is the fuel that muscles need to keep moving. Men who eat breakfast have more energy and endurance. They're also less likely to gain fat than men who skip the morning meal.

Pump up with protein before and after workouts. Men usually get enough protein from their diets, but you may need more if you're trying to move up to the next neck size. The best time to supplement with protein is about a half hour before training, and again a few hours after. Doing so will minimize the breakdown of proteins already present in muscle cells. More available protein means faster recovery and greater muscle gains.

Eat before bed. Assuming you're already in pretty good shape, go ahead and have a meal later in the evening—say, an hour before you go to bed. A lot of muscle-building protein breaks down when you sleep. Eating before bedtime will help maintain the peak protein levels that you need for increased size and strength.

Eat after bed. Don't just check your e-mail when you wake up in the middle of the night; drink a protein shake. Your muscles will absorb the protein, and the extra calories will help kick you into a bigger size class.

Time your carbs. On workout days, get most of your carbohydrates an hour or two after training, with smaller amounts throughout the day. On non-workout days, you'll do better if you get most of your carbohydrates earlier in the day.

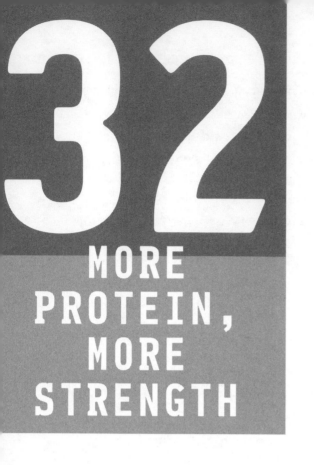

32

MORE PROTEIN, MORE STRENGTH

"Gotta get more protein"—it's a mantra among weight lifters. There are guys who suck down egg whites by the dozen, load up on supplements, and eat unbelievable quantities of beef.

Protein is an essential component for building and repairing muscle. You need quite a bit if you're hoping to put on size. But there is such a thing as overkill. Men who pound down 300, 400, even 500 grams of protein a day aren't going to get any bigger than they would getting lower—and saner—amounts.

HOW MUCH IS BEST?

There is a decent amount of research available that studies optimal protein intake. The answers are pretty clear-cut. Men who do serious strength training should try to get about 1.8 grams of protein per kilogram of body weight. Forget the conversions: Make it simple and get 1 gram per pound of body weight per day. If you weigh 180, that's 180 grams of protein.

That's more than the research says you actually need to build muscle, but the extra won't hurt, and it's an easy number to remember. Besides, a little extra protein has a fringe benefit. A high-protein intake suppresses appetite and can help strip surplus pounds from your frame.

If you're serious about getting in shape, and you have more than a pound or two of fat that you want to lose, consider getting anywhere from 25 to 40 percent of your total daily calories from protein.

THE DIFFERENT PROTEINS

Assuming that you're doing some serious lifting, and also assuming that you're serious about getting big, sooner or later you're probably going to take supplements. Forget for the moment that whole foods always provide better nutrition than isolated parts. Forget, too, that once your body's basic protein needs are met (which is easy to do with diet), the extra doesn't do a whole lot. The truth is, a lot of men like the convenience of protein powders. They can add some to their oatmeal or smoothie and instantly meet their meal macronutrient requirements.

If you want to twist your brain into a knot and don't feel like reading *A Brief History of Time*, try

Scientists have come up with all sorts of protein and dietary formulas for different stages of training. Here's a sample mix.

- Pre-workout: Combine 20 to 40 grams whey protein with 1 teaspoon each of leucine, taurine, and glutamine.

- Post-workout: Combine 20 to 40 grams whey protein with 1 tablespoon each of leucine, taurine, and glutamine. Add 1 teaspoon of creatine, and between 40 and 80 grams of carbohydrate.

- At bedtime: Combine 30 to 40 grams of a casein-based or time-release whey protein with 1 teaspoon each of leucine, taurine, and glutamine.

getting through some of the discussions about different kinds of protein. Everyone quotes research studies (usually inaccurately), and everyone is convinced that one particular brand or ingredient is superior to all the rest.

Forget the hype. All protein sources build muscle and aid in the repair process. There are some differences, though, so it's worth taking a look at the choices.

WHEY. The current "King of Proteins" among lifters, whey is the liquid left over after making cheese. It has several benefits. It mixes easily in most liquids, is easily digested, and contains most of the amino acids that you need. As a bonus, it contains glutamyl-cysteine groups, substances that the body uses to make antioxidants—free-radical fighting compounds that protect against heart disease, some kinds of vision loss, and even Alzheimer's disease.

The downside to whey is that it's relatively low in the amino acids arginine and glutamine. Manufacturers of whey protein powder have started to fortify their products. Unfortunately, this adds to the cost of an already high-priced protein.

CASEIN. Some lifters swear by this milk protein because a recent study indicated that it's anti-catabolic; that is, it prevents the breakdown of muscle-building protein in the body. This is only partly true. Casein is digested more slowly than whey protein and maintains higher amino acid levels in the blood for a longer period of time. It's not yet known whether it truly promotes less catabolism, or whether it promotes faster gains in size or strength.

Still, it does have some advantages. It's fairly high in the amino acids glutamine, tyrosine, threonine, and arginine. It moves relatively slowly through the digestive tract, which may allow for better absorption of amino acids and growth factor hormone.

One problem with casein-based protein powders is that the quality varies tremendously from manufacturer to manufacturer. Consider the instant, nonfat powdered milk that you can get at the supermarket. It has protein, sure, but just about all of the valuable amino acids have been wrecked (denatured) in the manufacturing process.

An equally serious problem, from a lifter's point of view, is that most casein proteins are low in branched-chain amino acids and high in lactose. The low content of branched-chain amino acids makes it more difficult to replace amino acids lost during exercise, and the high lactose is a problem for those who are lactose intolerant.

EGGS. Remember Rocky gulping down a yummy glass of raw eggs before his morning run?

For a long time, raw eggs, especially the whites, were considered an essential food group for building size. The down side is that raw egg whites contain avidin, a protein that binds to biotin, a B vitamin, and keeps the biotin out of your system. Supplement manufacturers did their part by coming out with egg white proteins without the avidin.

By all means, eat more cooked eggs. Even if you scoop out the yolk, which is high in fat anyway, egg whites supply all the necessary amino acids. Forget egg white protein powders: There's no evidence that they do much of anything.

SOY. Soy proteins are a hot research topic right now. They're high in branched-chain amino acids, glutamine, and arginine. Some athletes claim that the amino acids in soy help them maintain adequate nutrition when they're dieting. There's some evidence that soy protein can lower thyroid levels. This may be especially critical for guys trying to lose weight.

As with other legumes, however, soy is low in methionine, one of the essential amino acids. So it needs to be combined with other proteins for adequate nutrition. Most of the research on soy proteins, incidentally, has been done with the Supro brand. That's the brand to look for if you're using a soy protein.

WHICH ONE TO USE?

Keep in mind that whey, casein, and soy proteins all have good benefits. (There's a lot of interesting research on milk protein isolates, so that may be the next wave.) For now, whey and casein complement each other, while soy offers benefits that casein and whey don't.

So why not a combination? If you use a protein powder, you can mix your own, using equal parts of each.

TIMING COUNTS

The type of protein you choose is just one part of the equation. When you take it is another.

The latest evidence indicates that ingesting protein immediately before a workout is much better than immediately after. Since whey releases amino acids into the bloodstream rapidly, it makes sense to use a whey-based protein powder right before a workout. Casein, on the other hand, releases amino

TASTY AND QUICK

Today's protein powders are a lot more palatable than the products of yesteryear, but that doesn't mean you'll necessarily want to pound them down straight. It's easy to make a tasty shake that adds a few other essential nutrients.

For example, blend a scoop of whey protein with 2 cups fat-free milk, a tablespoon each of leucine, taurine, glutamine, a banana, and some ice.

Crave something sweeter and thicker? Make the same shake, only this time mix in some instant sugar-free banana pudding. About 1 tablespoon thickens the shake and really enhances the flavor.

You can also try flavored protein powders. For example, mix strawberry whey protein with fresh or frozen strawberries. Use your imagination and try different fruits and flavors—but be smart. You'll get more of a nutritional pop when you use whole fruits instead of overly sweet, and nearly fiber-free, fruit juices.

acids more slowly, and *may* inhibit protein breakdown—a plus when you're trying to gain maximum size—over a period of 3 hours.

Here's a protein program you may want to try:

• Combine a whey protein isolate with the amino acids leucine, taurine, and glutamine.

• Take it immediately before lifting. As you hit the weights, amino acids will be coming into your blood. With each muscle contraction, amino acid uptake is stimulated. The muscles get all the amino acids they need to synthesize protein, and possibly reduce protein breakdown.

• Immediately after training, take the same mixture, and add plenty of carbohydrates, along with a tablespoon of flaxseed oil and some fruit.

• If you're trying to gain weight, consider adding a protein drink at night. Use a sustained-release whey or a casein-based protein powder, spiked with extra taurine, leucine, and glutamine.

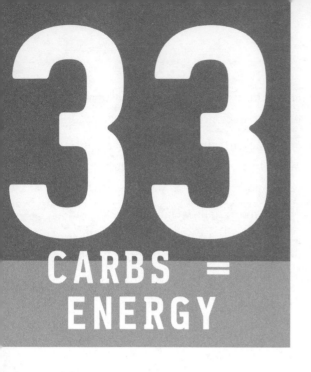

33
CARBS = ENERGY

Ever since the Zone and Atkins diets topped the bestseller lists, carbohydrates have been blamed for—well, just about everything. Never mind that study after study has shown that you need high-carb foods to control weight and prevent diabetes and other diseases. Carbohydrates are equally important from a hard-body perspective because they pack your system with the energy that you need to complete a hard-core workout. Unfortunately, until the low-carb craze goes the way of a hundred previous (and equally ineffective) diets, millions of guys will continue to avoid them. And pay the price.

Strictly speaking, the human body doesn't require carbohydrates. But it does require the vitamins and minerals that are mainly found in high-carb foods. You can't be strong if you don't get these nutrients. For that matter, you can't expect to stay healthy. Most men need to be getting more carbs, not less. It's the only way to put on muscle, develop endurance, and give your cells the gas that they need to keep going.

MORE CARBS, MORE POWER

Carbohydrates are one of the three macronutrients that supply the body with energy (the other two are protein and fat). All carbs are either sugars (oligosaccharides), starches, or fibers, or a combination of the three. Sports nutritionists advise men to get between 40 and 60 percent of their calories from carbs. There's a good reason for this, especially if you're serious about putting on size.

Carbohydrates are crucial because of the way they're broken down and stored in your body. The carbs you eat are stored in the form of glycogen, a substance that the muscles use for fuel. Unlike protein or fat, carbohydrates in the form of glycogen are stored directly in muscle tissues, where it's immediately burned during exercise. If you don't have enough glycogen in your muscles—along with backup stores in the liver and blood—you'll fatigue long before you nail a decent workout.

Keep in mind that starches and sugars, even though they're both forms of carbohydrate, don't have the same effects on your body—or on your workouts. The so-called simple sugars, such as the white stuff in the bowl next to the coffee pot, are immediately absorbed into the bloodstream. They provide a quick surge of energy in a blast of calories, but the energy doesn't last. That's why starches, also known as complex carbs, are a better choice. Foods in this category, such as pasta, legumes, vegetables, and other "whole" foods, are absorbed relatively slowly into the blood, giving long-lasting energy without any more calories than that tablespoon of sugar.

Keeping your muscles stocked with energy requires that you constantly top off your carb tank. If you don't get enough carbs, and you exercise regularly, before too long your glycogen level will essentially be in the basement at the start of every workout. You'll hardly have enough muscle energy to initiate a movement, let alone complete some tough sets.

Here's another reason to include plenty of carbohydrates in your diet. They influence the body's metabolism of key chemical compounds and hormones, including testosterone. Since testosterone plays a key role in muscle metabolism and muscle growth, you want plenty of it floating around in your blood when you need it. Studies suggest that a high-carb diet, one that limits fat intake to about 20 percent of total calories, may cause measurable boosts in testosterone. More testosterone means more energy, more strength, and, if you keep lifting, significant gains in muscle size.

HOW MUCH IS ENOUGH?

One of the first steps in your maximum muscle plan is to figure out how much carbohydrate you need. The best way to get a good estimate is to work backward: First, figure out how much protein and fat to include in your diet. Everything that's left is carbohydrates.

Here's an example. A 175-pound man probably gets 3,177 calories a day. Since a gram of protein has 4 calories, and a man this size needs about 175 grams of protein daily, his protein calories add up to 700.

Now, you have to subtract out the fat. This same

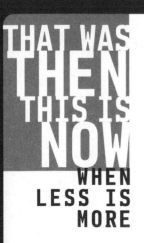

THAT WAS THEN, THIS IS NOW: WHEN LESS IS MORE

Carbohydrates used to be classified as either simple (for example, table sugar) or complex (a sandwich on whole-wheat bread). Nutritionists still use these terms, but a newer classification scheme is the glycemic index. It rates carbs by how quickly they raise blood sugar levels.

This is an important concept to understand. Carbs with a high glycemic index blast into your system and, after an initial rush, cause your energy to crash. Lower-rated carbs, on the other hand, creep into the blood. They give longer-lasting energy and exercise endurance.

A store-bought cupcake with strawberry icing probably has a glycemic index somewhere between 73 and 83. A bowl of muesli cereal, on the other hand, will be in the low 40s. Natural, whole foods, such as fruits, vegetables, and whole grains, invariably have acceptably low glycemic numbers, while processed sweets and snacks will be in the upper ranges.

Here's a good rule of thumb: Foods with a glycemic index of 70 or higher won't do you much good, and may set you back. Those with glycemic numbers of 55 or less will stick with you, no matter how long you're at the gym. They're the ones to eat most.

guy, if he follows some pretty tough guidelines, only gets 25 percent of his calories from fat. Multiply 0.25 by his total daily calories (3,177) and you get 794 calories from fat.

Now, he has the numbers he needs to figure out his daily carb quota. Add the daily protein calories (700) to the daily fat calories (794), and subtract that number from his total daily calories (3,177). You now have 1,683 calories left over for carbohydrates. A gram of carbs has 4 calories. Divide 1,683 by 4, and you get 421 grams (about 15 ounces) of carbohydrates a day.

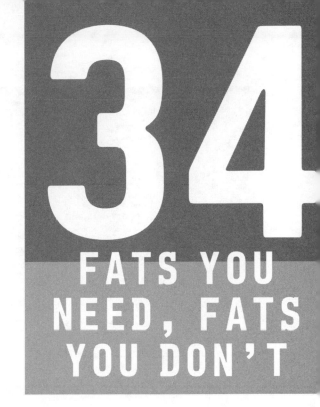

34

FATS YOU NEED, FATS YOU DON'T

F at isn't your enemy. Not only is it acceptable to eat, it's *required*— for energy, for nutrition, for good health.

Which isn't to say you can stuff a candy bar in your mouth or polish off a box of doughnuts and still maintain anything resembling a decent build. A gram of fat has roughly double the calories of an equal amount of protein or carbohydrates. Too much fat will make you fat. And some fats greatly increase the risk of diseases you don't want to get.

That said, the food cops have gone overboard in labeling fat Public Enemy Number One. You can think of fat as a family of related nutrients—some you need to avoid, others will make you healthier. It's worth knowing the difference.

FATS YOU NEED

Besides being a source of energy, fat is used in the production of cell membranes and eicosanoids, hormonelike compounds that help regulate blood pressure, heart rate, blood vessel constriction, and blood clotting, among other things. Fat is a natural insulator that keeps you warm. It dissolves fat-soluble nutrients, such as vitamins A, D, E, and K, and makes them available to cells. From a fitness point of view, moderate amounts of fat can actually help you maintain a good weight because fat provides a sense of fullness (satiety) after meals.

So, which fats do you need most?

MONOUNSATURATED FATS. Think cooking oils, especially olive, canola, and peanut oils. Avocados and most nuts are the foods with the highest amounts of monounsaturated fat. For once, scientists are unanimous. Men who replace some of the harmful fats (see below) in their diets with monounsaturated fats have lower levels of harmful, LDL cholesterol. They have a lower risk of heart disease and diabetes. They tend to live longer.

When you're working out to gain size, there's another reason to get more monos. They slightly increase levels of testosterone, the hormone that's integral to muscle growth, and which also fuels libido and sexual performance.

POLYUNSATURATED FATS. Like the monounsaturated fats, they help maintain healthful cholesterol levels when they're used to replace saturated fat in the diet. The polyunsaturated fats include vegetable oils, such as corn, sunflower, and cottonseed oils.

OMEGA-3 FATTY ACIDS. Found mainly in seafood and flaxseed, the omega-3s are among the healthiest fats you can eat. They've been linked to everything from heart health (they reduce the tendency of blood to form clots in the arteries), to less muscle soreness (by inhibiting the effects of inflammatory chemicals), and even to less depression.

Salmon, mackerel, herring, and other cold-water fish have the highest levels of omega-3s. Flaxseed is loaded with them, and you can get small amounts from soybean and canola oils.

FATS YOU DON'T NEED

If you were able to shrink yourself down to the size of a red blood cell and take a cruise through the pipes in an average American adult, you'd see a scary sight: fatty deposits on the blood vessel walls. These deposits (plaques) can seriously narrow the waterways leading to the heart. That means less blood flow, less oxygen to cells, and, in severe cases, a much higher risk of a heart attack.

You have saturated fat to thank for this ugly scenario. Mainly found in red meat, poultry, butter, and whole milk, saturated fat is the stuff that sends your cholesterol north. It increases your risk of cancer as well as heart disease. It's among the main *preventable* causes of disease.

If you want to stay on the planet for as long as possible, stay away from saturated fat. Doctors advise limiting the total amount to no more than 10 percent of total calories—and less is better.

The only other fat that you really have to worry about isn't a natural fat at all. It's called trans fat, or trans-fatty acids. These are fats that are created in laboratories by adding hydrogen to vegetable oil. This process, called hydrogenation, makes fats more solid and less likely to turn rancid. Research has shown that trans fat is even worse for your heart than saturated fat. Avoid it at all costs.

Shortenings and some margarines are among the main sources of trans fat. Check the label: If you see the words "partially hydrogenated," you're looking at trouble. Processed foods, such as doughnuts and french fries, also tend to be high in trans fat.

Beginning January 1, 2006, food manufacturers will be required to list the amount of trans fat on nutrition labels. No one really knows if there's an acceptable level. For now, the word from docs is "zero." Don't eat them.

KEEP IT HEALTHY

Entire books have been written about minimizing fat in the diet. That's way too complicated. You can easily shift your dietary balance from bad to good fats with a few simple approaches.

- Sauté with olive oil instead of butter.
- Use olive instead of vegetable oils in salad dressings and marinades. Use canola oil when baking.
- Munch nuts rather than potato chips or crackers with trans fat. You can fill up a little more with peanut- or other nut-butters. Spread them on celery for a ready-to-go snack.
- Top sandwiches with avocado instead of cheese.
- Got a hankering for steak? Go for it—but no more than twice a week. The rest of the time, eat fish or other foods low in saturated fat.

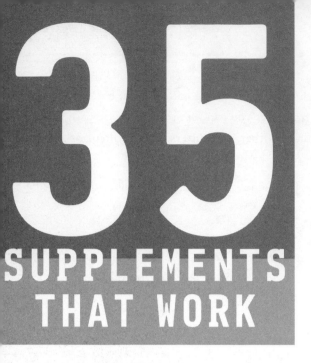

35 SUPPLEMENTS THAT WORK

There are thousands of dietary supplements on the market—supplements for increasing energy, boosting aerobic endurance, accelerating post-workout recovery. And, of course, increasing size—and we're not just talking about muscle size.

Before you pull out your wallet and slap down big bucks for a product that promises something like "Instant Blast to Pure Power!" there are a few things you should know about supplements.

- The Food and Drug Administration, the federal agency that oversees over-the-counter and prescription drugs, has little power to regulate the supplement industry. If people aren't dropping dead after taking a particular supplement, the FDA is unlikely to get involved—even if those horse pills don't contain a single molecule of the active ingredient listed on the label.

- Supplement manufacturers don't have to prove their products are effective before bringing them to market. Scientific studies that prove they work? Some manufacturers invest in research. Most don't.

- Supplements are expensive. Some muscle-building "systems"—impressive-looking assortments of bottles filled with pills meant to be taken up to six times a day—can wind up costing $100 a month or more, even when the active ingredients are basically what you'd get in a chicken sandwich.

- The vast majority of supplements are worthless. Even when they contain the exact mix of ingredients listed on the label—and a lot of them don't—they're unlikely to do what the manufacturers claim. In fact, they're unlikely to do much of anything except give you expensive urine.

So much for the caveats. If you take the time to actually read the labels and sort through the various claims, you can find a *few* supplements that really do make a difference. Will they "blast" you to huge size in 2 weeks, or give you that ripped look no matter what you eat or how often you work out? No. But they can be a useful adjunct to a well-designed workout plan. Here are the main ones.

ANTIOXIDANTS

There's no such thing as "pure" energy. Whether you're talking about the engine in your Honda or the machinery inside your body's cells, there's always waste. An unfortunate by-product of normal metabolism is something called oxidative stress. Cells in your body generate trillions of biochemical reactions daily. In the process, they also generate free radicals, unstable oxygen molecules that have lost an electron. These volatile molecules cruise through your body, trying to stabilize themselves by stealing electrons from other molecules. When they succeed, they create still more free radicals—and healthy tissues are damaged in the process.

Anything that increases metabolism, whether it's pumping iron or running on the treadmill, increases free radical production. This oxidative stress diverts energy from muscle building to muscle repairing. It also slows the rate of recovery after hard workouts. The only way to slow the process is with antioxidants—substances in foods or supplements that block the free-radical cascade.

Scientists have identified thousands of antioxidants. They still aren't sure which are most effective for combating oxidative stress. Nor are there any simple tests you can take to determine precisely which antioxidants are low in the blood and need to be replenished. That's why it makes sense to take multi-antioxidants—either individually or in a combination supplement.

Plan to eat, or plan to fail. The best source of antioxidants is a well-balanced diet. Especially when you're doing serious training, eat at least five servings of fruits and vegetables daily. They contain every one of the antioxidants your body needs, in a form that's probably more effective than what's available from supplements.

For extra insurance, take the following supplements with breakfast, and again with the last meal of the day.

- Vitamin C: 250 to 500 milligrams
- Vitamin E with mixed tocopherols and tocotrienols: 400 IU
- Alpha lipoic acid: 300 milligrams
- Coenzyme Q_{10}: 30 to 45 milligrams

You'll notice that we aren't recommending beta-carotene, N-acetylcysteine (NAC), or selenium. These are superb antioxidants, but they're much easier to get in the diet than from supplements. Sweet potatoes, carrots, and other orange or yellow vegetables supply all of the beta-carotene and other carotenoids that you could possibly need. If you are taking at least one scoop of whey protein (especially Immunocal) daily, then you don't need to supplement with NAC. Selenium is easy to obtain as long as you eat nuts, vegetables, fish, and dairy foods. An ounce of Brazil nuts, for example, dishes up 840 micrograms of selenium. That's a very healthy dose.

BRANCHED-CHAIN AMINO ACIDS

There are three of them: L-leucine, L-isoleucine, and L-valine. They're naturally occurring molecules that the body uses to build proteins. Most men don't need to supplement with branched-chain amino acids because they're readily available in the diet. However, men doing high-intensity, high-volume workouts might benefit from supplements because preliminary research suggests that they may help sustain muscular strength and stamina by enhancing protein synthesis in liver and muscle cells.

Serious lifters often take branched-chain amino acids because they appear to help repair muscle microtears and enhance recovery after hard workouts.

The optimal dose hasn't been determined. The standard recommendation is to take 1 to 5 grams daily.

CREATINE

It's the grandfather of muscle-building supplements. Everyone involved in the exercise industry has heard of or used creatine, or at least known other men who used it. Why has everyone gone berserk over creatine? Because it's the real deal. It's one of the few supplements that has been rigorously tested and proven to work.

Studies show that men who take creatine gain weight and increase strength more readily than those who don't take it. It has also been shown to speed recovery time and give men more energy during workouts. Creatine allows lifters to accomplish more work. If you can normally complete 8 reps while benching 225 pounds, for example, you might be able to increase the reps to 10 when taking creatine.

One of the main goals of weight training is progressive overload. Creatine helps with this in a number of ways. It helps to build muscle, which allows the use of heavier weights. It provides prolonged energy, so you can lengthen the time you spend under tension. It enhances recovery, so you can exercise more often.

Creatine may also act as a cell volumizer, meaning that your muscle cells retain more water. This can generate increased protein synthesis and minimize protein degradation. At the same time, it increases glycogen synthesis. Glycogen is essentially muscle fuel. More glycogen means a higher capacity for workouts, which in turn means more muscle growth.

Small amounts of creatine are present in meats; you'd have to eat about 10 pounds of raw steak to get the weight-training benefits of supplementation. The recommend dose is typically 2 to 5 grams daily. Trainers usually advise men to start with a "loading dose" of 15 to 30 grams, divided into two or three daily doses. Take this dose for several days, then drop down to the maintenance dose.

Other important points about creatine:

Take it with high-carb meals. The combination may increase creatine's effectiveness by up to 60 percent. A recent study found that athletes who took creatine with carbohydrates ran faster, jumped higher, and gained more muscle mass and strength than those who took creatine alone. The carb-creatine combo also appears to improve anaerobic (weight lifting) performance by 30 percent.

Drink a lot. Creatine draws water into your muscle cells. This is good because it makes muscles larger. Get a few extra glasses of water or sports drink daily.

Choose a supplement that contains sodium. New research shows that creatine is more efficiently absorbed when it's combined with sodium. The combination is also less likely to cause an upset stomach, a common side effect of creatine supplementation. Don't bother with creatine supplements that include sugar. They're not as well absorbed as the sodium-combo supplements.

Take creatine breaks. Studies show that the body adapts rapidly to creatine. The benefits slow or stop after about 6 to 8 weeks. Plan to take it for 8 weeks, stop for 6 to 8 weeks, then start taking it again.

ESSENTIAL FATTY ACIDS

These include the omega-3 and omega-6 fatty acids—nutrients that the body can't produce on its own, and which have an enormous range of health benefits, including heart-disease prevention, less joint pain and inflammation, and possibly improved lipolysis, the breakdown of fat that can result in less visible flab.

Essential fatty acids (EFAs) don't have the same powerhouse effects on weight training as creatine, but because they reduce inflammation, they may help you recover from workouts more quickly.

The most important EFAs are the omega-3s. In the diet, you can get plenty of omega-3s from fish. For supplemental amounts, take flaxseed oil (1 tablespoon for every 75 to 100 pounds of body weight), fish oil (2 to 3 grams daily if you're on the lean side, or 6 to 9 grams if you're heavier), and extra-virgin olive oil (2 to 4 tablespoons daily).

GLUTAMINE

It's an amino acid that is found in large amounts in skeletal muscle. Doctors use it to help patients recover from surgery. Glutamine is commonly used in the fitness industry because it's a very effective anti-catabolic that helps prevent muscle breakdown. In other words, it helps men maintain more muscle mass, and it helps restore glycogen stores to muscles even in the absence of carbohydrates.

That last point is interesting because so many men these days are on low-carbohydrate diets. Forget for the moment that the last thing you want to do is cut back on carbs when you're trying to build muscle. Millions of men follow these diets anyway because they're relatively effective, at least in the short run, for losing weight. By combining glutamine with protein, you can aid muscle recovery after workouts without loading up on high-carb foods.

Glutamine also appears to inhibit the tissue-damaging effects of free radicals. It's a cell volumizer, and it also stimulates the release of growth hormone—good news when you're trying to build muscle fast.

Plan on taking 10 to 20 grams on workout days and 5 grams on your off days.

HMB

Many of the world's top athletes take HMB and are seeing dramatic results. Short for beta-hydroxy beta-methylbutyrate, it's a relatively new supplement that is a metabolite of leucine, one of the body's essential amino acids.

HMB's main role is the synthesis of muscle tissue. It appears to increase the rate of protein utilized for muscle growth, while decreasing the atrophy, or breakdown, of muscle tissue. A recent study showed that men who took HMB daily for 3 weeks gained three times more muscle on the bench

HOW IMPORTANT IS A MULTI?

Sure, a multivitamin/mineral complex isn't the kind of flashy supplement that will impress anyone at the gym. Take one anyway. If you don't, you're setting yourself up for failure.

Men who are always getting sick—with colds, flu, whatever—can't train consistently. Taking a good multi will strengthen immunity and also help with energy levels and muscle recovery. In some cases, it can slightly improve strength, as well.

Few supplements are cheap; by comparison, a multivitamin/mineral complex is a steal. Don't get the bargain-basement brands, however. They usually derive their minerals from oxides, which are poorly absorbed by the body. Better-quality supplements get their minerals from more absorbable aspartates and amino acid chelates. They're worth the extra money.

press than men taking a placebo. That's an incredible gain.

Other studies suggest that HMB enhances strength and endurance, accelerates fat loss, and increases lean mass. One small study found that men who took 3 grams of HMB daily for 4 weeks during a heavy training program—3 days a week of aerobic workouts and 2 of weight training—had dramatic drops in harmful LDL cholesterol. At the same time, they showed significant strength gains in the leg press, lat pulldown, and biceps curl.

If you're looking for a muscle-building edge, consider HMB. The recommended dose is 3 grams daily, in combination with regular lifting workouts. Take it before training or just before bed for optimal results.

You need water just to keep your body running. And when you exercise and lose water through perspiration, you have to put it back. If you don't, you lose efficiency in circulation, nutrient delivery, work capacity, and thermoregulation. At the same time, you lose a lot of carbohydrates during endurance activities that last more than an hour. Carbs are not only a source of energy but also—you guessed it—water.

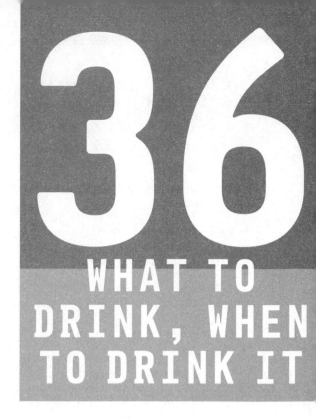

36
WHAT TO DRINK, WHEN TO DRINK IT

This gets us back to the question of how much the average guy really needs

to be drinking, and how often. If you drink normal amounts of fluids throughout the day, you aren't going to suddenly dry up in the course of a 30-minute workout. If you're thirsty, you should drink. If you're tired of lifting, taking a drink of water is as good an excuse as any to take a break. But you don't really need it. Your body's reserves will easily carry you through.

SWEAT MORE, DRINK MORE

Now, let's assume you're working up a good sweat. Maybe you're lifting heavy and fast, or you're running on the treadmill for an hour or more. The combination of exercise and heat stress can cause your body to lose as much as 2 liters of water an hour. When you're sweating that much, you lose sodium as well as water. Sodium is the electrolyte that stimulates the thirst mechanism. Low sodium means less

thirst—so you might not know that you need water even though your supplies are running low.

That's a good argument for doing the frequent sip thing. Fluid requirements vary widely from person to person, so there are no hard and fast rules to follow. The best way to figure out how much to drink is to figure out how much you lose, and the best way to do that is to weigh yourself before and after exercise.

The basic rule is "ounce for ounce." For every ounce of weight lost, drink an equal amount of fluid. During really hard exercise, drink even more—up to 50 percent more than you're sweating out.

A drink of water can only do so much, however. If you're exercising in high heat and at high intensity, and you find that your body weight loss exceeds 4 percent of your original weight, don't count on water to bail you out. You need to reduce the intensity and duration of your exercise.

WATER OR SPORTS DRINK?

The perennial debate is whether you'll do better spending the extra money and drinking a sports beverage when you exercise, or if you should just stick with Mother Nature's recipe and chug plain old water. There are (no surprise) good arguments for both.

- Water is readily available and a lot less expensive. In terms of thermoregulation and survival, water won't let you down.

- The American College of Sports Medicine recommends adding carbohydrates to water when you're exercising for longer than 1 hour. Specifically, it calls for getting 30 to 60 grams of carbohydrate per hour, in a liquid concentration range of 4 percent to 8 percent. That's what you'll get in most sports drinks.

- A sports drink that contains sodium tastes better and will also enhance your body's ability to retain water. Sodium stimulates the thirst mechanism that may be depressed after a heavy workout, so you'll be reminded to drink more.

The bottom line seems to be this: If you eat a healthful diet and normally drink six to eight glasses of water a day, you'll have all the fluid stores you need to get through an average workout. Drink more if you're thirsty, drink less if you're not. Your performance won't change one way or the other. The electrolytes lost in perspiration are easily replaced in a normal meal.

On the other hand, if you're exercising hard for an hour or more, drink throughout your workout.

A carb- and sodium-fortified sports drink will help keep your muscles fed and your energy high.

A HEALTHY HYDRATION PLAN

Whether you prefer beverages such as Gatorade or just plain water, you still have to make an effort to eat nutritionally balanced meals and drink fluids throughout the day. This will prime your body with the nutrients and electrolytes that you need for peak performance.

Here are a few other points to keep in mind.

Check the labels. Most of the sports beverages on the market contain the appropriate mix of carbohydrates and plain water—but some don't. Read the label to make sure you're getting at least 30 grams of carbohydrate, and no more than 60 grams. Forget the supersaturated carb solutions: They delay water entering your system and can actually cause dehydration.

Prepare your body prior to exercise. You don't want to walk into the gym with a fluid deficit. Try to drink about 17 ounces of fluid 2 hours before you work out.

Keep sipping if you're working hard. Since the thirst mechanism isn't all that precise, you can't depend on it to tell you when to drink during tough workouts. Take a drink at the end of every few sets—more if you're still thirsty.

Don't float your boat. Studies have shown that maintaining a *hyperhydration state* by drinking bucketfuls of water does no more for heat regulation or sports performance than maintaining a normal fluid balance, or *euhydration.*

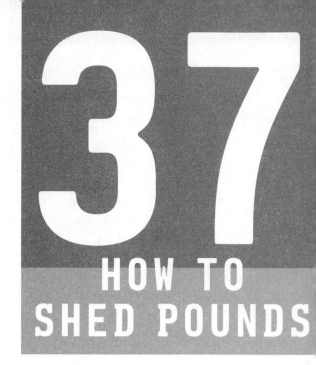

37

HOW TO SHED POUNDS

The average man has about 30 billion fat cells. Individually, the cells may not be visible to the naked eye. But put them together and you wind up with one lumpy, naked guy eyeing you contemptuously from the bathroom mirror.

Each of us is born with a genetically determined capacity to make fat cells. Their primary purpose is to be a reservoir of energy. The problem is that most of us deposit far more than we withdraw. That's a great idea if you're talking about banking, but not when it comes to fat. Well-fed fat cells can increase a thousand times in volume. They can also multiply.

Unless you attack fat cells from two directions—cutting off their food supply and burning more calories with exercise—you'll become just one more statistic in America's burgeoning weight problem.

It's not quite that simple, of course. If it were, we'd all be as thin as whippets. The devil is in the details. Cutting calories is tough in a culture that's all-food-all-the-time. Spending hours at the gym? Finding time isn't easy, especially if you're loaded down with the kinds of responsibilities required to put food on the table, let alone have a normal kind of life.

Where do you even start?

ESTIMATE YOUR ENERGY NEEDS

It's easy enough to figure out how many calories you should be getting in the course of the day. This is information you have to know if you're planning to drop a few pounds. Otherwise, it's like throwing darts when you're blindfolded and turning in circles—and someone keeps moving the board. Direction is everything.

For starters, multiply your weight by 16. This tells you how many calories you need to maintain your current build. So, for example, a 200-pound guy needs 3,200 calories a day. If that same guy wants to lose weight, reduce that amount by 20 percent, for a total of 2,560 daily calories. That's all there is to it.

Well, not quite. You also have to decide where that calorie deficit is going to come from. There are 3,500 calories in a pound. To lose 1 pound per week, you need to drop 500 calories a day. You have three choices:

• Burn 500 calories with exercise.

• Consume 500 fewer calories in your diet.

Most weight-loss plans recommend exercising at a moderate pace for 40 to 90 minutes. If you're pressed for time—and who isn't these days?—you can accelerate the process by boosting exercise intensity. For example, you might burn 220 calories by exercising for 30 minutes at 50 percent of your top heart rate. You can boost that burn to 332 calories by exercising at 75 percent of your max.

In other words, upping the intensity allows you to burn about 50 percent more calories in the same amount of time.

• Split the difference by getting 250 fewer calories in your diet and burning 250 more calories with exercise.

The third approach is by far the most effective. Studies show that men who simultaneously exercise and diet are more likely to reach their desired weights—and then maintain the weight loss—than those who depend only on diet or only on exercise.

SWEAT TO BURN

Resistance training can help you lose weight, and not only because you torch calories when you're lifting. Exercise builds muscle, and muscle is metabolically more active than fat. Putting on muscle is like putting a bigger engine in your car. It sucks extra fuel even when you're going the same distance.

Aerobic exercise is even better. The body burns fat most efficiently when you elevate your pulse to 70 to 80 percent of its resting rate—by swimming, biking, fast-walking, and so on. In addition to burning fat, aerobic workouts boost metabolism—upping your RPMs, as it were. When your motor idles faster, you burn more fuel.

For serious weight loss and fitness, you'll want to go beyond the aerobic minimum of 20 minutes, three times a week. But you don't have to go very far past this point.

Hit the middle ground. You don't have to be an aerobic fanatic to lose weight, but you can't depend on being a weekend warrior, either. The body burns fat most efficiently in aerobic sessions that last 40 to 90 minutes, exercising at a moderate pace that kicks your heart rate up to 50 to 65 percent of its top rate. Do this 4 or 5 days a week, and you're going to see the difference.

Expect the best—and prepare for the worst. It happens to everyone: You cut back on desserts, quit eating fatty foods, and sweat buckets in aerobic workouts. "Easier than I thought," you tell yourself, as you phone in a pizza order and blow off your workout for the day.

Uh-oh. That early weight loss may have felt great, but it was misleading. Within a few weeks, the needle on the scale invariably seems to stop moving—or actually creeps upward. What went wrong?

It's a common phenomenon. For many men, the heavier they are, the faster they lose weight initially. Then the weight loss slows w-a-a-a-y down. This is physiology, so expect it. Don't get discouraged, and don't give up. Keep up with your aerobic workouts. The pounds will continue to come off, even when it happens more slowly than it did at first.

Start slowly. It's true that intense exercise burns calories faster than long, slow stuff. But if you're 40 pounds overweight and haven't exercised since the Clinton administration, speedwork on the track is not for you. Start slowly. Begin by building your cardiovascular health. Take 10-minute walks before breakfast, at lunch, and again before dinner. Then work your way up, slowly, to roughly an hour of long, slow distance—a brisk walk, a moderate run or bike ride—three to five times a week.

Follow the 10 percent rule. It's natural human tendency to overestimate our abilities while underestimating our weaknesses. But when you're trying to lose weight—and stay uninjured—it pays to be careful.

For every year that you let yourself slide, figure that you'll need to add a month of easy-effort workouts (say, running at half-speed) three times a week to get back in shape. Don't increase your training time or mileage by any more than 10 percent a week.

Do less more often. Research has shown that three 10-minute sessions of exercise provide about 95 percent of the cardiorespiratory benefits of a continuous 30-minute session. That goes for weight loss, too. A calorie burned is a calorie burned, whether it's burned in three, 10-minute sessions or all at once.

EAT TO LOSE

Unless you've been in a coma for the past 20 years, you already know the weight-loss basics: Cut back on fats, meats, and sweets, and eat more grains, beans, fish, fruits, and vegetables. We all know this. Yet most of us don't do it.

One survey found that, while we're supposed to be eating 5 to 9 servings of fruits and vegetables a day, we actually eat closer to 3½ servings. And when you take women out of the picture (they tend to eat more of the good stuff than men do), only about one in five of us is eating as many servings as we should.

Meanwhile, we're eating a lot more meat and other fatty foods. This is serious stuff. Not only because these eating habits tend to make us fat, but also because they predispose us to the chronic diseases, including diabetes, heart disease, and even cancer.

So what can you do about it?

Cut the cow chow. This might seem contrary to the barbecue gene that resides in most every man, but it's by far the most effective way to reduce your intake of calorie-dripping fat. Like it or not, you need to eat less of the cow and more of what the cow eats.

Pack in beans and grains. They're among the best sources of fiber. Fiber is one of the most filling substances in the diet. Men who eat more grains and beans naturally take in fewer calories from meat and other high-fat foods.

Distract your taste buds. There's no question

DON'T BE DENSE

All foods have a certain number of calories within a given amount (volume). Some foods, such as desserts, candies, and processed foods, are high in energy density. This means that a small volume of that food has a large number of calories.

For example, just a half cup of mixed nuts has 438 calories. Alternatively, some foods, such as vegetables and fruit, have low energy density. In that same half-cup serving, raw broccoli has just 15 calories, and a half cup of cubed cantaloupe has 28 calories.

that switching to a low-fat diet after a lifetime of chowing on butter, sour cream, and other delectable fare can give you the sense that something is, well, missing. Like flavor.

Adding a jolt of spices to your food can help make the transition easier. Instead of sour cream, slather Mexican salsa on your baked potato, or drop a few chili pods into a low-fat stew.

Never skip breakfast. For one thing, it gives you the energy to get through the morning. You'll have food in your stomach, so you'll be less likely to graze on vending machine junk or overeat at lunch. George Washington University researchers found that people who skipped breakfast actually burned 5 percent fewer calories than those who got three or more meals a day.

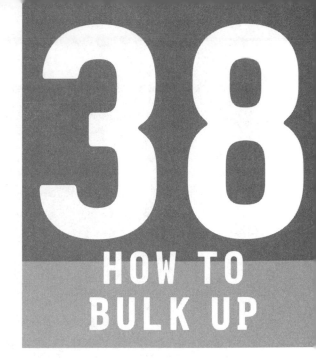

To get bigger (meaning to get more lean muscle, not just more weight), you have to take in more calories than you burn. That seems pretty obvious, yet men are notoriously vague about how many calories they consume. You've probably heard some guy claim that he eats all the time, but somehow his superfast metabolism must prevent him from putting on size.

He probably does eat a lot—sometimes. Inconsistent calorie intake isn't going to shift your frame from lean to bulky, no matter how much you occasionally shovel in. If you kept a food-intake record, you'd find that you might

pack in 4,500 calories one day, and as little as 1,500 on another. Your weekly average is probably just enough to maintain your current weight. That's fine if you're looking to keep the status quo. It doesn't work if you're trying to bulk up.

You burn a lot of calories when you lift. That's obviously one part of the equation you don't want to change. The part you can change is calories-in. You'll probably need to eat more—a lot more—to get where you want to be.

FUEL FOR SIZE

Before you start tinkering with what you put on your plate, you need to figure out how many calories you actually need. Probably the easiest equation is to multiply your weight by 16. A 200-pound guy, for example, needs 3,200 calories a day just to stay alive and maintain his current build. If he wants to

put on size, he'll need to up that amount by about 20 percent—for a total of 3,840 daily calories.

Depending on your current weight and lifestyle, you'll need to adjust the numbers up or down. If you only get to the gym once or twice a week, and aren't very active in between, you'll need fewer calories than someone who lifts hard and never seems to sit still.

Your goal should be to gain one-quarter to one-half pound a week. Don't try to gain faster than that—this isn't a race. A man who gains more than half a pound a week is probably accumulating more fat than muscle.

All calorie sources aren't created equal. Sure, you could pack in more calories by wolfing down candy bars. But if you do this long enough, you'll get big in all the wrong places. What you want to do is find the right balance of *macronutrients:* protein, carbohydrates, and fat.

THE BULK-UP PLAN

Suppose you weigh 200 pounds, and you take in 3,840 calories a day. For maximal size, you'll be getting 160 grams of protein, 107 grams of fat, and 560 grams of carbohydrates—preferably spread across six daily meals. You'll load up on real food—not merely protein bars or meal replacement drinks.

Here's a sample 1-day plan.

Meal 1

2 whole eggs—scrambled, poached, or soft- or hard-boiled
1 cup fat-free milk
1 cup cooked oatmeal (prepared with water, or use the cup of milk)
1 tablespoon flaxseed oil mixed in with the oatmeal
$\frac{1}{4}$ cup raisins, as a snack or mixed in with the oatmeal
$\frac{1}{2}$ cup mixed frozen berries, as a snack or mixed in with the oatmeal

Meal 2

6 ounces chicken breast
2 cups salad, using spinach or other dark, leafy green vegetables, along with onions, peppers, or other vegetables. Add 1 tablespoon olive oil, and vinegar to taste.
$\frac{1}{8}$ cup shredded cheese in salad
1 apple
1 banana
1 orange

Meal 3

6 ounces tuna or lean meat
1 sweet potato, baked
2 cups stir-fried vegetables, cooked in olive oil
1 ounce almonds or peanuts, as a snack or added to stir-fry
1 cup blueberries or strawberries
1 cup orange juice with pulp

Meal 4: Immediately Post-Workout

2 scoops whey protein
1 cup fat-free milk
18 ounces grape juice

Meal 5: 90 Minutes Post-Workout

2 scoops whey protein
1 cup fat-free milk
18 ounces grape juice

Meal 6

2 cups plain yogurt
$\frac{1}{2}$ cup raisins
2 ounces mixed nuts
1 cup berries or other fruit

Pack in the protein. Research shows that men who lift weights need more protein than those who are sedentary. This makes sense because muscle tissue requires protein both to repair itself and to grow. As a rule of thumb, plan on getting 1 gram of protein for every pound of body weight. This is actually more than you need, but it's well within safe levels, and the extra amounts will help you put on extra size.

Get plenty of carbs. Forget the trendy, low-carb diets. If you're trying to build muscle, you need plenty of rice, bread, fruits, vegetables, legumes, and other carbohydrate-rich foods. Anywhere from 45 to 65 percent of your total calories should come from carbs. Consider the hypothetical 200-pound man who's on a muscle-gaining diet of 3,840 calories a day. He'd need to consume about 560 grams, or roughly 20 ounces, of carbohydrates a day.

Reach a smart fat balance. Until fairly recently, all fat was cast in the same negative light. The research is clear that a diet high in *saturated* fat—found mainly in red meats and processed foods—increases your risk for just about every major disease. But there are plenty of healthful fats out there: olive oil, the fats in fish, and so on. Most experts advise getting about 25 percent of your total calories from fat—in the example above, about 107 grams daily.

Timing counts. Most lifters know from experience that they tend to stay in their peak fitness zone, and maintain top-flight energy, when they eat five or six smaller meals a day, rather than the traditional three squares. A study that followed the eating habits of boxers found that men who ate six meals daily while on a weight-loss diet preserved more muscle mass than those who ate two meals. The same is probably true of men who are in size-maintenance or muscle-building mode: more meals will give you greater gains than fewer meals, even when the overall calorie count is equal.

Eat after exercise. Laboratory studies show that rats given a meal immediately after exercise put on more bulk than those that eat several hours later. In humans, the essential amino acids that you get from foods stimulate protein synthesis—and more protein in the blood means better muscle repair and greater potential increases in size. In addition, the combination of carbohydrates and protein, eaten after lifting, stimulates insulin release. Post-workout insulin decreases the breakdown of muscle proteins.

Add protein-carb shakes. This is a good time to add a supplemental drink to your diet. Studies show that a protein-carb shake, taken right after exercise, and again 1½ to 2 hours later, is optimal for serious lifters. A ratio of three parts carbohydrates to one part protein is ideal. Of course, if you're training your butt off to put on extra size, you'll need some extra carbs. A ratio of 4:1 is probably a good choice.

POST-WORKOUT FUEL

Research shows that your body craves nutrients after lifting. To facilitate muscle growth, you should be getting 75 to 100 grams of carbohydrates within an hour or two after your workout. This roughly translates into a good-size plate of pasta, or a plateful of whole-grain salad, or a sweet potato or two. At the same time, tuck into some high-quality protein. A protein-enriched shake with 40 to 50 grams of protein will give your muscles the nutrients they need to repair and keep growing.

INDEX

BOLDFACE PAGE REFERENCES INDICATE PHOTOGRAPHS.

UNDERSCORED REFERENCES INDICATE BOXED TEXT.

Joshua Wartman
Cell: 613 531 1040